CANCER
CUREOLOGY

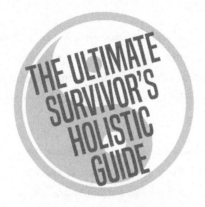

THE ULTIMATE SURVIVOR'S HOLISTIC GUIDE

**INTEGRATIVE
NATURAL
ANTI-CANCER
ANSWERS:
THE SCIENCE
AND TRUTH**

DR. STEVEN A. VASILEV MD

21st Century Patient-Centered Cutting Edge Integrative Comprehensive Cancer Care vs. Old School Cancer Treatment

The Choice Is Obvious.

Cancer Cureology introduces a new 21st-century integrative paradigm of cancer care where you are at the center of attention, not cancer by itself. While cancer treatment almost always requires some combination of Western techniques, it is equally important to actively support the body, mind, and soul during and after treatment. These mainly natural strategies are crucial to prevent cancer, to reduce symptoms during and after treatment, and to proactively do everything possible to help prevent recurrence.

Cancer Cureology is not a book focused simply on "alternative medicine." It is MUCH BETTER and much more far-reaching than that because it is a compilation of what is leading edge and what is most likely to help you! It is the background information for a five step anti-cancer integrative treatment and support system.

Cancer Cureology explores the scientific evidence to get at the truth behind natural therapies. 21st-century sciences such as epigenetics, nutrigenomics, and immune modulation form the basis for collaboration between mainstream and natural anti-cancer strategies.

Cancer Cureology sheds an authoritative guiding light on:

- The keys behind natural anti-cancer strategies
  - Reducing pro-carcinogenic inflammation and oxidative stress to anti-cancerize your body
  - Reducing tumor angiogenesis to starve cancers for nutrients and oxygen
  - Balancing hormonal influences to limit cancer progression
  - Stimulating and optimizing innate and adaptive immunity to naturally attack cancer cells
  - Epigenetically "silencing" cancer stem cells to make them dormant

- The five steps to achieving these strategies
  - Baseline anti-cancer nutrition and super-food support
  - Targeted supplementation
  - Psychoneuroimmunology and mind-body stress reduction
  - Rational anti-cancer detoxification
  - Lifestyle modification and exercise
- Selected "alternative" therapies that have scientific support
- Natural cancer and treatment-related symptom management
- And much more…

Cancer Cureology is indispensable to anyone who wants to survive and thrive after a cancer diagnosis. It can also help anyone who wants to prevent cancer in the first place.

If You Want To Get Your Free Cancer Cureology Anti-Cancer Five Step Summary Blueprint, Please Visit www.CancerCureology.com Now.

Dr. Steven A. Vasilev MD MBA FACOG FACS FACN ABIHM ABOIM

America's first & leading quadruple board certified integrative gynecologic oncologist.

Clinical Professor, David Geffen UCLA School of Medicine

Medical Director & Professor, Integrative Gynecologic Oncology

Providence Saint John's Health Center and John Wayne Cancer Institute

About The Author

Dr. Steven Vasilev MD, MBA, FACOG, FACS, FACN, ABIHM, ABOIM is a nationally recognized cancer surgeon, quadruple board certified in Obstetrics & Gynecology, Gynecologic Oncology, and Integrative & Holistic Medicine (two boards). Dr. Vasilev strongly supports patient-centered integrative oncology care as the 21st-century new gold standard. Given that the word doctor derives from the word docere, he firmly believes the most skilled doctor must also be a patient teacher and caring guide.

Dr. Vasilev is also a nationally known educator and clinical researcher. He has been on the faculty at multiple medical schools and cancer centers including USC, UC Irvine, and the City of Hope. He is currently a Professor at UCLA and John Wayne Cancer Institute in Santa Monica, California. He has trained over two hundred doctors in complex surgery and integrative cancer care. As an innovative master surgeon, he performs 90% of his surgeries using advanced minimally invasive laparoscopy and robotics.

As an author, he has published and contributed to hundreds of articles, research meeting abstracts, and book chapters. He also authored a textbook on the topic of scientific evidence based perioperative and supportive care.

Among many awards, Best Doctors® has listed him among the nation's top 5% of doctors for sixteen years running.

As a physician who also holds an MBA degree from the prestigious UCLA Anderson School, Dr. Vasilev has a keen sense of science-supported truth vs. marketing hyperbole. So, in practice and this book, he shares how to find the best evidence supported natural anti-cancer options. At the same time, he strives to keep your "B.S.-meter" tuned up to help you avoid useless and harmful treatments. As a true certified multidimensional and authoritative expert in both Western and Eastern natural approaches to cancer care, he forges an integrative path for the reader to follow towards surviving and thriving after a cancer diagnosis.

ALSO BY
DR. STEVEN A. VASILEV MD

Gynecologic Oncology:
Evidence-Based Perioperative and Supportive Care

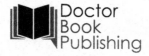

Doctor
Book
Publishing

Published by:
Doctor Book Publishing – An Imprint Of Deep Think Media
1775 Eye Street, NW
Suite 1150
Washington, DC 20006
1-800-704-3447

Cancer Cureology

ISBN-10: 1-942065-23-X
ISBN-13: 978-1-942065-23-4

DISCLAIMER

The author and publisher have strived to be as accurate and complete as possible in the creation of this guide. Notwithstanding that, we do not warrant or represent at any time that the contents within are accurate due to the rapidly changing nature of scientific advances and new knowledge.

While all attempts have been made to verify information provided in this publication, the author and publisher assume no responsibility for errors, omissions, or contrary interpretation of the subject matter herein. Any perceived slights of specific persons, peoples, or organizations are unintentional.

The materials presented are meant to be food for thought and seed for further research in the area of integrative oncology. It is written as more than a quick read but is not meant to be an authoritative textbook. Therefore, simplification is a necessary evil.

Like anything else in life, there are no guarantees of results made or implied herein. Readers are cautioned to rely on their own judgment about their individual circumstances to act accordingly.

This book is not intended for use as a source of medical advice for diagnosis or treatment. All readers are advised to seek services of physicians and other competent professionals in the healthcare field. If you have or have had cancer, work with an oncologist! Further, the author and publisher are not responsible for any injury or damage to persons or property related to any use of this work.

It is crucial for you to work with a board certified or board eligible oncologist for best chances for success. Also, please do not keep secrets from your oncologist if you are using any natural strategies. Sometimes natural support strategies can be employed safely and effectively during treatment, but in some cases, it can interfere with your mainstream therapy or even be dangerous due to interactions with medications, surgery or radiation therapy.

We are obligated to say that statements contained herein have not been evaluated by the Food and Drug Administration and are not meant to diagnose, treat or prevent any disease. Legally, only drugs, surgery, and radiation therapy can claim to do so.

This book is dedicated to cancer survivors worldwide, and in particular to those whom I have had the privilege to know personally and care for as patients.

If You Want To Get Your Free Cancer Cureology
Anti-Cancer Five Step Summary Blueprint,
Please Visit www.CancerCureology.com Now.

TABLE OF CONTENTS

I. Preface

"The best way to predict the future is to create it."

—*Abraham Lincoln*

Steve Jobs, one of the smartest magical thinkers and visionaries in the tech world of all time, turned out to be not so smart with his health. His untimely death from a very curable form of pancreatic cancer was highly avoidable according to almost all credible experts. What could have been a survivorship journey starting with a relatively simple and possibly life-saving surgery, followed by a carefully coordinated treatment plan which may have included mainstream "adjuvant" therapy plus natural integrative support was instead turned into a torturous nightmare that claimed his life. This included an ultra high-risk liver transplant in the late stages of his uphill battle, including mandatory cancer enabling immunosuppressive drugs required with transplants, as well as very exotic futile therapy which was all too little too late. Why did this happen? How did an otherwise brilliant man get so misled? We know that he regretted his choices in the end. However, we will never know how he got into the mindset of not wanting to be violated surgically and other rhetoric that is part of the dangerous drumbeat of the wrong and often lethal kind of alternative treatment pathway. There is a better way.

Right from the very beginning of my medical career as an oncologist, I was struck by three observations. First, although my patients were generally eager to accept my advice, it always seemed like I was handing out dis-empowering treatment options. In other words, I was either performing invasive surgery on my patients or doling out toxic chemotherapy or advising the use of radiation therapy. All of these carried a significant potential for complications and poor quality of life. In some cases, these were temporary, in others permanent. In all cases, this meant I was doing something to a patient, but the patient was not really engaged in any of it other than trying to recover and survive. The problem is that the tools to enhance such a recovery were by and large not part of the accepted standard of practice plan. In many cases, my patients adapted, made do and did their best to survive both the disease and the treatments.

Observation number two was that many of my patients, largely unbeknownst to me, were seeking advice elsewhere in an attempt to take back some control of their life regarding mindset, symptom abatement, natural "alternatives" to improve their survival chances and so on. It has since been well documented that up to 80% of cancer patients seek natural, complementary or "alternative" support sometime during their survivorship journey. However, after I became aware of this and engaged my patients in a discussion about what they were seeking and getting, I was very dismayed by the quality of what was too often being offered to them by dubious practitioners with meager credentials. This ranged from rather benign but costly recommendations to take fistfuls of useless and expensive remedies to dangerous propositions that brought some to the brink of death from "alternative" treatment. This motivated me to explore the possibilities and breadth of rational natural complementary, holistic support. I wanted to make sure my patients were helped rather than hurt by absurd treatment and support recommendations. What followed was a re-birth of my interest in nutrition and natural health solutions that predated medical school.

Unfortunately, there is a third observation that occurred and had reoccurred. I found that despite having in-depth conversations with patients about all aspects of integrative cancer support, some chose to ignore such discussions and resort to various cockamamie ill-conceived treatments anyway. In some cases, the selected treatments were *very* dangerous with no prayer of working. In other cases, they were undertaken during mainstream therapy, the combination of which could have been lethal. Why? Of course, desperation sometimes leads to inexplicable behavior and actions, but there was more to it than that. I often found that such patients truly believed they were being presented with very legitimate "alternative" science based therapies. In other words, they thought these were real alternatives that were proven and truly effective, just like mainstream options. They simply thought that I was unaware of them being a mainstream doctor and that my supposed ignorance was because I was part of the Big Pharma medical establishment or something to that effect. Most importantly, they had no idea that many of these "alternatives" were dangerous, unproven and some even completely disproven. So, I was stuck with the ugly realization that patients sometimes view the MD degree and mainstream oncology training as a badge of "*dis*honor" or a vote of "no confidence" when it comes to natural, integrative, "alternative" and complementary support.

Some of the "options" that are presented to unwitting patients are done so by a range of slick marketers to deluded naive individuals untrained in how the human body works. In some cases, they are actually MDs that clearly slept through many classes and subsequently received very little if any postgraduate training in oncology. Worse, some of these docs know that they are spewing garbage but continue to do so for profit. In my view, those that prey on desperate cancer patients in such a twisted and ill-conceived manner should be charged with criminal activity. Thankfully, some are.

As an outgrowth of the above observations, I would implore you to be mindful of one thing. One can argue about what practitioners can safely help people stay healthy and out of trouble. However, once you are sick with a potentially lethal disease like cancer, you need someone who has studied cancer in-depth and was trained by a legitimately accredited institution to treat cancer. This means at the center of your team there should be a trusted board certified or board eligible (completed training) mainstream oncologist. You should also be open and frank with your oncologist and not play cat and mouse regarding what you may be doing on the side because you can hurt yourself by inadvertent reactions between natural and mainstream therapies. If you are not under the care of an oncologist you can trust and communicate with, find another one. If this does not positively resonate with you, it would be best if you put this book down and read no further.

Think about it this way. You would not hire a plumber to fix your computer. You would not hire a criminal litigation attorney to be your warm and fuzzy marriage counselor. Now, more than ever before in your life, it is time to find and then trust the physician expert you have retained to help get you through this. This is not the time to consider contrary advice from non-physician family members, friends, accountants (CPA), lay hobbyists in health care or the like. Some individuals who act as "experts" even purport that they have "done research" on how to beat cancer naturally and say they can, in fact, cure you. They may have learned a thing or two from Googling things or reading, or even attending some less than well accredited "school," but that does not an expert make. Let me ask you this. If you wanted to learn a martial art, would you go to someone who has learned a little about it by reading or watching video as part of "distance learning," or would you go to a multiple level Black Belt who has spent decades practicing the art they are about to teach you? Similarly, even if they are well-meaning, many alternative cancer "experts" do not have the in-depth knowledge and expertise to understand truly what it will take to help you beat cancer. Your life hangs in the balance. Don't choose wrong.

As a gynecologic oncologist, even considering the mainstream medical world alone, I have always practiced medicine in an "integrative" sense because in my specialty we are trained in a combination of surgery and the use of chemotherapy and radiation principles. Today we are also using next generation cancer specific "biologicals" that will soon eliminate toxic chemotherapy. In other words, in our specialty, we have more than one tool to fight cancer with, which is not the case for most other oncology specialties. By adding integrative, complementary, holistic medicine to this equation, I simply stacked more on to this patient-centered notion that there are multiple tools for each problem.

It is usually not just surgery, and not just chemo and so on that will help you beat cancer. It is a mixture of treatment strategies to get the best patient-centered outcome, which includes holistic, integrative support. If you find an integrative oncologist that you can work with, that is the ideal scenario in my opinion. Someone who has mainstream and natural treatment information integrated into their brain, running through the same brain neurons, is most capable of advising you about the best combination of therapies. However, as you will discover, if you do not have such an individual near you, there are other options that can work very well.

This book is about action and lots of it. It sets the bar high for your role as a crucial active partner in your battle to live, survive and thrive against cancer. Your oncologist is one side of the puzzle, and you are the other in this system. Think about it. You are the most vested partner in this fight. It is *you* that needs to live and beat cancer, not your oncologist.

This book is also unique, and there is nothing else quite like it out there. Why? Because it is *not* a collection of false promises and kooky loony tunes alternative cures that are somehow being withheld from you, hawked by unqualified doctors and other dubious practitioners. It is not a collection of hype-filled junk and calls out those who propose such treatments, and the reasons why. Rather, it is about truth and Mother Nature's science-supported options to improve your survivorship.

At the same time, this book calls on those mainstream doctors who are in the dark and missing the boat on the intent of holistic, integrative cancer care to wake up. Cancer is a disease, but in treating the disease, there is much that can be done to proactively correct "root causes" for cancer and thereby contribute to quality of life as well as the best-known chance for longevity. While we cannot always find the exact root causes of cancer in any given individual, we do know the main lifestyle choices and environmental exposures that contribute to cancer overall. Seeking these out and reversing them if possible is a very low-risk proactive proposition. The alternative is passive hopeful, wishful thinking, which is disempowering, depressing and quality of life lowering by definition. Mainstream oncology focuses almost exclusively on treating the disease. There is much to be said about the benefits of patient-centered natural and complementary support, focusing on symptom reduction and overall health improvement. You need both mainstream anti-cancer therapy and natural integrative support! In fact, scientifically based integrative holistic cancer care should be considered the new de facto standard of practice as we move forward.

The notion of "scientifically based" should pique your interest. As doctors, we all have success stories, and some are truly at the unexplainable miracle level. However, it is one thing to parade a handful of success stories around that are only based on casual observation, especially when some of these are not well documented to be true. It is quite another, and several magnitudes more powerful, to talk about scientific studies that look at hundreds and thousands of people in each study, statistically well controlled for important variables. These types of studies do not always exist, but when they do, this is *very* compelling proof. I have sought out the best scientific evidence to help you decide what you should do and how accurate and supportive research is about certain treatments. I will refer you to the Appendix of this book multiple times if you want to learn more about how scientific "proof" is created.

In all walks of life, science dictates, or at least helps explain, how things work. We know that round wheels work better than square wheels, and we are aware the Earth is not flat. How did we find out? This is all based on science. To understand how the body works is also based on science. Some people ignore science. For example, a Flat Earth Society still exists. You are certainly welcome to your choices, but if you are of the mindset to ignore science, then it may be best for you to return this book as it will not resonate with you and I cannot help. Parenthetically, for those of faith, we are not talking about scientific issues that put religion or faith at odds with secular science. Rather, use of science in the manner I am talking about is applicable whether you believe in evolution or an existence based on Almighty God as a Creator. In either case, there is a path you can take that is more likely to help you than not, beyond faith or hope.

This book can serve as a bridge between your mainstream oncologist and natural integrative options that are scientifically supportable rather than dubious. If you combine what is described in this book with mainstream therapy, with your oncologist being on board, you are most likely to have the best outcome as measured by better quality of life and possibly improved longevity. If on the other hand, you tried to combine your mainstream oncologist's efforts with that of an "alternative" snake oil salesman's set of recommendations you will have a more challenging and possibly dangerous time. It is that simple! It's the difference between supportable plausible combinations of patient-centered care vs. woo-woo pseudo-science based care that is just not going to help you and can actually hurt you.

This book is about forging ahead with the best possible strategies combining mainstream and natural anti-cancer methods and therapies. Using these you will achieve results in improved quality of life before, during and after treatment. As you will see, developing science also strongly suggests you may significantly increase your longevity. In other words, this combined strategy gives you the highest possible chance of beating cancer and living longer with a better quality of life throughout. Every individual is different, and every cancer is different so that the results will vary. However, compared to sitting idly by and passively letting things be done to you, you will see a proactive approach unfold that you just can't afford to ignore. Are you in? Join me on your journey to live, survive and thrive. Your life may hang in the balance.

It follows that this might be the single-most crucial and eye-opening truthful information guide you will ever find about overcoming and preventing cancer, either up front if you are at high risk, or recurrence if you are a survivor. Please keep in mind that "prevention" can be effective but it is not foolproof. Just like you can generally prevent traffic accidents by being a prudent driver you can help to avoid cancer by prudent lifestyle and nutrition choices. You can't prevent all accidents, and you cannot prevent all cancers, but you can do your level best to do your part.

You are about to be introduced to the basics about such concepts as epigenetics, nutrigenomics, and single nucleotide polymorphisms. You will discover how your interface with the environment influences cancer occurrence and recurrence. You will then find out what you need to do to correct some leading root causes of cancer and how to take effective action to help prevent and overcome cancer to every extent possible. Once you realize why cancer occurs and recurs, related to "cancer stem cells" and tumor dormancy, you will have the keys to your success using the best-known strategies to defeat cancer beyond clinical remission after mainstream therapy. The information outlined in this book is science based, not voodoo and woo. Some things are proven, some are strongly supported, and some are plausible, and this is how ethical science-based integrative medicine is practiced. The best available scientific evidence, not anecdotes and tall tales or miracle results, is what drives the content in this book. Once you appreciate the power of this, you will be far better informed about what your choices really are. References are provided if you would like to explore concepts presented in this book in more depth, but keep in mind that even these only scratch the surface of the credible information available. There is also plenty of published *in*credible (meaning *not* credible) information, for which reason there is an Appendix that provides valuable clues as to why all scientific proof is not created equal.

Discovering that you or a loved one has cancer is utterly terrifying. All the same, once you understand the causes of cancer and learn how to reverse those root causes, you or your loved ones will have a better fighting chance of regaining health and beating cancer. Regrettably, despite the very best mainstream treatment and potent natural techniques, we still can't help everybody survive. Some cancers are extremely aggressive and don't respond to anything very well. However, there are survivors of EVERY cancer, no matter how aggressive. So, statistics may suggest the average course of the average patient, but statistics can also be irrelevant to a personal cancer battle because everyone is an individual. You may as well try everything YOU can to contribute personally towards a successful anti-cancer fight. As long as any individual utilizing these strategies has enough time left so that these plans may start to work, they can help their personal anti-cancer outcome and survivorship.

I realize that there will be a criticism of this book as "*too something*." Perhaps it might be perceived as too incomplete, too simplistic, too moderate, too complicated, too extreme or too little documentation or some such thing. I can only offer that this book is meant to be as factual as possible and food for thought, as well as a nidus for more research in discovering your best personal path. It is intended to be readable, yet as authoritative as possible for some of the top options, without being a 10,000 page textbook in unreadable medicalese. The references provided, as well as the Appendix on how scientific evidence is created, should help those that want to delve into greater depth on any given topic.

Anyway, if you are just starting standard medical treatments, have just finished them, or just trying not ever to get cancer, you will discover your best shot to improve your quality of life safely and possibly your survival chances is by applying what you are about to discover.

I will repeat. This is about action. Specifically, it's about your action. Take it, survive and thrive.

II. About The Author

Rather than read this book as an instructional guide written by some doctor, you might want to think of this book as a meeting of paths. Your path meets mine as an integrative oncologist who has treated many thousands of cancer patients and as one who has also been personally touched by cancer several times. Ideally, there is a resonance that can develop during a meeting of paths: a connection if you will. I believe that patients do better when they "connect" with their doctor, at least a little bit, beyond just blind consumption of advice and treatment. There is quite a bit of science that backs that up. While I can't connect with you like I can with my private patients, what I am trying to get across is that you should seek this out in your doctor-patient relationship because as hard as this might be to achieve, the better your outcome is likely to be. This is also true of having an interconnected support network that you may or may not have around you. Allow me to elaborate a bit because it will give you a better idea of where I am coming from. In my opinion, this is critical to your success.

The standard doctor-patient relationship in oncology is built on what has been labeled a Cartesian model of healthcare. This means a "one problem with one direct solution" approach that works well for acute emergency or urgent care of a problem. For example, you break a bone and the orthopedic surgeon fixes it. You get an infection with a particular bacterium, and you get the antibiotic prescribed that works best to get rid of it. This does not work well when trying to prevent disease or while treating chronic degenerative disease like cancer. The typical cancer treatment paradigm mandates a more holistic and ideally a personalized approach. There is no single cancer-defeating "magic bullet" and there never will be because cancers are different, and the people that are affected by it are even more diverse. In fact, part of the perceived "failure" of the war on cancer is that while we have identified magic bullet drugs to cure many diseases, this has not occurred in treating cancer. As you will see, this does *not* mean that we are losing or have lost the war against cancer, but rather that parts of the care process have just not been very evident. Cancer is now being diagnosed earlier, less morbid and ever more effective treatments are being developed, fewer side effects are being experienced and in most situations quality of life filled survivorship is ever increasing. However, there is a component that can add to prevention or quality of life after diagnosis or possibly even length of survivorship. This is the component of "connection" on a spiritual, mental and emotional level to supplement physical treatment in humanistic integrative holistic cancer care.

Cancer, like many other degenerative diseases, has a certain component of stress as part of its root causes. Stress leads to adverse hormonal responses that affect epigenetic-mediated change, activation of bad genes and suppression of good genes. Stress is just the beginning of a downward spiral that can lead to depression, obesity, and generalized chronic inflammation which in turn can spawn cancer cells. We know that stress-related visits account for 70-90% of doctor's office visits. So this is a huge issue to be aware of for primary cancer prevention, better outcomes during treatment and in the tertiary prevention of recurrence. In essence, the constant chit-chat between your genes and the environment extends to psychologically mediated effects. A toxic psychology can be just as damaging as any toxins we breathe, eat and drink. Also, through the emerging science of psycho-neuro-immunology, we know that your immune system can be suppressed in a similar way, potentially leading to cancer because of breaks in immune surveillance and possibly immune editing.

Connection with parents, in marriage, with friends, and in the community is also known to reduce stress and leads to greater optimism and better health. This is especially true if the emotion of love or power of spiritual awareness and faith is in play. Connection and belief in your doctor lead to better outcomes as well. It is called the "clinician effect" and critical in the healing process. Voltaire once said: "It is the physician's job to amuse the patient while nature cures the disease." Of course, today's doctors have a better set of tools to help prevent and treat diseases with. However, on a molecular level, this valuable augmentation of the healing process is based on reversing the stress hormone response and immunologic suppression which influences cancer growth or regression. This mind-body type of connection even acts at the level of gene expression, through epigenetics. You will learn much more about this in the chapters that follow. Optimism, giving and receiving love, healthy spirituality and really all forms of connection are all part of integrative holistic cancer care.

My core philosophy in writing this book and with my private patients is "informed choice." My mission is to get the truth to you regarding the best of "mainstream", "natural" and "complementary" options. It burns me up when I see self-proclaimed "experts," who are anything but, hurting people by hawking miracle cures and nonsense remedies to people who are in an extremely vulnerable time of their life. To every extent possible, it is my mission to get the truth to my patients and the greater readership of this book.

What exactly is the truth? Well, based on Mother Nature's laws of science there is a lot that we know about how the human body works. We do not know "everything" but we do know enough to say what is most likely to work based on 21st century scientific understanding. Mind you, while "double-blind placebo-controlled clinical trials" are the gold standard for determining which treatment is best, the lion's share of mainstream medical practice is not at that level. The good news is that Mother Nature's sciences (like anatomy, physiology, biochemistry, genetics, epigenetics, etc.) do not discriminate between mainstream or natural. Something is either likely to work or not based on how it affects the human body that functions within the parameters set by these sciences. Just like it makes no sense to plan a trip around a flat Earth, it is useless to plan a treatment based on nonsensical concepts of how the body works.

Something is either plausible or not, even before it gets to a "proven" level or not. Armed with that knowledge, rational practitioners explore and review the best solutions for you, mainstream and natural. This growing wave of medical practice is called "Integrative Medicine" and, in the case of cancer, "Integrative Oncology." This approach will increasingly bridge the gap between mainstream and natural as we move into the era of "personalized medicine". We are not there yet, but inching closer and closer to truly individualizing treatment at the cellular, molecular and genetic level.

OK, now finally a little about me. I have been in practice for over 25 years. I am deeply involved in teaching, research, and have been writing on advances in health care in both mainstream and natural areas.

I have a traditional allopathic medical degree from the Keck School at the University of Southern California, where I was elected to the Alpha Omega Alpha national medical honor society. I completed my residency and fellowship training at the USC-Los Angeles County Women's Hospital and the USC Kenneth Norris Comprehensive Cancer Center. So, I am board certified by the American Board of Obstetrics and Gynecology in both Obstetrics and Gynecology and in Gynecologic Oncology, which is a sub-specialty in women's cancer care. I am also board certified by two boards in Integrative and Holistic Medicine.

Over the last 25 years, I have taken care of patients just like you in all possible settings. I have taught and been a faculty member at three major universities and cancer centers, including the City of Hope Comprehensive Cancer Center in Duarte, UC Irvine, USC and UCLA, where I am currently a Professor. I have been listed nationally in *Best Doctors* for sixteen years running. I also have an MBA from UCLA, a top business school, which you might think has absolutely nothing to do with this book and fighting cancer. Fast forward to Chapter 17 to discover how vital this is in delivering my message of truth to you.

We could go on, but all of this is not the most important part because this book is about you, not me. At the end of the day, the most important part is that I have taken care of patients just like you for many many years. During this time I have reviewed, researched and practiced a lot of integrative science based solutions. So, while all these credentials hopefully prove that I am whom I say I am, you will see that what I mainly have to offer to you are personal solutions for many problems. Theses are solutions that are most likely to work. Alternatively, if there is no good solution, you will find out why and where to look for at least some help in reducing the impact of the particular problem. Even more importantly, I have made a lot of important observations about what CAUSES conditions like cancer over the years. In the end, prevention wins out! Primary prevention is best, but many of the same principles can arguably be applied toward prevention of recurrence.

Finally, as far as background is concerned, my training is not entirely mainstream medicine, called allopathy. I also attended chiropractic school, which I left after I realized that my full scope of practice to help patients would be limited. At that point, I had already been involved in advanced cancer research and care. Anyway, chiropractic school planted a seed to keep my mind open to alternative and complementary care options. Before and after that I spent years of extra time taking advanced University level courses in nutrition and biochemistry. All of this diverse background and training helps me help you separate truth from fiction and realistic integrative hope from quackery. You should know what is most likely to help you and what the risks are before making an educated decision.

On a personal note, my interest in integrative health care, and cancer care in particular started 36 years ago when my dad died of cancer. I watched a very painful but thankfully brief battle that did not include what I consider to be a holistic approach to give the best chance for not only beating cancer but also maintaining quality of life. All of my training has at its core the credo of helping patients achieve a shot at cures, while at the same time trying to provide tools for maintaining their spirit and soul.

Cancer touched me personally again when my mother-in-law was diagnosed with an aggressive type of liver cancer. While she did not seek out integrative oncologic care formally, her path was positively facilitated by using nutritional support and complementary modalities such as Tai-Chi. Although I saw a far more holistic approach to her medical care, it was still not at the level that I think should be the new standard of integrative holistic cancer care.

Hence, based on the above personal experiences, along with advising countless friends who have been diagnosed with cancer of the years, and having taken care of thousands of cancer patients, I offer you this book as a guide. I hope it will somehow soften the harsh realities of cancer being in your life and give you the best opportunity for quality of life enriched survivorship.

Here is what just a few of my patients, past and present, have to say:

"Quite literally this man saved my life many times over. Through thick and thin he never gave up on me, including expertly performed difficult surgeries to get through my multiply recurrent ovarian cancer over the last 15 years."

—L.B.

(LB Addendum by Dr. Vasilev: Unfortunately cancer ultimately claimed her life after 18 years of battling with it. She enjoyed life to the fullest and was one of the most upbeat people I have ever known. She helped many overcome fears of treatment and the disease and was simply a fantastic person. It was an honor to know her and to be her doctor. May she rest in peace.)

"Dr. Steve is an understated, compassionate person. Sixteen years ago after being told a third ovarian cancer surgery (OC) was impossible I was introduced to Dr. Steve in California by another OC survivor. He thoroughly evaluated my medical history, health, scans and labs and gave me confidence surgery would be successful. Dr. Steve's surgery saved my life at that time which allowed me to witness the birth of eight grandchildren through the years."

—C.J.W.

"Dr. Vasilev's superior skill is matched by his willingness to spend as long as it takes to explain things, his compassion, and great bedside manner. He skillfully carried out very complicated surgery when required and steered me away from it when it was not. The end result is that I'm alive 12 years later, including the ovarian cancer recurrence scare about six years ago. Over the past decade, he has also introduced integrative natural health guidance into his practice which has made the overall treatment package that he can deliver better than anyone else out there. It has been a blessing and a great privilege to have Dr. Vasilev as my Doctor. Without him, I wouldn't be here to write this."

—E.S.S.

"Dr. Vasilev is the kind of doctor you can trust with your life. In September 2006 I was told I had a very aggressive form of ovarian cancer and six months to live. My husband and I were overwhelmed, confused, terrified, and seeking a cure for my ovarian cancer. Then we met Dr. Vasilev, and we have never looked back. Doctor Vasilev immediately put our minds at rest, he gave us a direction, introduced us to all our options and guided us through the decision-making process making himself available through office visits, emails, and phone calls to answer all our questions. Doctor Vasilev has seen us through seven recurrences in nine years. Each time he has been innovative in his way of thinking and applies his arsenal of knowledge in developing his treatment plans. He integrates western and alternative medicine using the best of both to ensure that his patients handle their diagnosis with the best possible care and whenever possible, that they recover healthier, wiser, and better informed

than before their diagnosis. I wish that every cancer patient could have a Dr. Vasilev in their corner."

—M.P.

"Dr. V was the only physician with a different approach to my diagnosis in the beginning, and I trusted him. Thank you for your constant guidance over the past seven years. You have supported me with difficult chemo choices and choosing 'outside the box' therapies. You have performed difficult surgeries and continue to support me in pursuing additional therapies needed to keep me going on this journey. And my family….we are constantly reassured to have you by our side."

—E.D.

"I am a 48-year-old mother and a 2x Cervical Cancer survivor. I have been in full remission for 16 years after distant recurrence. I am so grateful for my life today, and I attribute my amazing and fulfilled life to Dr. Steven Vasilev. He was so instrumental in the success of my radical hysterectomy done laparoscopically and has been by my side every single step of the way for all these years. I am always able to rely on him for anything I need to maintain a cancer-free lifestyle. His knowledge, understanding and expertise on all facets of clinical trials, current chemotherapy drugs as well as his resources and knowledge of Eastern vs. Western medicine has been astounding and well respected. To have Dr. Vasilev as part of my continued excellent health is beyond what I could have imagined when I was originally diagnosed. He proves over and over again how very fortunate I am every day to be living life to the fullest, cancer free!"

—A.R.

III. Introduction To Integrative Oncology

Integrative oncology augments cutting edge mainstream therapies with complementary and natural approaches to improve outcomes in treatment by seeking to alleviate side effects, improve overall health, improve mindset, possibly improve cancer cure rates, and enhance quality and length of life in survivorship. The focus of *legitimate* integrative practitioners is to concentrate on the BEST options and discriminate between completely implausible disproven therapies and plausible or proven treatments. This guide focuses on the complementary natural aspects of integrative cancer care, but also touches on cutting-edge mainstream treatment option concepts. The two must work hand in hand for optimal results.

The key is involvement of scientific principles to determine what works, what doesn't, what is plausible vs. implausible and what is of most benefit vs. potential harm. As such, the term "alternative" is not a very good name because it has tended to include a garbage can of treatments that have been "dreamed up" by less than qualified people. Having said that, some therapies that have been called "alternative" are in reality plausible or proven natural based treatments. The problem is, sometimes it is all but impossible to discriminate between the two unless you are a pretty sophisticated health professional who understands not only how the human body works but also how and why cancer develops and the proven science behind that. It ideally requires sophisticated investigation to determine the difference and help you with choices between viable options. This discrimination can be extensively facilitated by a trained integrative oncologist who genuinely understands cancer as well as natural integrative approaches to fighting disease and achieving wellness. Alternatively, this can be accomplished by an integrative oncology team that works in close cooperation together. The results are NOT as good, and can be dangerous when supporting integrative practitioners do not communicate with your primary oncologist.

In many countries, the principles of integrative medicine have been the standard of care and are taught in medical schools and post-graduate residency programs. In the United States, this was slowed by the Flexner Report which was a rather narrowly focused big-business funded and government supported attempt to feature mainstream medicine advancement. It was published over one hundred years ago in 1910. Integrative natural science approaches were vilified and all but disappeared from cancer treatment for the better part of a century in the United States. Now it is on a comeback trail and is more evidence supported and patient-centered than ever before.

Integrative oncology seeks to involve the following rationally in cancer care, and more:

- nutritional treatment and support
- structured exercise program support
- natural health products such as vitamins, minerals, and botanicals
- detoxification support
- acupuncture and acupressure
- meditation and other mind-body strategies
- music therapy
- aromatherapy
- touch therapies such as massage
- fitness and stress reduction therapies such as yoga
- putative and veritable energy medicine

To some extent there is a convergence, or coming together, that is accelerating between mainstream and natural anti-cancer strategies. It has long been recognized that certain foods, herbs, and micro-nutrients have medicinal properties. The list is long and includes vital medicines such as antibiotics, some mainstream anti-cancer agents (e.g. Taxol), and commonly used daily medications like aspirin. As we learn more about the interaction between the environment and our physiol-ogy, our biochemistry and our genetics, we see an ever – broadening opportunity to gain and maintain health. The trick is to determine what degree of artificially stripping out biochemicals and nutrients from a plant is beneficial vs. consid-ering the incredible synergies that Mother Nature built into what we eat and drink in whole foods. In some cases, these stripped out ingredients or nutrients become refined and concentrated pharmaceutical drugs. However, they are also developed and marketed as natural nutraceuticals of variable purity, strength, and quality. Both of these can bring good or harm, or a combination thereof. However, as you will soon discover, in the case of cancer, bags of supplements are no better than bags stuffed with drugs.

As we come to understand the biochemical makeup of macro and micro-nutri-ents, we can better appreciate the power of whole food as medicine. While this is a much better preventative than cancer treatment strategy, there is no question that you can help your body fight cancer using natural support.

Many other complementary and natural approaches are easy to recommend simply because their risk is so very low and the potential benefit is so great. For example, how can one argue against laugh therapy to help get through treatment? In other cases, while we do not completely understand the treatments, we have scientific evidence that they work as is the case with acupuncture and acupressure to relieve pain and nausea. Also, and of critical importance, the risk of these treatment types is also very small. They are literal "no-brainers".

On the other hand, some natural and complementary treatments need further review. It is essential to understand that levels of scientific evidence from such studies vary widely in quality and degree. But not everything can be or should be subjected to a clinical trial, which represents the highest quality of clinical evidence or proof that something works. For example, do we ever need to per-form a randomized clinical trial to determine if using parachutes reduces the risk of death when jumping from an airplane? NO! It would be idiotic to throw half the people out of the plane without a parachute and the other half with a parachute. We already know what would happen. We know there is plausibility that parachutes prevent death from falling out of an airplane based on the sci-ence of physics. In other cases, observational epidemiologic data is sufficient. For example, there were never any large randomized clinical trials to prove that the Pap smear helps prevent cervical cancer. Yet, it has become accepted as the standard of practice on the strength of overwhelming epidemiologic evidence and is a lifesaver for millions of women. Finally, even if the therapy is only theoretically beneficial, it is worth considering if the risk is acceptable. However, if the risk to you is high, caution and informed consent are critical. To learn more about evidence scientific realities and how things are proven to be effective, please review the Appendix.

One thing is crucial to understand about integrative oncology. No ethical and credible integrative oncology practitioner would ever recommend forgoing life-saving surgery or mainstream therapy in favor of using an unproven or disproven "alternative" treatment when there is a real hope for a cure or substantial prolongation of good quality life.

There are those out there who are polluting the concept of integrative oncology by illegitimately combining mainstream and "alternative" therapies that have no prayer of working. These charlatans are usually not trained in cancer biology and are toying with your life with unproven or disproven brainstorms (read brain fart) or far-fetched ideas. Always dig deeper when looking at your options.

When effective mainstream therapies exist, and someone elects a treatment that is squarely in the "we know this does not work" or the "we have no idea if this works" category, he or she may be risking his or her life. If one elects to follow that path, it is certainly their choice. All I can say is that there are a lot of unqualified charlatans out there selling such treatments as "effective," so buyer beware! Sometimes these bonafide kooks sound extremely convincing with scientific jargon and quote studies as if they were real experts on the subject. However, please keep your brain's internal "bullshitometer" awake. If it sounds too good to be true, if there is too much being said about "secrets *they* don't want you to know about", or if they are going completely against what the rest of the international scientific community is saying, you should probably be at least a little skeptical. Finally, look at the source. Is it credible? Really? Take an objective closer look, because your life is on the line.

It is one thing to be thinking out of the box and being open to new ways to approach a problem. It is quite another to be slinging useless treatments at people. That is what the scientific research process is all about; to be constantly searching for what is new and what works. Those of us who are active in clinical research are constantly asking questions about a better way. Along that path, if we can help patients and survivors with quality of life and naturally contribute to strengthening their body against cancer and other disease, this is also a great goal.

While radical nutritional therapy can influence the progression of cancer, in the overwhelming majority of people (i.e. 99.99999%) when cancer is diagnosed it is beyond this being a reasonable approach as the only treatment. On the other hand, as a primary prevention strategy, of course, nutrition and lifestyle are crucial. Whether this translates to lengthening and improving the quality of survivorship after mainstream therapy remains to be seen, but there is encouraging data in this regard. So, after cancer seems to have been controlled or eradicated, considering lifestyle modifications is very prudent, and I highly recommend it. It is low risk and may very well save your life.

A comment or two is in order about conspiracy theories and "the establishment" or "government/FDA" or other bad guys who are supposedly not allowing access to cancer cures that are somehow being hidden from public view. For this to occur, the entire world, including communist China, all socialist countries, and all capitalist countries would have to be in cahoots. Further, the tens of thousands of healthcare workers, including doctors and research scientists around the world, who study and treat cancer would all have to be crooks and wish ill will on you. Furthermore, even if this were true, all whistleblowers out there working for Big Pharma or the government and FDA would have to remain quiet. Does this sound a little far fetched? Well, it is. That is not to say that there are never "bad people" in the mix, and that profit motive is not counter-productive in some cases. However, the same could be said about charlatan snake oil salespersons who are trying to sell you on alternative therapies that just have no prayer of working. This book aims to provide a balanced viewpoint for you to consider in your journey to survivorship.

True integrative oncology may help you in an even broader sense that you may not realize. By empowering and engaging yourself to take control of your body and defeat cancer, the fact that you ever came down with cancer may be a sort of blessing in disguise. That may sound incredibly weird but bear with me as I have seen a lot of fantastic personal transformations that go beyond beating cancer.

I think anyone would agree that beating cancer is a very powerful personal achievement. We do not wish cancer upon anyone. However, once you have actively beaten it (i.e., you participated in your own cure), you have proven something to yourself and others. A person who is in control of defeating their illness, regaining their health and achieving happiness in survivorship is a very strong person indeed. That person is in a far better position to control their destiny than one who takes a passive approach. So, as odd as it sounds, by beating cancer you rise to a level above most of those around you. You are special or are destined to be. Engage and help heal yourself and others.

This book contains MANY actionable steps for you to consider, focusing on the crucial core ones. There are many more but, if you focus on what is presented herein, it will take you at least 80% of the way to success in survivorship.

Finally, think long term. This book is about transformation, from diagnosis to thriving in survivorship. It is not about quick fix natural "magic" anti-cancer bullets. Take as many steps as you can and you will be surprised how fast you will start to see results. Those who do not know about these actions or don't follow them will take notice and probably ask about what you are doing. So, you have an opportunity to not only improve your own life but also to help others in their journey.

There seems to be quite a confusion about the various types of non-mainstream medicine. Although there are some similarities and overlaps, there are also some important differences.

Integrative Medicine

The American Board of Integrative Medicine defines integrative medicine as the practice of medicine that reaffirms the importance of the relationship between practitioner and patient, focuses on the whole person, is informed by evidence, and makes use of all appropriate therapeutic approaches, healthcare professionals, and disciplines to achieve optimal health and healing. Integrative oncology is an extension of this definition to address the whole person (body, mind, and spirit) with cancer. It means we use the best available evidence from all productive areas to treat not only the disease but also the person with the disease, which is more important in the long run. Note the "evidence-*informed*" part vs. "evidence-*based*" which is a more commonly used concept in mainstream medicine. To those that know the roots of this, the original intent of the evidence-based medicine notion was the same as evidence-informed. In other words, we should simply use the *best* available evidence to make informed decisions.

In the mainstream world, the definition of evidence-based medicine has become somewhat perverted into the notion that only randomized controlled clinical trials evidence is worth anything. This is known as Level I evidence. The fact is that, at least in oncology, only about twenty to thirty percent of mainstream therapy is based on Level I data. So, it is ill advised to chastise complementary and even some alternative practices for lack of Level I evidence. It's sort of like the kettle calling the pot black. On the other hand, both "evidence-based" and "evidence-informed" is a far cry from "seat-of-the-pants" medicine where practitioners make things up as they go along, or perpetuate something that started that way. This distinction can lead to the difference between your long happy survivorship and premature death.

Alternative Medicine

We already touched on this term in the introduction. This entire pseudo-medical area is very misleading just in the name alone. The word "alternative" strongly implies something is a valid evidence based therapy that can be used *instead* of mainstream Western medicine with similar results. This is not the case. Whether or not you believe that something is plausible, or should work, the treatments that are sequestered into this area of "alternative medicine" are usually unproven or even disproven. If you were somehow convinced that you should take an alternative treatment suggested by a doctor on his or her word alone, or based on a few anecdotal testimonials, without any sound scientific evidence, please consider the following. If you have a good chance of cure based on mainstream treatment, you may be literally throwing your life away on alternative unproven or disproven therapy.

If you have an advanced and probably incurable or recurrent aggressive cancer, you should be thinking about risk vs. benefit of any treatment. It is true that mainstream treatment may make you sicker than the disease, at least temporarily, but most often this is not the case. However, if nothing is likely to help according to your oncologist, this is the only circumstance where choosing a low toxicity unproven but plausible alternative therapy instead of doing nothing makes some sense. On the other hand, consider that mainstream treatment may still give you months or years of quality filled life, even if no cure is possible. Talk to your oncologist about the hard questions and risk vs. benefit of treatment.

Accepting alternative therapy can be like playing the lottery. Just because your neighbor or co-worker won, it is *highly* unlikely that you will get the same result. You may be lucky because there are miracle cures no matter what treatment is used. However, miracles happen even less often than lottery winners are created.

Functional Medicine

This is another relatively new term and a paradigm which overlaps solid artful science-based medical practice, incorporating the principles of integrative medicine. Practitioners of functional medicine try to involve the patient in a partnership as part of a systems-based approach to get at root causes. This means spending more time listening to patients and getting at the complex interaction of genetics, environmental exposure, lifestyle choices and the like. It is patient centered and in my view is the very definition of a good integrative oncology approach, incorporating the best of Western medicine and natural support.

Complementary Medicine

This word implies using something together to complement or help another therapy. By the way, a good test for your internal "bullshitometer" is if you see someone is offering "complimentary" therapy rather than "complementary." That signifies that they not only have a poor command of the English language but probably are not reputable practitioners either. Complimentary just means "free."

There is a broad range of complementary therapies that are used with mainstream treatment to improve wellbeing and reduce symptoms. Encouraging evidence shows that complementary strategies may improve chances for survival by reducing the risk of recurrence. When used with or after mainstream therapy, even a low risk plausible "alternative" treatment is reasonable to consider. This is not the case for high-risk alternative therapies, of which there are many, even though they are peddled as kinder and gentler. We cover the most common ones in this book and note if they are proven, unproven, disproven or flat out dangerous.

What doctor(s) should I be working with?

First of all, please make sure they are legitimately trained doctors in something or are closely working with a legitimate oncologist. Keep in mind there are "diploma mills" out there and the person sitting in front of you claiming they are a doctor, may not be one. It's scary, seems far-fetched, but it is true. It is especially true if you seek cancer care outside of the United States in a third-world country. There are good doctors everywhere, but the percentage of charlatans is higher in a system that is not well organized.

Anyone who is not a bona fide medical allopathic (MD) or osteopathic (DO) doctor may be a highly valued member of your cancer-fighting team, but they cannot lead it. Beyond the MD or DO degree, you *must* have a board certified or board eligible (meaning they are in the process of certification but completed all training) mainstream oncologist involved. In fact, you may have different types of oncologists involved: surgical, medical, radiation, pediatric, gynecologic, neurologic, and so on. Oncologists are the most extensively trained doctors in the biology of and best current treatment options for cancer. Without one, you have a 99% chance of not getting your best shot at a cure. It is as simple as that.

On the other hand, oncologists are often not trained in integrative support, which includes complementary medicine and nutrition. Ideally, you should find a fully trained integrative MD or DO oncologist. However, integrative oncology physicians such as myself are hard to come by. If you can't find one nearby, then find an oncologist who works with integrative providers as part of a team, not just one who loosely refers and does not communicate well with them. Integrative providers may be nutrition professionals, naturopaths, acupuncturists, chiropractors, nurses or non-oncologist MD or DO medical doctors who focus on integrative medicine.

Teamwork is great but DO NOT let anyone but an MD or DO oncologist guide your mainstream anti-cancer treatment. For example, there are plenty of family practice doctors out there who run "cancer clinics". These physicians may even be "board certified" in family medicine, or emergency medicine or something other than oncology but they are not adequately trained to help you defeat cancer as the primary provider. Naturopathic oncologists (ND) can be an outstanding valued member of your team, but they do not have the experience in mainstream oncology to lead or even advise on that aspect of care. If you are going to work with a naturopathic doctor, seek one who has a FABNO designation. This means they have undergone additional training and certification in oncology as a Fellow of the American Board of Naturopathic Oncology.

As far as mainstream MD or DO oncologists are concerned, keep in mind that levels of expertise vary. Just like you can have a good lawyer or not, or a good mechanic or not, you may or may not have the best oncologist either. Part of the equation is whether or not you can connect with them. This is *subjective* but important. However, the other critical *objective* part is that some are more in tune with advances than others. This is not something a Specialty Board or State Medical Board can police for two reasons. First, the doctor may be satisfactory but not great. They may have demonstrated basic competence, but that is all. As far as Specialty Board certification is concerned, if your doctor was certified back in the 1980's or so, they may have never picked up a book after that or read a single new study, because they do not have to recertify periodically. Those that were certified in the 1990's and later do have to demonstrate at least basic competence regularly. Also, although it is awkward to say, some of those folks who work for State Medical Boards are not always the sharpest tools in the shed. There is no 100% way to be certain that you have the best doctor for your needs, but the less there is a connection, the less there is good communication and the less discussion there is of cutting edge options, the more you should be seeking a second opinion.

Please consider that it might not be prudent to follow the advice of physicians who have had their license revoked or suspended or who have been disciplined by their State Medical Board for unethical practices. This is way below the most basic level of competence. It's scraping the bottom. I have even seen such physicians claim that they are "stepping out of the box" against the "cancer establishment" for *your* benefit. Nothing could be further from the truth. This is plain loony toons. These physicians simply have no idea about what they are doing and are in effect experimenting on you with their "ideas", should you choose to let them. While it is always reasonable to *think* out of the box and come up with new treatments via research, *acting prematurely* out of the box with ill-conceived, scientifically implausible, unproven and potentially dangerous treatment is not what a credible physician should be doing.

There is another emerging trend. Since integrative medicine and integrative oncology have become more accepted by mainstream doctors, and they are in demand, it has become a money-making and marketing opportunity. So, seemingly everyone is out there putting up a sign that proclaims they are an "Integrative Cancer Center" or clinic. However, when you look at the people involved, the same warnings that we just covered apply. Are there fully trained MD or DO oncologists involved? Are they really involved and knowledgeable or are they just signing off on things their integrative staff says without understanding if these complementary, alternative and integrative modalities will help or possibly hurt you? Ideally, are the oncologists themselves board certified or trained in integrative medicine? Is it really a team or is it just a "slap on" smorgasbord of integrative type services with no real coordination? Dig a little deeper to see what the level of qualifications and teamwork is.

Lastly, in addition to getting the *kooks* completely out of the kitchen, it is also a good idea to identify the main trusted physician you will be working with and not have too many credible *cooks* in the kitchen either. Having too many doctors bending your ear at the same time will lead to more confusion and possibly undermine trust. Having confidence in your doctor has been proven to influence your outcome strongly. Choose wisely and limit "doctor shopping" after you find someone whom you connect with that is verifiably well credentialed.

Section I
Cancer Causation and Your Body

We will start by answering some frequently asked questions and follow with some "should ask" questions that you may not have thought of. I try to do that in a number of the chapters where it applies.

CHAPTER 1
WHAT IS CANCER?

Cancer is a group of diseases involving abnormal cell growth that escapes normal regulation and programmed cell death (apoptosis) with the potential to invade or spread to other parts of the body. In other words, healthy cells know when to die, make room for new ones, and respect boundaries. They know how to behave in an orderly fashion, being replaced only when needed. Cancer cells overgrow and invade, or burrow into, healthy tissues. This invasion can be local, creating a primary tumor or growth, or can be secondary tumors or metastases that spread to other parts of the body through the bloodstream and lymphatic system.

Only 5-10% of cancers are primarily heritable or genetic in origin. On the other hand, a commonly quoted statistic is that 35% or so of cancers are based on environmental factors. Well, if that is the case, what about the 50-60% in the middle? It is far more likely that 90-95% are mainly due to environmental factors based on a lifelong interaction between poor lifestyle choices and pro-carcinogenic epigenetic and genetic factors. This delicate interplay between what I would call "bad environment" and "weak genes" is incompletely understood. However, more and more evidence is pointing towards bad environment cancer causation.

Cancer is not caused by only one thing. The causative factors include diet, chronic inflammation, obesity and lack of exercise, some oncogenic viruses and parasitic infections (mostly for specific cancers usually in the third world), exposure to chemical toxins called carcinogens, excess radiation exposure, and hormone imbalances. The genetics, epigenetics, biochemistry, physiology, anatomy and other sciences studying carcinogenesis and spread, show cancer causation to be an exceedingly complex issue.

Our understanding of cancer has grown by leaps and bounds and is eons ahead of what we knew when President Nixon declared the "War on Cancer." However, cures or prolongation of life in many cancers remains elusive precisely because we now know cancer is not one disease with one cause.

We also know that cancer is *not* the result of, or related to, the following disproven or isolated concepts:

NOT always due to bad genes you can't influence (in 95% of cases)

NOT a fungal overgrowth or a result of fungal infection

NOT the result of your body being "too acidic" per se

NOT an iodine deficiency, or any other single nutrient deficiency

NOT from one particular isolated toxin like Mercury amalgam

NOT due to vaccinations (in fact some alternative practitioners use dubious vaccinations wrongly in treating cancer)

NOT due to scars

NOT spread by exposure to air during surgery

NOT due to a deficiency of so-called "vitamin B-17", which is not a vitamin

….and so on.

There are many other ill-advised alarmist "causes" of cancer that are proffered out there by alternative "merchants of doubt". Such individuals seek to undermine and create conspiracy theory angles rather than be proactive and help cancer patients find the best scientifically proven or at least plausible integrative cancer care options out there.

We cover some of these erroneous concepts in greater depth and provide specific recommendations. Don't waste your time chasing these notions. Focus on the scientifically proven or plausible approaches we present and you will get far better results without wasting time and money. Remember, unscrupulous charlatans with marketing expertise are very good at what they do. They often fly "real-looking" but bogus credentials and use scientific sounding jargon. They can sell ice to an Eskimo. Don't fall for slick hype and ludicrous scare tactics like "the cancer establishment is trying to poison you, and your doctor is only in it for the money". That is a slap in the face to literally millions of researchers and physicians worldwide that are trying to find better answers for you every day. Don't get me wrong. There are bad apples in every walk of life, but it is not a norm or organized conspiracy in healthcare.

How Did I Get Cancer?

The question of "how did I get cancer" always comes up. Many people falsely assume that they came down with cancer because they were dealt bad cancer-causing genes that they couldn't do anything about. It is true that we are born with a varying number of what you might simplistically call "bad" or "potentially bad" or "weak" genes. However, the interaction of environment that we create for ourselves with these genes is well within our control. With lifestyle modifications, you have a lot of influence on activating good genes and suppressing bad genes. The problem is that we do not have gene-specific accurately targeted strategies yet, only generic ones. Gene targeting precision medicine is already here but mostly in clinical trials. It is not yet standard of practice for most cancers. Having said that, you are already more in control than you might think. Whether it be from carrying too many extra fat pounds or eating too many processed foods or working too closely with toxins, or overexposure to hormones, these can all help activate bad genes. However, you can also suppress these and activate good genes by assessing your surroundings, changing your lifestyle, reducing inflammation and getting into better shape. In this way, you are closer to getting at the root cause of your cancer.

There is a theory that we all develop cancer cells every day and that our immune system takes care of that most of the time. This is called immune surveillance and immune editing but is not completely understood. The problem with this theory is that many people are on immune suppressive drugs after an organ transplant or for autoimmune diseases. Their cancer rate is much higher, with about 5-6% of transplant patients coming down with cancer within the first few years. Overall the risk can be two to three times compared with those who have not had a transplant and did not require immunosuppressive medication. However, *most* do not get cancer despite a chronically suppressed immune system. The truth about immune-surveillance and editing is very complicated, but it guides us towards the importance of staying away from disease, drugs or environmental factors that can be immune suppressive and cancer promoting.

For you to have come down with cancer, some significant changes have occurred in your body related to a breakdown of genetic cellular control due to environmental factors (mentioned above) which have overwhelmed your immune system. You now have an invasive malignant tumor which has either been diagnosed physically or by scan and has been biopsy proven to be cancerous. Assuming the tumor is at least one centimeter (about half an inch) in size, this means billions of cancer cells now threaten your life.

After The Diagnosis: What Now?

Cancers grow at a variable rate, but some can kill within months. To eliminate a cancerous tumor growth, you need rapid industrial strength treatment. This may include removing it surgically, or killing the cells that make up the tumor with radiation or chemotherapy, or newer so-called "biologic" agents. While natural support for your body with diet, supplements, lifestyle changes and the like are crucial to your success in the long run, they are not potent enough strategies to eliminate a rapidly growing cancer at this point. For example, obesity is an inflammatory cause of cancer in many cases. As you also know, weight loss is not easy and done right, takes time. Getting into awesome shape and not just losing a few pounds, can take months if not years. Meanwhile, since the root cause of obesity-related inflammation is not reversed, cancer keeps growing and will kill you well before you can get into fantastic shape.

The time for primary prevention has passed when you are diagnosed with cancer. However, as is covered in this book, your attention to root cause correction is vital to the quality of your survivorship and reducing your risk of recurrence as much as possible. The scientific explanation for this is probably at the level of something called the "cancer stem cell" which may or may not be eradicated by mainstream therapy. However, stem cells may be strongly influenced by lifestyle and natural support, as you will soon learn. While you can work on strengthening your body and making it as cancer-proof as possible all along, first things first. You need to eliminate or radically push back those billions of cancer cells in your body, and this can only be accomplished by mainstream treatment.

So, if mainstream therapy is so good, why are we not "winning the war on cancer"? Actually, we are, and the results are rather impressive. However, we are all stepping on our own tail along the way as humans, which impedes our forward progress. What do I mean by that? Winning the war with fewer cancer diagnoses and more people alive after a cancer diagnosis depends on both prevention and treatment. Prevention is made up of screening tools and lifestyle choices. In those populations that have availed themselves of screening recommendations and have committed to prudent lifestyle choices, cancer rates are way down, and cancers are being detected much earlier when they are more amenable to curative treatments. This part of the war on cancer is definitely being won if you are making proper lifestyle choices. We know what those choices need to be. If you choose correctly, you are highly likely to win. It is as simple as that.

The other important part is the treatment options themselves, especially when cancer is more advanced. Let there be no mistake. We have wonder-drugs and wonder therapies on the surgical and radiation side compared to the 1970's. The advances have been spectacular! However, those that ignore or don't have access to screening or who have descended into an abyss of cancer-causing lifestyle choices, come in with advanced cancers. Too often, in addition to cancer, people are in poor overall health and have other very debilitating disease like obesity, diabetes, hypertension and so on. Obesity and diabetes lead to increased risk for cancer. It's a snowball effect, all based on chronic inflammation. Unfortunately, the number of people oncologists see in this multiple disease category is rapidly increasing. At this point, the oncologist is too often faced with a disaster scenario to fix, and the end result is a predictable "too little too late".

Oncologists are not God. Honestly, I am surprised we are squeaking out a steady improvement in survival despite the situation we just covered. If this group of patients was treated today with treatment options that were available 40 years ago, they would all be dead. So, we are steadily advancing and making wondrous discoveries and inroads to better cancer treatment and support. However, society *must* fundamentally alter their lifestyle choices behavior and diet. Also, much work needs to be done in the areas of food industry practices and regulation of toxin-producing industries.

In summary, the increase of advanced cancer in multi-disease patients is over-whelming the phenomenal advances in the "cancer industry". I put that in quotes because although there is a profit motive in everything these days, this is not a nefarious industry complex of people-hating money-grubbing researchers and doctors condoned by the FDA in trying to keep cancer alive as a "business disease". That thought process deserves a loony-toons badge and a sharp whack to the side of the head. Credit should be given where it is due, and the bigger problem of why we are not curing more cancer because of worsening population health should be addressed. Everyone contributes to the war on cancer if it is to be won, and this starts with you!

Why Does Cancer Recur?

Conventional time-honored scientific wisdom has held that cancer cells become resistant to chemotherapy during treatment, and a resistant clone of cells develops which never gets eliminated. This is very variable between cancer types and the sensitivity of any given cancer to chemo is variable right from the beginning. However, in those cases where cancer appears to be gone after treatment based on scans, blood tests, and examination, a microscopic clone of resistant cells may be left behind. This may be a few cells or even hundreds or thousands of cells, but they are too few to be detected by any blood test or scan. Eventually, depending upon how aggressive the cancer type is, the visible tumors grow back. In some, it can be weeks and in others many years.

Recently, so-called "cancer stem cells" have been identified in numerous types of cancer. These are not the rapidly dividing aberrant cells that make up the bulk of a cancerous tumor or growth. They are far fewer in number and are resistant to chemotherapy and radiation because they do not replicate very rapidly. They are probably also the cells that break off from primary tumors and spread or metastasize to grow additional tumors in the body. These cells have been detected in the blood stream and are called "circulating tumor cells" or CTC's. Although it is not clear, the evidence suggests that they are cancer stem cells in transition. If a very early cancer is removed surgically, the offending stem cells may go with it, before they circulate, which explains cures after surgery alone. What's critical is that this assumes the cancer was removed before any stem cells have had a chance to access the vascular or lymphatic circulation. The problem is that this is impossible to know at the time of surgery and is the reason why some patients with "early cancer" where the surgeon announces "we got it all" end up suffering a recurrence. Actually, by measuring circulating tumor DNA fragments, we are now able to very precise about whether or not the surgery "got it all". This is a research tool, but will soon be standard.

Research is very active in this area of stem cells, but the concept is not universally accepted. It's certainly not yet utilized in clinical practice and counseling of patients. However, it plausibly explains why some cancers recur while others do not and why some more readily metastasize than others. It also offers an avenue towards potentially natural epigenetic prevention or risk reduction, whether it be primary prevention or secondary prevention of recurrence. You are about to discover how to do this.

Environmental toxins and nutrients can either negatively or positively affect these stem cells where chemotherapy and radiation fails. This is part of the scientific basis of "getting at the root cause of cancer" in order to be cured. This goes far beyond what mainstream medicine can do to minimize cancerous tumor growth and produce remission because there are no medications which reliably suppress cancer stem cells and induce tumor dormancy. As you will soon discover in this book, by avoiding carcinogenic toxins and by leveraging anti-cancer nutrients, you will have another weapon against cancer under your direct control.

Top Seven Innovative Strategies To Prevent And Attack Cancer

You may or may not believe that mainstream cancer therapy is a lifesaver. You may be a dyed-in-the-wool natural alternative therapy believer to the exclusion of mainstream medicine's "cutting, poisoning and burning", which is an irreverent and, in my strong opinion, unwarranted dig against surgery, chemotherapy, and radiation. It does not matter because there is a convergence and overlap between evolving mainstream therapies and natural methods that bolster your body to become cancer resistant or even cancer-proof. It's all based on scientific principles of how the human body works and how cancer develops and grows.

Mother Nature's science has shown us how cancer can be defeated. It is just that our tools are not perfected yet, and each cancer is a little different. As we move into the future, we are learning how to attack cancer from more angles, and what follows are the top seven ways currently known to science. These are subjects of intense research. All these strategies go beyond removing a tumor surgically, or killing more cancer than healthy cells by a brute force approach inherent in chemotherapy and radiation. The risks and benefits of mainstream cancer therapy are discussed later in this book, but first here is a quick overview of where we are headed and which of these can already be targeted to some extent using natural approaches.

First, to prevent cancer in the first place we need to do everything possible to limit toxin exposure, increase our ability to resist toxins we cannot avoid, and strengthen the function of "good" tumor suppressor genes in our body. We also need to maintain as strong an immune system as possible, reduce insulin resistance, and reduce chronic inflammation. Finally, we need to manage sex hormones to prevent certain cancers and reduce stress hormones to help to avoid all cancers. All of this makes a hostile environment for cancer, so in effect, you are cancer-proofing yourself to every extent possible based on known contemporary scientific principles.

We know that to defeat rapidly dividing and growing cancer cells in tumors we need to get them to recognize that they can't live forever, which means we need to limit their life by inducing apoptosis or programmed cell death.

Then, to prevent recurrence directly, cancer stem cells and circulating tumor cells must be kept in a state of dormancy or reverted back to normal. As you will see, this is plausible and doable in the lab but not completely proven in the clinical setting. However, if it's easy, cheap, not dangerous and healthy for you, it is still reasonable to consider.

Finally, to help avert recurrence, your body must be made as hostile towards cancer cell growth as possible, just like we do with primary prevention. You undoubtedly have heard both fact and hype about "cancer-proofing" your body and it is hard to tell the difference unless you are a savvy health care professional or bona fide scientist or both. The truth is that you can very likely enhance your cancer resistance but there is no proven one-size-fits-all solution, and it is not 100% effective. Having said that, it is still well worth the effort.

The above is a tall order, and we do not have a red pill or blue pill to accomplish these tasks, at least not yet. However, the good news is that while we wait for high-tech targeted solutions, Mother Nature has some good options to improve our chances of avoiding and beating cancer. These strategies are based on key targets which you can influence naturally using diet, important supplements, specific types of exercise, targeted herbals, and stress management on a mind-body and spiritual basis.

Cancerous cells and tumors can either be eradicated or placed in a state of dormancy using a combination of the following strategies:

1. Reducing oxidative stress, thereby reducing cancer cell genetic instability and inducing apoptosis or programmed cell death

2. Reducing abnormal expression of genes through epigenetics

3. Affecting cell surface to internal signal transduction

4. Reducing abnormal cell to cell communication

5. Reducing tumor angiogenesis

6. Limiting invasion and metastases

7. Stimulating innate immunity to limit immune evasion

In this book, we will be covering all of these strategies. However, as you will see, while drugs might target one of these at a time, natural approaches will target multiple strategies at a time. For example, nutritional recommendations might affect cancer by epigenetic effects as well as by reducing angiogenesis and influencing cell signal transduction. Quite a complex example is that the very important phytonutrient genistein has a positive epigenetic effect, is a protein kinase inhibitor and reduces signaling effects of IL-10. Wow! That's a mouthful. The point behind my mentioning these technical details is that this book is chock full of the very best scientifically based recommendations for fighting cancer, but you do not have to know exactly how each of them works unless you want to dig deeper. For that purpose, multiple references are provided, and you can go even deeper by searching http://pubmed.gov. However, the main point is for you to appreciate the incredible complexity of the human body and cancer, in order to reject simpleton garbage "cures" out there that only raise false hope and provide no benefit.

CHAPTER 2
PREVENTION AND SCREENING

Unfortunately, I have taken care of many cancer patients over the years who "did everything right" with respect to lifestyle choices and still came down with cancer. So, while healthy choices are extremely important, cancer can occur anyway. Finding cancers early, or when they are in pre-cancer phases, becomes another goal of effective prevention.

There are several points at which prevention is important. The best is primary prevention, where the goal is to prevent any pre-cancer or cancer from developing in your body. Secondary prevention is defined several ways but often means preventing cancer from growing from a pre-cancerous condition. For example, cervical dysplasia is pre-cancer. When dealt with appropriately, invasive cancer is prevented. Lastly, there is tertiary prevention. At this point, cancer has already been diagnosed and treated. The goal is tertiary prevention of symptoms and ideally, if in remission, recurrence of the disease. The concepts raised in this book can be applied to all three points in time. However, it's crucial to understand that you have to work much harder for tertiary prevention of recurrence to be effective than primary prevention. However, at the very least, quality of life may be improved.

Prevention of cancer depends on two key elements. First of all, and most important are lifestyle choices. These are covered extensively in this book and are crucial to effective prevention. This is based on your environmental exposure and the food you eat directly "talking" to your genes through something called epigenetics. It is in your power to generally switch off pro-cancer genes and switch on anti-cancer genes. Can you switch on or off a specific gene using a particular food? The answer is maybe, but this is not understood completely at that micro level yet. You can however generically activate good genes and deactivate bad genes, and this is covered in more detail later in this book.

The second component to effective prevention is to take advantage of screening tests that are designed to find early cancer or even pre-cancer before there are any signs or symptoms. There are some controversies regarding best practices and best tools for this, which we will touch on in this chapter.

If you already have or have beaten cancer, you may or may not be predisposed to certain other cancers. However, one thing is for sure; you do not want to get *another* cancer after beating your first. I have known patients to have as many as seven cancers in their lifetime. That is NOT a club you want to belong to if at all possible. So keep up on recommended screening guidelines.

Guidelines for cancer screening are developed by expert panels from some organizations, based on science and statistics. The one most people are familiar with is the American Cancer Society (ACS). However, the US Preventive Services Task Force (USPSTF) also produces evidence-based guidelines. Both are often updated. Other specialty specific organizations also put out guidelines, but these are usually less robust or less detailed than the ACS or USPSTF. For example, the National Comprehensive Cancer Network (NCCN) prevention guidelines focus on breast, cervix, lung, colon and prostate.

While there are some differences between guidelines, they are not usually very substantial. The purpose of this section is to raise awareness of what is appropriate and what is not. However, it is not meant to be an exhaustive review of all screening guidelines. The point of this chapter is for you to make sure you are being checked at appropriate intervals with appropriate tests to minimize the risk that you will end up with a second cancer. For those readers who have not been diagnosed with cancer, this is even more important because primary prevention beats any kind of treatment offered for any cancer.

What is screening? Why do we screen for some cancers and not for others? Why do we start some at a certain age and why do we stop at any particular age? Why are some tests recommended every year and others five years apart? This is all based on scientific knowledge of how cancers develop, at what age they tend to develop, how long it takes for them to develop or cause harm and very fundamental statistical concepts. While we are not going to get into the very complicated statistical details here, it is crucial for you to know the core concepts or else you will not understand why the recommended testing is prudent for you. Without this understanding, you can very easily be misled by "alternative" propaganda or fanatical unsubstantiated ravings of "false-experts". Screening is not about opinions. It is about facts that are scientifically substantiated and statistically sound.

The goal is to use effective tools to find early cancer, or ideally *pre*-cancer. The screening must effectively reduce mortality from cancer while avoiding over-diagnosis and overtreatment for conditions that may be pre-cancerous or are cancerous but are very slow growing and not life threatening. The screening tools must be acceptable, with reasonably small discomfort and minimal risk of harm.

As far as why some cancers are screened for and others not, the answer is twofold. First, there may not be an effective screening tool yet, as is the case with ovarian and endometrial cancer. Second, the particular cancer must be prevalent enough (i.e. occur often enough) that screening for it would not be like looking for a needle in a haystack. Screening for low prevalence cancers means that many people would undergo unnecessary risk, pain or costs. Since the tests are not perfect, a significant number of cancers would still go undetected or worse be over-diagnosed.

There is another hard fact to face, and that is that resources are limited in health-care no matter how well the healthcare system is designed. With limited resources, the most prudent plan is to spend more money screening for cancers that we can more readily find and do something about to help the most people and risk harm in the fewest number of individuals. There is one other statistical reason why it is not prudent to screen for low prevalence cancers, and that's covered below.

So, how do we determine which tests should be used and how often? This is all based on research studies and very complicated statistical analysis. Contrary to what "alternative" naysayers suggest, these are not just dreamt up based on fly-by-night recommendations from the "cancer establishment" or based on who has the coolest new screening tool that might work because they simply *think* it might.

A crucial part of any research study, in this case for screening tool evaluation, is the statistical analysis. The analysis is done by statistics professionals who are charged with determining: 1) Is it possible that the difference or lack thereof between tests or treatments was based on a "flip of the coin heads or tails 50/50" chance alone, rather than a cause and effect relationship? 2) In the case of screening tool evaluation, how sensitive and specific is the test? These two words have very different meanings, even though they sound similar, but both are crucial. Sensitivity means how likely is it that cancer or pre-cancer will be found if it is there. Put another way, it is the ability of the test to identify correctly people who have the disease. Specificity means how likely is it that those without cancer or pre-cancer will have a negative test. Put another way, it is the ability of the test to identify correctly those people who do *not* have the disease.

Using the sensitivity and specificity of a screening test, one can take it a step further and determine the negative and positive predictive value. Negative predictive value means the proportion of people with a negative test who do not have the disease. Positive predictive value indicates the share of people with a positive test that actually have the disease. So, on the basis of these, you hear of a screening test having a false positive rate (i.e. test is positive, but nothing is wrong, which raises the concern of over-diagnosis) and a false negative rate (i.e. the test is negative, but the disease is actually there). Finally, if a type of cancer has a low prevalence, then the chances are very high that a positive test is really a false positive. This is the other reason that screening for low prevalence cancers is not a good idea with current technology.

The final statistical tidbit to understand is that the sensitivity of a test can be plotted on a graph against the specificity. This is known as a ROC curve and can help those who develop guidelines to see visually which tests have the best tradeoff between sensitivity and specificity and provides the overall accuracy of the screening test.

The above probably sounds like statistical mumbo jumbo and not very important, but in fact, it is *critical!* For example, if a test has a high sensitivity and low specificity, then it is very possible to get a false positive and put someone through a lot of unnecessary additional tests and even unnecessary treatment. Sometimes this treatment can be injurious and even kill people. A test that has high specificity but low sensitivity can lead to false negatives, which means a cancer may be present, and it was simply missed because the test is not that good. Obviously, this can lead to cancer growing and killing someone when it could have been detected earlier with a better test.

So, in reviewing the specific tests for different cancers and in looking at new tools, data from statistical analyses like these are crucial to determining if the screening test should be recommended or not. Even with the very best screening tests, there is going to be a risk of under or over-diagnosis. Lastly, tests can sometimes lead to complications, some of which can even result in death. So, the safest, highest accuracy tests are the ones recommended for you in the major screening guidelines out there.

Keep two critical things in mind as you read further. First, even the best current screening tests are not perfect. This means you may have something wrong with a negative test or may have nothing wrong with a positive test. Second, screening is designed just to raise a flag that something is not right or to reassure you that things seem to be all right. It is usually not a diagnostic tool. So, what is done after a screening test is positive requires some expert guidance. A positive test does not mean you are going straight to surgery or to chemotherapy or anything of the sort. It means more tests or possibly a biopsy is required to clarify why the screening test was positive. If the screening, like colonoscopy, *includes* a biopsy then, in this case, it may be diagnostic. But you would still need more testing to see if cancer has spread or is still local for optimal treatment planning.

If you did not understand *any* of the above, it's OK. The key point or EZ Button to remember here is that there is a lot of thought and science behind what screening tools are best and how often you should use them to prevent or at least reduce the risk of cancer.

Breast

Despite some controversies, which we cover here, there is no question that the best screening tool for breast cancer is mammography. Specifically, regular film mammograms are most often recommended. However, digital mammography is becoming more and more available with a possible benefit of delivering a little bit less radiation. Both are equally accurate.

Mammogram results are reported as BI-RADS (Breast Imaging-Reporting and Data System) categories, zero to six. Depending upon the category, a decision is made to continue screening regularly or do further testing such as MRI or ultrasound.

The overall lifetime risk of breast cancer is a little over 12% or about one in eight women. Some have higher risk based on family history, age at menarche and other factors. You can access a risk assessment tool called the Gail model online: http://www.cancer.gov/bcrisktool.

For average-risk women, starting mammogram screening at 40 years of age is a bit controversial and recommended by some guidelines and not by others. However, all guidelines agree that annual screening should at least be the norm after age 50. As far as an age to stop, this is also a bit controversial. The American Cancer Society and NCCN recommend screening to continue for as long as a woman is in good health. Others use 75 years of age as an arbitrary cutoff and some talk about screening until life expectancy is less than five to seven years. Of course, the problem with that is that it is usually hard to predict how long someone will live. These days, if you are following a lifestyle filled with great health choices you may easily live well beyond ninety. So make sure you are not sold down the river if you are healthy at any age.

Annual breast examinations may add to mammography in that they can detect palpable (i.e. physically felt) masses when mammograms miss them about 15% of the time. The problem is that the sensitivity for detecting cancer by examination is only 59%, and the specificity is about 93%. So, this means that breast exams cannot replace mammograms.

Formal breast *self*-examination, offered as a major part of screening in the past, has been replaced by the concept of breast self-awareness. In other words, the formal education of women to try to detect cancer using specific time intervals and techniques has been dropped because it did not help much. However, promotion of self-awareness of the appearance and feel of breasts with constant vigilance for change is prudent and highly recommended.

For high-risk women, it depends on what the reason for high risk is. This ranges from family history through various syndromes and BRCA mutations, among other factors. So, the recommendation is variable but calls for more aggressive screening starting earlier in life. This can be as early as age 25 and often includes the addition of MRI to mammography and breast examinations. So, make sure you know what your risk is. Communication with your doctor is critical for the right individualized screening plan.

So, what do you get from the above screening recommendations? How many lives are we saving? It is critical to know the benefits of screening for breast cancer to determine if it is worth the risks.

Critics say that mammograms can cause cancer by needlessly exposing people to radiation. They also say that mammography leads to too much over-diagnosis and consequent treatment that is unnecessary. Alternative practitioners propose the use of supposedly "better" tools like thermography that is purportedly harmless and is better at early detection. Let's see if they are right about any of these.

Analysis of thirty years worth of mammography screening data shows that deaths from breast cancer have indeed dropped, but the effect differs depending on age. A major analysis of multiple studies showed that mortality rate has been reduced by 15% in women aged 39-49, by 14% in women aged 50-59 and by 32% in women aged 60-69. Analysis of the four most high-profile large studies show that the death rate has been reduced from 14-48%, which is a pretty wide range but means that all studies point to the same conclusion. Having said that, it is still controversial as to how much of this effect is from finding earlier breast cancer through screening and how much is related to more effective treatment of breast cancer. The truth is probably somewhere in between, but no one argues that when you detect a breast cancer earlier, less treatment is required. So, the benefits of screening using mammography seem pretty clear and are based on international studies. One caveat is that despite statistics being vital in proving or disproving a point, sometimes the statistics are just plain poorly done and misleading in any given study. So, the fact that all the larger completely unrelated studies ALL show benefit is reassuring.

What about the risk of getting cancer from the exposure to radiation? First of all, let's put things in perspective. The amount of radiation one gets from a series of mammogram images is about 0.7 mSv. Milli-Sievert (mSv) is a unit standard of measuring radiation exposure. Typical background radiation from your surroundings per year is 1.5 to 2.5 mSv. So having a mammogram is equivalent to living on this planet with average sun exposure for about 24 weeks or less. If you work in an environment that uses radiation, as an x-ray technician does, your yearly allowable maximum exposure (measured by a safety badge) is set at 50 mSv. This is quite a bit higher and still considered reasonably "safe." However, there is no question that screening and any increase in radiation mean added risk. But, let's keep this in perspective. The increased risk per mammogram over background risk that everyone has is tiny at about 1 in 10,000 to 1 in 100,000 women. Over the years this can add up a little, but is still a slight increase in risk considering the significant benefits of catching cancer early. In the end, it is your choice after you carefully consider the risk and benefit.

What about over-diagnosis and harm from that? Studies show that if you have annual mammograms, your risk of having to get extra tests due to a false positive mammogram ranges from 20-50%. The younger you are, the more likely this is going to happen. However, other than the annoyance factor, if all tests are negative no real harm is done. The much bigger problem is that over-diagnosis of breast cancer occurs in about 1% to 25% of women, usually in the form of ductal carcinoma in situ which is very slow growing and not regarded as life threatening. Over the last 30 years of screening in the United States, the estimate is that about 1.3 million women were over-diagnosed. Another way to look at it is from a review by the Cochrane Collaboration which estimated that for every 2000 women screened over ten years, ten women receive unnecessary treatment for over-diagnosed breast cancer. This includes lumpectomy, mastectomy, and radiation therapy. While this sounds pretty unacceptable, hold on a second. The job of the mammogram screening is to raise flags and suggest that cancer is present. It is *not* a diagnosis and what physicians do with a positive result is extremely important. Jumping straight to surgery or radiation is most often not the right answer and is often the fault of doctors not following diagnosis and treatment guidelines. A recent study showed that needle biopsy, which is far less invasive, continues to be omitted in favor of inappropriate and more invasive excisional biopsy in far too many cases. So, the key message is that over-treatment is a risk of screening over-diagnosis but mostly occurs if the diagnostic and treatment guidelines after a positive screen are not followed. If you have a positive screening mammogram, a second opinion about what to do next is probably prudent.

In light of the risks, especially if you do not believe the benefits are worth it, what about other screening tools? Alternative practitioners often proffer the use of thermography as the answer. Thermography measures and maps the heat at the skin level of the breast using a specialized heat-sensing camera technology. The idea is that slight temperature changes, which are related to increased metabolism and blood flow, may be the sign of a cancerous tumor underneath.

While thermography is often represented as something new, it has actually been around for many years. This means there has been time to do many studies. These studies all show that this technology cannot detect breast cancer early, despite the good theory. In fact, thermography can detect only about a quarter of cancers found using mammography. Improvements in technology, using digital thermal imaging, has not led to better accuracy. It can be utilized as an adjunct to mammogram screening and is approved by the FDA for that purpose. This is because it measures the physiology of the breast and as such contributes to the understanding of overall breast health. So, the bottom line is that thermography is *not* a safe, effective alternative to mammography but can be used as an adjunct. The science on this is clear. Anything else is a matter of opinion, which may be based on misguided advice. Personal choice is an individual thing, but choosing wrong may be the difference between life and death. An extra year or two of undiagnosed cancer can mean a world of difference regarding curability.

This information is not supposed to be an exhaustive review of breast cancer screening. However, you should know that other non-radiation producing tests that have been proposed for screening are ultrasound and magnetic resonance imaging (MRI). Neither are replacements for mammography. MRI is very sensitive but can lead to over-diagnosis. Ultrasound is good for evaluating masses detected by mammography but is not sensitive enough as a screening tool. So, as with thermography, they may help in breast health evaluation but do not replace the mammogram for breast cancer screening.

Cervix

In developing countries without widespread screening, cervical cancer is the second most common cancer in women and the second most common cause of death due to cancer in women. While in the United States, where screening has been available since the mid 20ᵗʰ century, cervical cancer went from the leading cause of cancer death in women to fourteenth. For many years, the "Pap test" has been the mainstay of screening and the intent is not to find cancer but rather *pre*-cancer, which is called dysplasia.

We know that several strains of the human papillomavirus (HPV) are a key factor in the causation of cervical dysplasia and cancer. However, not everyone who gets infected with HPV gets cancer. In fact, only a small percentage do. In the presence of persistent infection and other cofactors such as smoking it predictably progresses from pre-cancer to cancer over five or more years. Because of this discovery, over the past decade, screening has included not only Pap smear review for abnormal cells on a microscope slide but also molecular testing for the presence or absence of high-risk HPV strains.

Screening guidelines have been refined over the past five to ten years based on better knowledge of this disease. We know that starting the screening before age 21 leads to many false positives and unnecessary biopsies and treatments. We also know that after age 65, assuming normal prior screening tests, no history of high-grade dysplasia over the previous 20 years and no high-risk sexual behavior, further screening does not help many women. Based on how long the disease takes to develop from normal to pre-cancer to cancer, screening is recommended every three years with Pap smears or every five years if using both the Pap smear and HPV test. It is very important to understand that the Pap and HPV tests are only meant to screen for cervical disease and not uterine or ovarian cancer. Occasionally, this type of screening will uncover vaginal or vulvar dysplasia, but that is uncommon.

The concept of HPV vaccination is socially controversial, and medically it is not a 100% prevention guarantee. While the vaccine targets the main cancer-causing HPV strains, not all possible cancer-causing strains are covered. Therefore, screening is recommended regardless of whether or not vaccination is accepted. Having said that, studies are already showing that vaccination is reducing the incidence of cervical cancer.

Finally, if a hysterectomy has been done for reasons other than cervical cancer or pre-cancer, screening after removal of the uterus and cervix is not required. Vaginal cancer is very rare and dying from it is even rarer.

The above cervical screening recommendations are for average risk women. If a higher risk exists due to immune compromise or other factors, more tailored screening is recommended. This requires a discussion with your primary care provider.

Colorectal

A person at average risk of developing colon cancer is someone who has no personal or family history of colorectal cancer, high-risk genetic syndromes, inflammatory bowel disease or adenomas (benign pre-cancerous tumors). Screening should start at age 50 unless one is black, in which case it should start at age 45 because of higher risk. In most cases, an age at which to stop screening is not agreed upon in current guidelines. However, because of how long it takes to develop colon cancer on average, it is often suggested that screening be stopped if the life expectancy is less than ten years.

There are seven methods currently in use for colorectal cancer screening and they are as follows:

- colonoscopy
- sigmoidoscopy
- fecal occult blood testing (FOBT)
- fecal immunochemical test (FIT)
- fecal DNA testing
- CT colonography
- double contrast barium enema

This number of options is unusual for a screening program. Usually, there are only one or a few options. Despite the choices, some are better than others, depending on your personal situation. Let's review them in order.

Colonoscopy is often considered the gold standard and is the screening method most often used. The benefit is that the entire colon is visualized directly and if a polyp or suspicious area is seen, a biopsy can be done at the same time rather than a second procedure. The downside is that you have to drink a large volume of relatively bad tasting liquid to "prepare" the bowel by clearing out all stool so that the colonoscopist can see the colon walls clearly. It also requires sedation. Otherwise, you would be very uncomfortable when the instrument moves inside you. This does not carry the same risk of general anesthesia, but it is a risk nonetheless. Also, in a small percentage of patients, colonoscopy can result in bowel perforation with the instrument, and that requires surgery to repair. Finally, while it is an excellent screening test, it is not foolproof. Up to 5% of cancer and up to 12% of pre-cancerous polyps or adenomas can be missed.

Flexible sigmoidoscopy is a junior version of colonoscopy, and only the lower half of the colon can be seen. While it is true that most colorectal cancers are in this area, up to 20% more cancers can be detected by looking at the entire colon using colonoscopy. The benefits are no need for sedation and less bowel preparation is required.

Stool-based testing such as FOBT, FIT or DNA testing does not require any instruments to be passed through the anus and inside of you. These can all be done at home using a stool sample you collect. These tests are not as sensitive as direct visualization using colonoscopy or sigmoidoscopy but are better than nothing.

CT colonography is a virtual colonoscopy whereby no instruments are placed inside of you, but you still have to go through the procedure of a CT scan, including swallowing some not-so-tasty contrast material. If anything is seen, a colonoscopy or sigmoidoscopy would still be required to look at and biopsy those areas. It is not as accurate as endoscopy and is not the preferred method of screening, but is considered an option.

Some guidelines include the double contrast barium enema as an option. This is a much older technology and is not as sensitive as most other tests. As a radiologic type of screening test it has been replaced by CT colonography.

Because of the differences in sensitivity, how often these screening tests are done depends on which one you select. Stool-based tests should be done annually because of the lower sensitivity, with the idea being if you miss it one year you may catch it the following year or two. Keep in mind that might mean an early cancer is growing inside of you for an extra year or two. In the worst case scenario, if the cancer does not bleed for a while, a FOBT screen may not find a cancer until it's in a late stage. Flexible sigmoidoscopy, CT colonography, and barium enema are generally recommended every five years. Colonoscopy can be done once every ten years.

If anything is suspicious but not diagnostic of cancer using one of the above, the next screening test may be recommended much sooner. Also, if you are high risk, screening is started about ten years earlier. This is something to discuss with your doctor for the best personal recommendation.

Prostate

Until recently, routine screening with the prostate-specific antigen (PSA) blood test was recommended. The problem is that PSA screening became the poster child of how overdiagnosis can cause much more harm than good. Many men underwent unnecessary radical surgery or radiation for no benefit. In general, this is a disease that progresses so slowly that most men will die of something else way in advance of getting into trouble with prostate cancer. This does not mean the prostate should be forgotten.

Guidelines recommend discussing the risk vs. benefit for screening between the ages of 50 and 69, for the average risk male. Any high-risk factors, such as black ethnicity, family history, or the use of 5-alpha-reductase inhibitors for enlarged prostate, should lead to a discussion with your physician at any age.

The two most common screening tools, usually used together, are the PSA blood test and a digital rectal examination (DRE). Indeed prostate irregularities, enlargement, and cancer will be found using these two tests routinely. However, 20-40% of prostate cancers diagnosed by screening are over-treated, and the over-diagnosis rate is somewhere between 20-60%. Research continues to determine a better screening process, but meanwhile, testing should be highly individualized.

Lung

Screening for lung cancer in high-risk individuals is a new development. Prior to 2011 medical research did not show any evidence of effectiveness. It is still not recommended if you are at low to moderate risk.

High risk is defined as follows:

- age between 55 and 74 years
- history of current or former smoking
- smoking history of at least 30 pack years
- smoking cessation of fewer than 15 years if former smoker

So, the risk of lung cancer goes up with age and especially after age 60. Beyond that, the more you smoke or smoked and the more recently that you quit, the higher your risk of lung cancer.

Obviously, if you smoke, the best plan is to stop smoking rather than continuing to smoke and undergoing screening. That is a no-brainer. However, if you have quit and fit into the above criteria, the only test available today that is proven to reduce deaths from lung cancer is a specialized form of CT scan called the LDCT. The sensitivity is about 94%, and the specificity is about 74%. This means there will be cancers missed, and there will be over-diagnosis of benign lung masses or indolent slow growing cancers as well. However, it is the best we have, and it is better than regular chest X-ray or sputum analysis for cancer cells. To get the best results, this test should be performed annually. Obviously, a yearly CT means increased radiation which can be cancer producing as well. So, it is best to discuss this with your physician to see if this screening makes sense for you.

Oral

Another area of new recommendations is screening for oral cancers in those who partake in tobacco, alcohol or both. The only screening tool recommended is a thorough visual examination of the entire oral cavity. No fancy tools or tests are recommended at this point. This screening recommendation is less than five years old, so studies show that approximately 80% of dentists but only about 13% of doctors perform this screening as part of an annual physical or dental exam.

Ovarian

Routine ovarian cancer screening is only recommended for those who have been diagnosed with gene alterations which put them at higher risk. This includes breast-ovarian cancer (BRCA) syndrome (40% lifetime ovarian cancer risk), Peutz-Jeghers syndrome (20% lifetime risk) and Lynch syndrome (9% risk). The background lifetime risk in women is one in seventy. The highest risk can be as high as one in two when there is a BRCA deleterious mutation. Long-term use of fertility drugs, personal history of breast cancer after age 40 with no family history, hormonal replacement, or endometriosis increases the risk minimally, if at all. Family history, especially first degree relatives, personal history of breast cancer before the age of 40, or Ashkenazi Jewish heritage with a personal history of breast cancer before age 50, increases the lifetime risk to approximately one in ten.

The only screening tools available are the CA125 blood test and transvaginal ultrasound. Anything else is still considered a research test, but a better combination is likely around the corner. For now, the problem with these tests and with pelvic examinations is that they are very inaccurate. The potential for both missing cancer and over-diagnosing and harming people is significant. It is not that these tests work any better in high-risk individuals, but given no good alternative it is felt that the slight improvement in reducing death from ovarian cancer in the high-risk group is worth the risk, time and costs involved. If screening is decided upon, the standard recommendation is a transvaginal ultrasound every six months, with or without a CA-125 blood level depending on age. CA-125 is an awful screening tool due to inaccuracy, but the older you are, the more it's reasonable to consider CA-125 in addition to ultrasound.

Overall the effectiveness of ovarian cancer screening is awful with today's technologies. Better tools are in the research pipeline, including ultra-sensitive circulating tumor DNA. The best approach is to get genetic counseling if you had cancer, have a family history of cancer or are high risk based on ethnicity, such as the case in Ashkenazi Jewish women. After that it can be determined if genetic testing is required and what to do depending upon the results. In some situations, you might want to consider prophylactic removal of your Fallopian tubes and ovaries. But this is individualized and is usually not recommended until after childbearing at approximately age 40 and depends on your personal history of cancer, family history and the exact type of gene mutation.

Pancreatic

Individuals without high risk have less than a 1% risk of developing pancreatic cancer, so screening in the general population is not recommended by anyone for all the reasons we covered in a low prevalence type of cancer. However, if you are diagnosed with pancreatic cancer, the results are usually very poor because it is generally diagnosed in late stages. Because of this, research has been ongoing to at least determine if there are high-risk groups and what type of screening should be offered in that setting.

Only about 10% of pancreatic cancers are related to genetic syndromes which are high risk. This includes people who have hereditary pancreatitis, Peutz-Jeghers syndrome, Lynch syndrome, BRCA2 mutations, and those who have familial atypical multiple mole melanoma. If you fall into one of these groups, your risk of pancreatic cancer can be as high as 40% rather than the 1% risk most people face. If you're not sure, this is something to talk about with your physician.

High-risk individuals have several screening options including a blood test called the CA19-9, a specialized scan called magnetic resonance cholangiopancreatography (MRI-CP), endoscopic ultrasound and endoscopic retrograde cholangiopancreatography. Endoscopic ultrasound is the most often recommended because it is probably the most accurate way to screen for pancreatic cancer. These are all complicated terms that you don't need to think about unless you are at high risk. Talk with your physician if you are high risk because then it can be a lifesaving move.

Skin

Non-melanoma skin cancers are rarely life threatening but can become so if left untreated and allowed to grow to a larger size. However, melanoma is a different story. Even a tiny melanoma can spread to the lymphatic and vascular system and metastasize early. The problem is that your average doctor is not very good at visually telling cancer apart from a benign discoloration or mole or even a wart. You could go to a dermatologist, but specialists are not always available. So, the only answer is to biopsy anything that looks suspicious. The downside is that if you have many skin changes as you get older, you may have to suffer through a whole lot of biopsies for no benefit.

It is prudent to have a whole body skin examination yearly after age 20, along with constant self-awareness scrutiny for new skin changes monthly. If you have already had skin cancer, especially melanoma, these recommendations are even more important. Once you have had a melanoma, the risk of a second primary melanoma is 4-8%.

Other Cancers

No other cancers are common enough or have adequate available tools for routine screening. Having said that, an annual physical examination is still recommended overall. This should include looking at any new changes, new symptoms or any related health concerns or questions. Keep an eye out for yourself and tell your health care provider about anything new.

Chapter 3

The Inflammation and Cancer Connection

Is inflammation good or bad? Well, as it turns out, it can be both. Inflammation in your body is a necessary and good response to acute injuries like viral or bacterial infections or even trauma from an accident. This is the part of your immune system that rushes in and tries to fend off the damage and start the repair process. The white cell and cytokine (small proteins essential to cell signaling) response leads to the familiar redness, heat and swelling like you might experience with an infected sore throat or a sprained ankle. However, this good process turns to bad when the white cells in the area do not go away and keep producing their caustic chemicals, including cytokines. If this keeps going, it creates a chronically inflamed damaged toxic area, like a cesspool, which starts to encourage abnormal cell transformation.

The concept that inflammation is associated with cancer is not new. It was Galenus who postulated this about 1800 years ago and Virchow confirmed it in 1863. However, which came first? Inflammation seemed to precede cancer development and was certainly present when cancer arose. Research has been ongoing in this area because it is still not 100% clear if cancer causes inflammation or the inflammation helps cause, or at least promote, cancer. The most recent data from laboratories at leading cancer centers shows us that both are probably true.

Chronic inflammation seems to block the ability of the immune system to restrain cancer growth. It does this in two ways: 1) inflammatory chemicals produced by our white cells are used by tumor cells to grow, and 2) the inflammation dampens the rest of our immune system response to cancer growth. It looks like cancer cells may acquire the mutations necessary to invade and metastasize only after they have access to the chemicals our body produces by chronic inflammation. So, in this light, keep in mind the theory that our immune system protects us by eliminating early cancer cells every day. This protection is inhibited by chronic inflammation.

So what is this cancer-promoting inflammatory cytokine cascade all about? Even before tumor cells begin to grow, when tissue is chronically inflamed, it produces cytokines including Tumor Necrosis Factor alpha (TNF-α) and interleukin-6 (IL-6) which help generate DNA-damaging free radicals. These initially come from the stromal support cells of normal but inflamed tissue and the immune cells that infiltrate the area. Other pro-inflammatory cytokines reduce apoptosis (programmed cell death), which starts cancerous abnormal cell growth and creates another source of cytokines. At the same time, the "good" anti-inflammatory cytokines like IL-10 as well as Transforming Growth Factor (TGF) inadvertently lead to increased immune evasion by the proliferating cancer cells. Still, other pro-inflammatory cytokines promote angiogenesis (new blood vessel growth) to feed the growing tumor, invasion, and metastasis. How bad things get and how fast tumors grow or spread, depends on the delicate balance of how these cytokines act in a pro – or anti-cancer fashion. Measuring blood levels of various cytokines, like IL-6 and IL-10, has been proposed as a way to measure tumor activity.

One pro-inflammatory factor secreted by tumor cells stands almost alone in importance. This is nuclear factor-kappa B (NF-kappa B). In many laboratory models, blocking this single factor makes cancer cells mortal again and able to undergo apoptosis. As we will discuss, common blockers are resveratrol and green tea catechins.

Figuring out the delicate interaction of cytokines is an incredibly complex topic. First of all, there are hundreds of cytokines. Second, the timing of when they are elevated or reduced in amount is crucial. Artificially turning off or increasing the level of a particular cytokine at the wrong time can be extremely counterproductive. For example, we know that the interaction of cytokines is similarly complex in overwhelming infection, known as sepsis. Sepsis is a much shorter and defined process that develops quickly and either kills or, with proper management, the patient survives. Well, we found out that by turning off what appeared to be "bad" pro-inflammatory cytokines at the wrong time, kills or accelerates death. In the case of cancer, this is a more prolonged series of events, but the results can be the same in terms of accelerating or retarding cancer development or progression. With the above warning in mind, treatment options involving blocking specific cytokine elevation or blocking cytokine cell surface receptors have to be carefully researched, planned and tested.

Going against all of this precise targeting of cytokine pathways are the now rather ancient findings of Dr. Coley, who in the 1800's proposed that tumor progression might be inhibited by generalized inflammation caused by acute infection. So he and his colleagues injected bone sarcoma patients with bacteria and induced severe infection (sepsis), which produced a cancer-fighting immune response. Unfortunately, the documentation was inadequate, so we really have no idea how effective this was. He was also working without much knowledge of the immune system back then, which makes his work very visionary and brilliant. However, it is safe to say that the knowledge base of immunology today is light years ahead of what was known then. Using 1800's technology and understanding for treatment planning today is very backward and dangerous. Some alternative practitioners still promote giving "Coley's Toxins" or "Coley's Vaccine" to cancer patients. This is kind of Neanderthal and is not really a vaccine as we know it today, but rather a bunch of dead bacteria particles meant to create generalized inflammation. Even Germany, which used to produce this for administration to patients, stopped doing so in 1990 because there was simply no modern science to support this generic approach. Nonetheless, inducing a targeted acute immune response to fight cancer is a hot topic of today's research, using today's knowledge of immunology. In fact, there was a recent study which showed that injecting an attenuated (weakened) form of Clostridium, a bacterium, killed tumor cells directly and indirectly by inducing an immune response.

From yesterday, through today and into the future, balance and timing of promoting and suppressing inflammation is central to prevention and treatment of cancer. So what causes chronic inflammation? Many things, some obvious and others not so obvious. Let's review some of these.

Chronic inflammation can be caused by viral, bacterial and parasitic infections. For example, we know that the chronic stomach inflammation caused by prolonged H. Pylori infection increases the risk of gastric cancer. Likewise, prolonged or repetitive uterine cervix infections with the Human Papilloma Virus (HPV) contribute to cancer. Finally, some parasites can lead to liver cancer, mainly in third world countries.

Conditions such as obesity and diabetes also cause an underlying chronic low-level inflammatory state. Pro-inflammatory cytokines such as Tumor Necrosis Factor (TNF) are elevated, among many others, leading to the cytokine cascades we just covered. The diabetes process itself as well as the adipose cells in obesity both contribute. This leads to cardiovascular disease and hypertension, Alzheimer's, dementia, as well as cancer.

Long-term exposure to toxins leads to chronic inflammation. As we will cover in the detoxification chapters, it is hard to get away from all toxins in this world. However, it is very worthwhile to do a "toxin sweep" of your home and work environment and see what you can cut out from breathing, eating, drinking and putting on your hair or skin. These toxins can accumulate in your fat cells, and you can end up being a walking toxic cesspool, slowly re-releasing these inflammatory toxins into your blood stream twenty-four hours a day.

Consuming certain foods, with sugar being at the top of the list, can be pro-inflammatory. Processed packaged foods and fast foods are laden with synthetic additives, sweeteners, and other pro-inflammatory substances. Wheat, gluten, alcohol and fried foods round out the short list.

Lastly, if you have inflammatory conditions or diseases like rheumatoid arthritis, lichen sclerosus of the vulva, periodontal disease, or hundreds of others, you may have an increased risk for certain types of cancers. Of interest, in some cases, these diseases lower the risk of other cancers. This is probably because of the delicate balance regarding activation timing and duration of the inflammatory response.

There is an entire chapter in this book devoted to non-traditional additional lab testing to help with treatment planning and following the course of cancer treatment effectiveness. This includes specific and generalized markers that monitor inflammation, such as C-reactive Protein (CRP) and an extremely sensitive version called hsCRP. Also, some of the cytokines (e.g. interleukins) are being scrutinized to see if they can help with diagnosis and monitoring of cancer treatment progress.

The bottom line regarding all of the above is whether or not we can use this information for primary prevention, treatment or prevention of recurrence. The answer is a resounding yes. You should be seeing a central theme develop in this book about anti-inflammatory diets and nutrients, anti-inflammatory supplements and even anti-inflammatory drugs. It is also prudent to look at your lifestyle choices and exposures and limit contact with anything that can cause chronic inflammation.

Chapter 4
Insulin Resistance

Insulin is a hormone which helps keep our blood sugar normal. When normal insulin function is impaired in tissues including skeletal muscle, liver, and fat cells, the condition is known as insulin resistance. At first, the pancreatic beta cells start to produce more insulin to counteract this resistance. This extra insulin helps drive sugar into cells and maintains normal blood glucose levels. However, after more time passes the pancreas loses its ability to work overtime and Type 2 diabetes develops. This differs from Type 1 diabetes, which is an autoimmune disease that develops early in life. It is due to lack of insulin production by the pancreas.

Elevated insulin levels, chronic inflammation, and high blood sugar, are all commonly seen in Type 2 diabetics. Current research suggests that this combination of problems may also lead to increased incidence of cancer, faster tumor growth, and worse outcomes. The exact molecular mechanisms behind that are very complicated, but let's cover the basics.

According to the China Study, the Mayo Clinic, and other leading research centers, a typical Western high fat and high glycemic index diet leads to obesity, diabetes, hypertension and may also be a major factor in causing cancer. The glycemic index (GI) is a ranking of carbohydrates on a 0 to 100 scale based on the extent to which they raise blood sugar levels after you eat. High GI foods are digested easily and quickly absorbed. They result in wide fluctuations in blood sugar and insulin levels. The biochemical processes that occur afterward are complicated but suffice it to say that this fluctuation of blood sugar and spiking insulin leads to fat storage and obesity. The state of being obese is a pro-inflammatory state, and this leads to cancer. Of course, this is extremely over-simplified, but this general risk connection is 100% proven for the following cancers and suspect in many more: esophageal, pancreatic, colorectal, breast, endometrial, kidney, thyroid and gallbladder. You can avoid high GI foods by looking up lists online and focusing on those that sport a low GI. Unfortunately, unlike Australia, in the United States, we have not started to put the exact GI number on food labels yet.

Having said that, the scientific evidence that glycemic carbohydrates themselves influence cancer is not conclusive. It is not clear whether it is the glycemic carbs or the insulin fluctuation or insulin resistance or the inflammation caused by obesity or what exactly is the primary event leading to cancer. There are only a few epidemiologic studies which have found a close or tight association between high GI food and cancer. Keep in mind that epidemiologic studies offer only association, not proof about anything. If that sounds confusing, read the Appendix on the topic of scientific evidence creation.

On a molecular level, research has strongly associated insulin and insulin-like growth factors (IGF) in the genesis, promotion, and growth of cancer. In fact, individuals with mutations in the growth hormone receptor (GHR) gene have severe GHR and IGF-1 (insulin-like growth factor–1) deficiencies. They have a much lower rate of diabetes and cancer because there are no receptors for insulin or IGF to attach to and force cellular changes. They also have less IGF produced. Normally, the hormone insulin can directly act as a growth factor for various cell types. It can directly stimulate multiple pro-cancer cellular signaling cascades and affect cellular metabolism. More importantly, it also causes an increased liver synthesis of free IGFs which act as "mitogens" and reduction of IGF-binding proteins in the liver, which further increases the total amount of circulating IGFs. Mitogens are biochemical substances which are required to help push cells through parts of the mitotic cycle. This results in their "mitogenic" effects of increasing cell division, replication, and growth. These same IGFs have an anti-apoptotic effect as well, which means they interfere with normal "programmed" cell death. This association has been demonstrated the best in colorectal cancer, based mainly on laboratory and animal studies.

There is also some research which supports the same relationship in breast, prostate, and pancreatic cancer. One can only assume that this likely affects many hormonally sensitive cancers. Insulin also reduces sex hormone binding globulin (SHBG) which increases sex hormone bioavailability. In this way, breast, prostate, uterine, ovarian and other cancers under the influence of sex hormones can be affected.

Going back to the obesity connection, we know that obesity is a chronic low-grade inflammatory state and is the biggest cause of insulin resistance. This inflammation leads to overproduction of pro-cancer molecules such as IL-6, free fatty acids, leptin and adiponectin, TNF-α, among others. As we already discussed, this increased inflammatory, oxidative stress actively contributes to cancer development and growth.

The story does not end here. There are still other ways that chronically elevated glucose found in pre-diabetes, metabolic syndrome and diabetes can help foster cancer. Glycation means the haphazard creation of new larger molecules by combining sugar with a protein or lipid molecule. This can occur external to the body (i.e. dietary or preformed) or internally, without the need for an enzyme in the process. The sugar can be circulating glucose in your bloodstream or standard table sugar sucrose or "natural" fructose from fruits or galactose, which comes from sources like sugar beets and dairy. This new molecule is called an "advanced glycation end product" (AGE), and can contribute to mutagenesis and genetic instability by causing nucleotide "mispairing" and abnormal DNA replication.

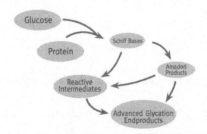

By Jasper Dijkstra (http://www.diagnoptics.com/) [CC BY-SA 3.0 (http://creativecommons.org/licenses/by-sa/3.0)], via Wikimedia Commons

As far as external glycations are concerned, you can avoid them by minimizing foods that have been "browned" or "glazed" such as French fries and many baked goods. Going a step further, glycation from cooking and baking with sugar can also lead to the formation of the carcinogen acrylamide. Worse, AGEs can be added directly to other foods like dark colored soda, barbecue meats, and donuts.

Internal glycation can occur to a small proportion of absorbed sugars, mainly fructose, and galactose. If you smoke, AGE formation increases. This becomes a bigger problem when more and more circulating blood sugar is present due to insulin resistance. In addition to the AGEs being formed, a byproduct of this reaction is highly oxidizing hydrogen peroxide (H_2O_2).

The good news is that you can assess the degree of glycation going on in your body by measuring glycated hemoglobin (HbA1c). This is a test frequently used to determine the average circulating blood glucose in the management of diabetes.

You can protect yourself against glycation and insulin resistance by doing the following:

1. Reduce sugar consumption, bearing in mind that there is no such thing as a completely "healthy" sugar. Natural fructose and galactose are ten times more likely to be glycated. There are obviously other health benefits to fruits and vegetables which contain fructose, so that is not a reason to stop eating them. However, you can pick and choose lower glycemic index foods, and limit excess sugar intake from sources such as junk and processed foods. Especially limit foods that are browned, glazed and have known AGEs added. Finally, eliminate high fructose corn syrup. If you need sweeteners in your life, consider stevia root.

2. Eat fruits and vegetables raw, boiled or steamed. Water helps prevent external glycation and AGE ingestion.

3. Drink water or tea instead of sodas which contain AGEs

4. Ensure adequate Vitamin D levels and intake. Pancreatic islet cells have Vitamin D receptors which, along with modulating the immune system and reducing inflammation, may help increase insulin secretion. Deficiency also leads to increased parathyroid hormone (PTH) levels, which leads to insulin insensitivity.

5. Supplement with carnosine and Vitamin B6, which inhibit AGE formation.

6. Maintain adequate magnesium intake through foods like dark leafy vegetables or seaweed, or supplements. The mechanisms of how magnesium

works to optimize blood glucose are not well worked out, but proposed mechanisms suggest it acts at the intracellular signaling level.

7. Calcium intake from all sources should be 1500mg to 2000mg per day. Normal calcium levels are crucial for many intracellular signaling pathways, including normal pancreatic β-cell function and insulin secretion. Under normal circumstances, this helps improve insulin sensitivity among many other health benefits. However, keep in mind that if your body does not process calcium well and if you have high blood levels, this worsens the situation. So, best to have your calcium levels measured. This illustrates the point that "more" is definitely not better regarding supplementation in most cases. You can easily get into trouble with too much calcium, just like you can with other supplements.

8. Vitamin K is helpful in multiple ways. It can help forestall insulin resistance, which is an anti-cancer effect. When you take vitamin K along with vitamin D and calcium, it can help prevent deposits of calcium in places that may lead to problems like atherosclerosis or hardening of the arteries. We need both K1 and K2. Good vitamin K sources include fermented foods like natto (fermented soy beans) and green leafy vegetables. Most of us have enough Vitamin K to keep our coagulation system working so that we don't bleed or bruise easily. However, higher levels are required for optimal functioning of your body. In this regard, we are all mostly deficient.

9. Metformin is a pharmaceutical but was derived from the herb Galega officinalis (also known as French lilac, Goat's Rue or Italian Fitch). You may be taking it if you are an early diabetic. If not, ask your doctor about it if your blood sugar level tests are abnormal (e.g. HbA1c or fasting glucose). Metformin reduces glucose production by the liver, impedes intestinal sugar absorption, and improves insulin sensitivity in peripheral tissues. Multiple research studies are underway to determine if adding Metformin improves treatment of various cancers.

10. Myo-inositol, D-chiro-inositol and D-pinitol are three related natural compounds which perform at least part of the actions Metformin has in reducing insulin resistance. These inositols can metabolically interconvert in the body, so taking all three is not required. Also, for example, D-pinitol

is present in legumes and citrus, so a supplement is not necessarily required. Myo-inositol may have some direct cancer preventive functions as well, notably in the lung.

11. N-acetyl-L-cysteine, berberine, chromium picolinate, alpha lipoic acid, and cinnamon have all been shown to improve insulin sensitivity in tissues.

WARNING! Please keep in mind the goal is to reduce persistent excess in circulating glucose and insulin. This is a healthy strategy and can have the anti-cancer effects described above. The goal is NOT to reduce your glucose to extremely low levels which can be very dangerous and put you into a shock state. In someone who has normal glucose regulation and no evidence of metabolic syndrome or diabetes, this shock state is not likely. However, if you are diabetic or even pre-diabetic, or don't know, this is a risk you want to avoid. Work with your doctor if you want to look into this and start with the basics of diet (e.g. reduce sugar and increase legumes) and exercise.

CHAPTER 5

CANCER IMMUNOLOGY

Introduction

Even if one takes an incredibly simplistic view of the immune system, it is *still* a very complex and robust combination of many different types of white blood cells, multiple antibodies, and an impressive array of cytokine biochemicals that work together like a symphony orchestra to protect us from foreign invaders.

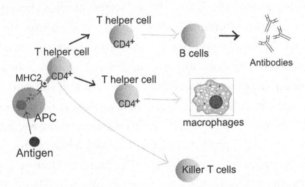

Häggström, Mikael. "Medical gallery of Mikael Häggström 2014." *Wikiversity Journal of Medicine* 1 (2). DOI:10.15347/wjm/2014.008. ISSN 20018762.

The theory of "immune surveillance", first proposed in 1909 by Erlich, has substantial evidence supporting the concept that your body is catching early cancer cells, recognizing them as abnormal, and regularly eliminating them. Likewise, the immune system may help limit the growth and metastasis of tumors that have escaped the surveillance. You will discover that there is a lot you can do to help your immune system prevent cancer or slow its progression. Keep in mind however that if a measurable cancerous tumor has appeared in a physical examination or a scan, your body is telling you that something went wrong beyond its ability to control through immune surveillance. It is reaching out for help and is signaling that you need some aggressive mainstream help to eliminate cancer and that you need to support your immune system better to help potentially prevent recurrence.

So, is it possible to naturally "boost" your immune system so you can defeat cancer? The answer is yes and no. Using natural means and lifestyle changes, you can significantly but non-specifically improve your immune system in some ways, but you cannot "boost" your immune system in a specific highly targeted cancer-fighting way using natural means. There are many exciting immune-modulating cancer-fighting targeted agents, "adoptive immunotherapy", "active immunotherapy" vaccines and other strategies in development. The critical point to understand is that the immune system is a million times more complex than the simpleton way it is often presented by some under-informed alternative practitioners. It is as far from "simple" as could be imagined. I do not mean to confuse you, but the following example illustrates how complex this can be.

For the past decade, there has been a big research interest in tumor infiltrating leukocytes (white blood cells, mainly lymphocytes) or TILs therapy. It is other-wise known as "adoptive immunotherapy." In fact, it is mainstream research but is quite "natural" in principle because it uses some of your very own lymphocytes to fight cancer. However, this requires some laboratory help. Your lymphocytes, as you are about to learn, can't recognize cancer very well and can't replicate to a high enough number to effectively fight billions of cancer cells which are present in even a small marble-sized tumor. They can't mount a strong enough anti-cancer targeted response. This is partly because cancer cells are an abnormal version of "you" and not completely foreign invaders, like bacteria. However, we know that patients with various cancers that have higher numbers of TILs in them seem to have a better prognosis. These favorable TILs include a smorgasbord of immune cells including (but not limited to) CD8(+) cytotoxic T lymphocytes, Th1 and Th17 CD4(+) T cells, natural killer cells, dendritic cells and M1 macrophages. At the same time, high levels of intratumoral CD4(+)CD25(+)FOXP3(+) regulatory T cells, Th2 CD4(+) T cells, myeloid-derived suppressor cells, M2 macrophages, and neutrophils are associated with poor prognosis.

TILs therapy has been pioneered in melanoma with very exciting results and is now being looked at in breast and other cancers. These white cells are retrieved from the cancerous tumors in your body, cultured in the laboratory to get very large numbers of them, and then reinjected into you to fight your cancer. A "super-charged" variation is called chimeric antigen receptor (CAR) T-cell therapy, where T cells are modified to express receptors unique to the particular form of cancer, enhancing effectiveness. The T cells, which can then recognize and kill the cancer cells, are reintroduced into the patient. Again, this is called adoptive cell transfer or adoptive immunotherapy, as opposed to active immunotherapy as seen with vaccines. Since your body cannot grow the huge number of TILs alone, it needs a little help. In principle, it is a very promising strategy to "naturally" kill cancer. This may seem to be complex and yet is vastly oversimplified. I hope you get the idea.

There are problems with toxicity because with today's version of this treatment you still have to use high doses of IL-2 (also "natural" to your body but in a much higher dose), or chemotherapy. It is not in widespread use even in melanoma yet, despite its apparent effectiveness. This is one of the ways we will be moving away from chemotherapy in the very near future, and this may indeed eventually become a kinder gentler but effective anti-cancer therapy.

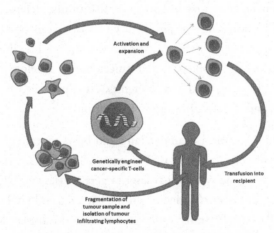

By Simon Caulton (Own work) [CC BY-SA 3.0 (http://creativecommons.org/licenses/by-sa/3.0)], via Wikimedia Commons

Meanwhile, short of participating in a TIL research study like this, or waiting for the future when this might be readily available, can you be proactive and naturally optimize your immune system, maybe even increasing meaningful TIL cells? Yes. Can you also get misled and be offered a bunch of "immune boosting" expensive junk that does not work? Absolutely! Many good things in life are free, and this is one area where this rings true. Most of what you can do to make your body as "cancer-proof" as possible by improving immune system health does not have to be expensive and can be almost free with diet and exercise modifications. Also, as you will discover in a minute, it is possible to overdo it with some supplements or botanicals and harm yourself through immune suppression when you think you are taking something to improve your immune system.

To really understand the immune system and the intricacies of almost daily new scientific findings, you need a Ph.D. in immunology. Tens of thousands of research papers and hundreds of textbooks have been written on this subject. In fact, by the time you read this, some significant advance may have made which is not noted here, or some other concept may have been proven or disproven. However, on the whole, the immune-supportive natural strategies that work are enduring and have been around for centuries. We are simply learning more about how they work, and can thereby guide you towards the best options.

For purposes of understanding what you can proactively do, let's oversimplify things. The extremely basic way to understand the immune system is that it is split into two parts: innate and adaptive. These two components work in concert. The innate system is your first line of general immune defense. The adaptive immune system is more targeted and evolved so that your body could protect itself from new "pathogens" that you come across during life, including various bacteria and viruses. The problem is that cancer, which develops from your own cells, is not as easily recognized as a foreign external pathogen like bacteria. We will cover innate and adaptive immunity in a second.

First, the following is critical to understand and bears repeating. Cancer is, unfortunately, part of you. Its origin is your own cells. So, as aberrant as the cells are, the adaptive immune system that laser targets viruses and bacteria based on easy identification of foreign "antigens" on the bacterial and viral surface, cannot target cancer cells as well. Transformed cancer cells do display foreign-looking antigens to a significant degree, and these come from tumor causing viruses, up-regulation or amplification of antigens to higher levels than normal and so on. The problem is that the types of tumor antigens (TA) displayed on cancer cell surfaces are not highly immunogenic, even if there are a lot of them. In other words, they do not stimulate a robust immune response like foreign antigens do, which are much more immunogenic.

There is a lot of research underway to help tag cancer cells and their surface antigens as being more foreign to make them more immunogenic. That is part of multiple mainstream "immunotherapy" strategies that exist today or are in various phases of research.

As exciting as this is, these types of immunogenicity-enhancing tagging strategies are largely not amenable to natural approaches. On the other hand, heading in the opposite direction, natural methods can epigenetically influence cancer stem cells, which are thought to be the source of rapidly dividing cancer cells in tumors, towards not looking or acting foreign or cancerous anymore. This epigenetic and nutrigenomic modification, which we will get to in a bit, may be an immunity-related natural cancer-fighting strategy, but it is not "immune boosting" per se.

Also, cancer creates an environment around itself, partly related to the inflammation we already discussed. This defeats immune surveillance and sets the stage for immune evasion. Cancer actively evades the immune system by producing significant amounts of immunosuppressive chemicals. This includes a myriad of substances and includes pro-inflammatory prostaglandin E2 (PGE2) and cytokines, like interleukin 10 (IL-10) and transforming growth factor-beta (TGF-β).

The following image depicts the balance between pro-cancer genetic changes, positive epigenetic forces and both tumor antigen (TA) dependent and independent immune response. This is vastly oversimplified and yet probably still looks utterly confusing. However, it gives you the core big picture of the push-pull or pro-cancer vs. anti-cancer molecular forces, with the immune system being at the center of the action.

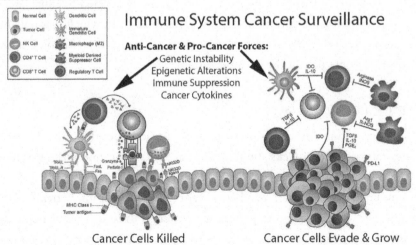

Modified from Frontiers in Oncology [CC BY 3.0 (http://creativecommons.org/licenses/by/3.0)], via Wikimedia Commons

Innate Immune System

The innate immune system is nonspecific in its response and is fully ready at birth to be the first line of defense. This system initially attacks and helps activate the adaptive system against foreign pathogens. Against cancer, this initial attack can be effective, but may be limited in the long run, and we will cover why. Also, it is far less effective in activating the adaptive system against cancer cells than against foreign pathogens.

Cells of the innate immune system include the natural killer cells (NK), natural killer T cells (NKT), macrophages, polymorphonuclear leukocytes (PMNs), mast cells which help regulate both the innate and adaptive immune systems, dendritic cells (DC) which are phagocytes that digest and present foreign antigens to T cells (they are the messengers between the innate and adaptive immune systems), and cytotoxic T lymphocytes. Cytokines such as tumor necrosis factor (TNF) and multiple interleukins (IL) are also part of this system. Also, there are thought to be damage associated molecular pattern molecules (DAMPs) which can initiate an immune response or feed it and keep it going. These can be released from the inflammatory response areas between cells (extracellular matrix) and from dying and necrotic tumor cells, including proteins from their nucleus and cytoplasm.

All of the cells mentioned above and the myriad of DAMP and other effector molecules interact with each other and with the adaptive immune system to kill cancer cells. Some of these components can be naturally boosted to enhance the anti-cancer response, most notably natural killer (NK) cells, which you remember is one of the TIL types of cells. However, before we get to what you can do, let's cover the other part of the immune system.

Adaptive Immune System

The adaptive immune system is much more sophisticated in that it can remember previous pathogen attacks and therefore can attack the same pathogen more quickly if it were to attack again. So, in the case of cancer, it would be great if your immune system could remember cancer cells after the primary treatment is over and then attack it again to prevent a recurrence. This does occur naturally, but the effect is not robust enough to reliably prevent recurrences. Having said that, this is being very actively researched because it is probably the best possible laser targeted way to eliminate cancer without affecting healthy cells at all. Virtually all other approaches carry a risk of damaging normal cells, from toxic chemotherapy to radiation. Even completely natural methods, where too much of a nutrient could actually damage normal cells, carry a risk of harm.

Components of the adaptive immune system include cytotoxic CD8+ T cells, helper CD4+ T cells, gamma delta (γδ) T cells, antibody-producing B lymphocytes, five types of antibodies (Ab), multiple interleukins (IL), interferons (IF), and the complement cascade. There are many more components.

While you can optimize your total immune system through healthy habits and nutrition, and possibly enhance immunosurveillance for wayward cancer cells, you cannot specifically or directly boost the adaptive arm using natural methods to a high enough level to kill tumors which already contain billions of cells. You can naturally but indirectly stimulate some cancer-fighting components of the immune system and reduce cancer mediated immunosuppressive effects. Having said that, while we wait for results from hot areas of immunotherapy research, what can you do now?

Immune Optimization

So, now that we reviewed the basics, how can we optimize the immune system to ward off or fight cancer and help prevent recurrence? For starters, the focus should be to reduce immune suppression. Immune suppression may be cancer induced, treatment induced, overall health induced, and even stress and psychologically induced. We know that cancer creates an environment which blunts the immune response, and there is little you can do about that other than fight cancer using all the means in this book to support mainstream therapies. Also, unfortunately, until we develop more targeted biological agents and chemotherapy, the cancer-fighting treatment itself usually does not do your immune system any favors. You can't significantly reduce treatment-related immune suppression naturally but you can boost and support your immune system in a number of ways.

First, to complete the picture of reducing immune suppression, doing everything you can to get into the best health possible and reversing inflammatory conditions such as metabolic syndrome, insulin resistance, diabetes, and obesity is key to long-term survivorship. Of course, that is a tall order if you are in the middle of treatment, but every little bit helps and should become a huge priority if you have completed treatment or are only trying to prevent cancer. Another immune suppressing influence on your body may be related to toxins you are exposed to. This is covered thoroughly in Chapter 16, and you should consider those daily detoxification measures strongly. Finally, stress and depression are very common these days with or without having cancer. The resulting adverse hormonal changes (i.e. high cortisol) and negative mind-body connection can strongly influence the degree to which you suppress your immune system. There is an entire field dedicated to the study of this called psycho-neuro-immunology, which forms at least part of the scientific basis for the mind-body connection. So, do whatever it takes to relieve stress and depression. More on this topic can be found in Chapter 19.

Now, moving to active optimization of your immune system, our first line of defense against the world of toxins and infectious invaders is the intestinal system. In fact, the greatest mass of lymphoid tissue in your body is located in the intestine and is called the gut-associated lymphoid tissue (GALT). It stores many immune cells such as T and B lymphocytes and is part of the bigger mucosal associated lymphatic system (MALT), which contains 80% of the immunologically active cells in your body. The nutrients in your diet affect how the MALT functions, directly and in an indirect way that you may not have ever thought of. We will get to the fascinating indirect way in just a bit, but directly the MALT and intestinal wall require healthy nutrients, minerals, and antioxidants to function properly just like any other tissue in your body. In short, the baseline for how 80% of your immune system works is set in your intestine.

As already mentioned, one pro-inflammatory factor secreted by tumor cells and chronically inflamed cells is almost exclusively critical in its carcinogenic role. This is nuclear factor-kappa B (NF-kappa B or simply NF-kB). NF-kB is activated in most human breast cancer cells and, over the past ten years, has been the target of novel biologic agent development. In fact, it turns out that many mainstream chemotherapy drugs inhibit NF-kB, a fact that was previously unappreciated. This is a massive convergence with the many natural substances which also inhibit NF-kB. These are likely preventive, inhibit cancer progression and help prevent recurrence by this natural pathway. Natural NF-kB blockers, among many, include turmeric, kaempferol, procyanidins and sulforaphanes.

How does this tie into the intestinal barrier and MALT? Well, an unhealthy gut leads to leaky gut syndrome which leads to local as well as systemic inflammation and activation of NF-kB. There are so many moving molecular parts to this that it boggles the mind. However, this is a very plausible but still theoretical connection of leaky gut and cancer development. A healthy intestine, from the standpoint of both preventing leaky gut and keeping the MALT optimized, is key to anti-cancer success.

How does one prevent a leaky gut syndrome? It largely has a lot to do with the "microbiome", which includes the trillions of bacteria, archaea (primitive bacteria), viruses, and fungi that colonize the human body. They outnumber us almost 100 to one, and we co-exist with them in a commensal, symbiotic relationship, which means we get along for mutual benefit. We provide a safe host environment like the skin, the mouth, the intestine, and vagina, and provide them with nutrients. The microbial organisms reciprocate by helping process the nutrients we take in, protect us from pathogenic organisms (i.e. harmful bacteria, viruses, and fungi that cause illness), and help us regulate and mature our immune system. This mutually beneficial delicate balance can be thrown off kilter, and we fall into a state of "dysbiosis". For example, disease or the toxins and harmful nutrients we take in or even the antibiotics we use to cure infections can cause the microbiota to be dysregulated, disrupt normal immune system function and predispose us to all sorts of disease locally in the intestine and in general. This includes leaky gut which can lead to inflammation locally and in other areas of the body, resulting in inflammatory bowel disease, autoimmune disorders, asthma, both type 1 and 2 diabetes and cancer.

Much has been written about stimulating natural killer cells (NK) to fight cancer, and this is an ongoing area of active mainstream research. This special type of lymphocyte, which bridges the adaptive and innate immune system, was initially described approximately four decades ago. It is not clear how many NK cells need to be clinically activated to be effective against cancer, especially against solid tumors. Developing useful therapies on this basis has been elusive. However, for example, the flavonoid component from the seeds of Astragalus complanatus (FAC) has been shown to influence NK activation in cell preparations. Arginine, a semi-essential amino acid, can do the same. Both animal and small human studies have shown that enzymatically modified rice bran (EMRB) can significantly increase NK activity. Enzymatically modified rice bran is produced by exposing crude fiber from rice bran to enzymes isolated from the Japanese culinary mushroom, shiitake (*Lentinula edodes*). So, it seems that for the moment, the only way to activate NK cells outside of research studies is through natural substances. Again, it is not clear if this activation is enough compared to what biological agents and immunotherapy of the future may offer, but for now, this is a low risk and potentially high reward way to boost your anti-cancer fight.

In general, many adaptogenic herbs and nutrients, which we have touched upon in general already, may favorably and nonspecifically affect the immune system. Astragalus, reishi, maitake and shitake mushrooms, Panax and Siberian ginseng, and Echinacea all have such effects.

Whether adaptogenic non-specific or specific, the following micronutrients are key to a model healthy immune system. Relative deficiencies of selenium, iron, zinc, copper, vitamins A, B6, C, D, E, and folic acid are known to affect markers of immune response in the laboratory test tube. How much each one affects actual immune response in animals and humans is not as clear. But what's the downside? The only real risk with making sure you are not deficient in any of these is overdoing it and taking megadoses. I repeat this many times in this book. More is not usually better and can be very harmful. For example, higher doses of zinc act as a well-known immune suppressor. Too much Echinacea has been shown to cause anaphylactic shock, especially in those with ragweed allergies. The key strategy is to maintain a delicately balanced interplay of all micronutrients in supporting immune function.

Exercise

Scientists who study the beneficial effects of exercise have identified a lot of cytokine pathway activations, white cell count alterations, beneficial interleukin changes, and differences in certain antibody levels. There is a lot of intriguing research but no reliable conclusions about the extent of clinically measurable direct anti-cancer immune effect.

Nevertheless, at the very least, exercise promotes blood and lymphatic circulation which is healthy because this mobilizes the immune system components more efficiently. Also, exercise is overall anti-inflammatory in nature. There is of course inflammation initially, but it is rapidly counterbalanced by anti-inflammatory cytokines and pro-inflammatory cytokine inhibitors, which persist. We know that in certain cancers, notably breast cancer, exercise improves survivorship. There is scientific evidence that the best form of exercise might be "burst training" or "interval training", which is made up of multiple sets of aerobic or resistance training from twenty seconds to two minutes in duration. Of course, before engaging in such intense exercise, a warm-up routine is essential not to strain or tear muscles, ligaments or tendons.

Sleep

The International Agency for Research on Cancer (IARC) classified "shift work" with disruption of normal circadian rhythms as a probable contributor to the development of cancer. Also, multiple studies have shown that extremes of total sleep deprivation and rapid eye movement (REM) sleep deprivation significantly influence the immune system, specifically altering white blood cell type percentages (e.g., CD4+, CD8+, and NK) and cytokine levels (e.g., IFN-g, TNF-a, and IL-1). Clearly, there is a connection between poor sleep and various acute (e.g. infection) and chronic diseases, including cancer. However, everyone is different, so it's hard to say that eight hours is better than five hours of sleep or anything that concrete. However, the going thought is that approximately seven hours of restful, consistent and uninterrupted sleep is optimal.

Melatonin

Life, stress, cancer, cancer treatment and a slew of other factors make it easier said than done to get seven hours of restful sleep on a consistent basis. Most folks immediately reach for the medicine cabinet and seek sleep aid prescriptions. In the end, it is possible that a powerful medication may be the only thing that works. However, if that is true for you, it should be considered an extremely temporary solution. The health and immune benefits of drug assisted sleep are not as clear. So, before going to that extreme, consider the more natural solution of melatonin.

In the face of stress and cancer, natural secretion of melatonin is impaired. So, supplementation may be a useful sleep aid, plus you get many direct anti-cancer benefits. Melatonin is an antioxidant and helps cytotoxic T lymphocytes function while directly inhibiting cancer cell proliferation through multiple mechanisms including epigenetic influences and anti-angiogenesis. Particularly in combination with astragalus, the anti-cancer effect of IL-2 can be potentiated.

Melatonin can also lower toxicity from chemos such as cisplatin, etoposide, anthracyclines, and 5-fluorouracil, and reduce neurotoxicity, nephrotoxicity (kidney), myelosuppression, mouth sores and cardiotoxicity. The downside is that it is a potent antioxidant, and your oncologist may have a problem with that. So, discuss this before starting to take melatonin. To help alleviate this concern, studies show that at least at one year, survival rates are better in many cancers when melatonin is taken. As a sleep aid, a starting dose of 5mg should suffice. Sometimes even half of that placed under the tongue to dissolve (sub-lingual) can lead to restful sleep. Toxicity seems to be very low and doses at high as 30-50mg per day have been reported in studies.

Stress Reduction

Most people have heard that the stress hormone cortisol is an immunosuppressant. However, cortisol dysregulation is but one of many adverse events in stress-induced immunosuppression. It is hard, if not impossible, to remove stress from your life. However, the good news is that direct anti-stress intervention predictably lowers all the markers of immune suppression. Even subtle stressors, like lack of support, worsens cancer prognosis. For example, one of the earliest studies in breast cancer patients showed that higher levels of perceived social support led to greater NK cell activity. On the other hand, patients who reported more stress related fatigue and depression demonstrated lower NK cell activity. There are a kazillion studies looking at psychoneuroimmunology in disease. The bottom line is that stress reduction, which also reduced depression and anxiety, should be a Holy Grail mission for anyone trying to initially prevent, beat or prevent recurrence of cancer. Stress reduction is an active process from yoga or tai-chi to laugh or music therapy. It is not about passive consumption of anti-depressant or sedating medications.

Calorie Restriction

Calorie restriction (CR) has a number of health benefits. Studies in mice show higher NK cytotoxicity and 60% longer survival from artificially induced cancers. Even though these are spectacular results, this is a mouse model not a people model. But hold on, preliminary research suggests caloric restriction may enhance chemo effect and is known to potentially be a cancer preventative in humans. Also, the ketogenic diet in principle is largely carb calorie restriction, and is being actively researched in various cancers after showing some benefit in brain tumors. CR may affect the increased death of T-reg cells, which improves the balance of good anti-cancer CD8+ T cells to the bad pro-cancer Foxp3+ T regulatory cells. So, it looks like there is an immunologic basis for the anti-cancer effect of CR. As far as active intervention, resveratrol and metformin can help induce CR.

The caution is simple. First of all, caloric restriction does not equate to starvation. That would be overdoing it. Also any caloric restriction in a cancer state is a dangerous proposition since cancer is a "wasting syndrome". Going on a prolonged fast or severe caloric restriction can be extremely detrimental for multiple reasons. Do not try any caloric restriction unless under doctor's supervision and under specific circumstances. Preferably all treatment should be completed and you are in good overall nutritional balance before trying this.

Mushrooms

Beta-glucans, such an lentinan, from yeast, algae, bacteria, and fungi of various types are well documented to boost the immune system. But the main mechanism for this is unclear and probably multifactorial. Beta-glucans are known to enhance T-helper cell function, stimulate interleukins and interferons, and activate natural killer cells, among other effects. In the laboratory they can synergize with chemotherapy agents such as taxanes. They have also been shown to prolong life in a study of patients with advanced gastric and colorectal cancer who were also on chemotherapy. However, if you take it as an extract supplement it can interact badly with non-steroidal anti-inflammatory drugs like ibuprofen and aspirin. Also maitake extract can interact with warfarin (Coumadin), increasing its effectiveness and bleeding risk. Again, erring on the side of food sources turns out to be safer. The best sources are reishi, maitake and shitake mushrooms, although allergies have been reported. In addition, Maitake D fraction specifically can potentiate both the innate and adaptive immune systems through additional mechanisms. From more exotic mushrooms like Cordyceps and Trametes versicolor to the lowly white mushrooms you see in the grocery store there is a steadily growing dataset which suggests mushrooms should be part of standard cancer care, like it is in Japan.

Cannabinoids

There was some concern in the 1990's in AIDS patients that marijuana could be immune suppressive. However, quite a few studies refute that and generally support multiple positive immunomodulatory effects. If anything, more recent animal studies show that this negative effect may be due to tetrahydrocannabinol (THC), the psychoactive part of marijuana. Keep in mind that there are multiple cannabinoids in the marijuana plant and some have greater beneficial effects than others. Perhaps the most actively studied one in the area of cancer and the immune system is cannabidiol. Also, to address those who simply do not like the way marijuana makes you feel, most of the cannabinoids do not have a significant psychoactive effect. Medicinal cannabinoids are becoming more readily available, beyond the prescription medications such as Marinol® (dronabinol) which is mainly for nausea and appetite. We are talking about potentially immune modulating and anti-cancer cannabinoids here and one cannabidiol vendor that seems to be ahead of the game in quality and expertise is CV Sciences (http://CVSciences.com), formerly known as Canna Vest.

Turmeric / Curcumin

Although curcumin is the main active anti-cancer immunomodulatory component of turmeric, it is not the only one. The effects of turmeric on T cells, B cells, NK cells, macrophages, NFκB and more, are very broad but all favorable. Although it is easier to pick up a curcumin pill in the store, the bioavailability of curcumin is not good. The best recommendation is to find natural turmeric root, grind it up, mix in black pepper or piperine for better absorption and put in on your food. Although turmeric is also not readily absorbed, in all likelihood it is better because the other components in the root were placed there by Mother Nature for a reason.

In general, if you have biliary problems, stomach ulcers or are prone to kidney stones, you may have to minimize or avoid turmeric or curcumin. Also, it can interfere with metabolism of certain chemotherapy drugs that use the liver p450 system to metabolize the drugs. Metabolism may include activation of drugs or clearing them from your body or both. So it can either limit chemotherapy effectiveness or increase toxicity because of delayed clearance from your body. Examples include Taxol® and Cytoxan®, which are very common chemotherapy agents. These effects are more likely to occur with supplement doses rather than dietary intake of the root or spice. Speak with your oncologist or pharmacist.

Other immune boosting foods, supplements and botanicals you might want to consider and look into further are: Ubiquinol (Ubiquinone CoQ10), lycopene, green tea (EGCG), garlic, resveratrol, quercetin, capsaicin, andrographoloid, flavonoids, genistein, omega 3 PUFA, monoterpenes, and plant sterols.

To reiterate what I touched on in the beginning, the immune system is extraordinarily complex. I hope you got a feel for this from this discussion. It is extremely foolhardy to load up with a handful of mega-dose "immune stimulant" supplements and think you are doing the right thing. You may be harming yourself by accidentally suppressing your immune system. Furthermore, the details of the immune system can vary from individual to individual and differ as to how it attacks different cancers. Many natural compounds can affect the immune system, directly or indirectly, positively or negatively and the balance between harm and benefit is not possible to accurately determine. In other words one can overdo something and severely shoot themselves in the foot. It is prudent to simply pick the main immune-active substances and use them mainly in a dietary dose as opposed to a pharmacologic supplement dose, while carefully avoiding immunosuppressive substances found in the toxins in your food and environment. We will cover the topic of rational ongoing anti-cancer detox later in this book.

CHAPTER 6
HORMONES AND CANCER

When hormones are mentioned, people usually think of sex steroid hormones like estrogen, progesterone, and testosterone, or thyroid hormone, all of which are part of the standard endocrine system. However, hormones are more generally defined as chemical substances produced by your body, usually but not always by a gland (e.g. thyroid), that regulate and control the activity of other organs and cells. This is very broad and correctly suggests that there are many more hormones in your body, working in a delicate balance, as well as those you are exposed to in your environment. The ones that are produced in your body are crucial for life and act in a finely tuned concert. They help control processes such as digestion and metabolism, growth, reproduction, heart rate, temperature control and more. There are more than fifty known main hormones, and you will soon discover the critical ones when it comes to integrative prevention and treatment of cancer.

Some endogenous hormones (those produced by your body) are inflammatory and incite or support cancer development. Others actively protect you from cancer. But hormones have to work in concert and within normal body function levels. They can go out of balance, with some being produced in excess relative to another, causing harm.

Hormone Excesses And How They Occur

One way by which excesses occur is by taking in extra hormones or substances that have a hormonal effect in our diet or from our environment. That's our next topic.

External or exogenous hormones that you digest as a food substance (e.g. hormones given to cattle or sheep to accelerate growth) or are exposed to from various chemicals in your environment (xeno-hormones) can be part of the reason for hormonal imbalance and damaging endocrine disruption. This disruption can be pro-carcinogenic.

Xenohormones can be natural or synthetic. The most common subtype are xeno-estrogens which can attach to estrogen receptors and stimulate growth in cancers that are driven by estrogen. While the U.S. Department of Agriculture (USDA) does not allow hormone use in raising pigs, chickens, turkeys and other fowl, they are allowed in cows. So, you can find them in dairy products. These hormones are either the residual of administered growth hormones, insulin-like growth factors (IGF), or increased sex hormones from cows found during pregnancy and milk production. Of course, the official position is that these hormone amounts are not enough to cause concern in humans, but this is a tenuous and debatable position. Among chemical sources of xenohormones, there are various forms of plastic, including some food and water containers. But the list is very long and includes many things we put on our hair and skin or are exposed to in daily life, like household cleaners, air fresheners, insecticides and weed killers. You can search the Environmental Working Group site for more information on this topic (http://ewg.org).

Breast, gynecologic, prostate, thyroid, colorectal, stomach and pancreatic cancer are most often thought of as "hormone dependent." But developing science suggests more and more cancers are affected by hormones, not like previously thought, and some more than others. This is a developing story but is one of the potential "imbalances" that you need to pay attention to no matter what cancer you have.

"Balancing" Hormones And Hormone-Like Messengers In Cancer

The concept of hormone balancing usually addresses balancing sex steroids like estrogen and progesterone, and is a little over-hyped. But the principle is simple. Is there an excess or deficiency of a hormone or hormones that can cause harm, specifically increase the risk of cancer or create an environment in which cancer thrives? From the perspective of cancer prevention and anti-cancer support, the following are some of the key hormones and hormone analogs that need to be "in balance."

Estrogen

Estrogen deficiency may lead to symptoms of menopause such as hot flushes and mood swings, but will not be pro-carcinogenic. Estrogen excess or dominance can be. Beware that if you have an estrogen sensitive cancer, increasing estrogen to help with menopausal symptoms may not be in your best interest. It does not matter if it is a synthetic or a bio-identical natural estrogen. It can harm you in this situation because by and large cancer does not discriminate between synthetic and natural. However, it is sometimes possible to use plant or phytoestrogens to help with symptoms and that's discussed below.

Naturally reducing estrogen levels is possible using exercise to reduce body fat and through diet. Your fat cells produce a weaker type of estrogen called estrone. This is usually not a problem unless you have a lot of fat cells producing a lot of estrone. Also, losing body fat increases sex hormone binding globulin (SHBG) in your blood stream, which binds sex steroid hormones like estrogen and androgen and does not allow an excess to get to hormonally sensitive organs. So reducing body fat is a solid longer-term strategy to reduce estrogen dominance or excess androgen for that matter.

We know from epidemiologic studies that consuming soy products may reduce breast cancer risk. This is still controversial, but excluding the argument to avoid soy products because they are largely GMO, there are two mechanisms of action that support this. First, phytoestrogens do bind to estrogen receptors in hormonally sensitive tissues like breast, prostate, and the uterus. But they are much weaker estrogens than endogenous estrogen coming from the ovaries or fat cells. By attaching to estrogen receptors they can block the action of the stronger, potentially cancer stimulating, estrogens circulating in your body. The other mechanism of anti-cancer action is that phytoestrogens are anti-angiogenic, blocking blood vessel formation to developed or forming cancerous tumors.

Although not yet proven, dietary fiber may reduce the risk of numerous cancers. One way that this may happen is that the fiber may bind excess hormones, like estrogen. By binding hormones, fiber does not allow them to be reabsorbed from the intestinal tract. Cruciferous vegetables, like broccoli and cauliflower, can also bind estrogen and increase excretion in the stool.

In women, during the premenopausal years, estrogen and progesterone are under a delicate and highly orchestrated balance involving other regulatory hormones.

They cycle predictably under normal circumstances. For many reasons, you may or may not be in a state of normal circumstances, and it is beyond this book to go into the complete endocrinology of estrogen. In the postmenopausal years, ovarian estrogen production drops like a rock, usually leaving a state of progesterone dominance for a while. With time, progesterone levels also drop. However, depending upon the amount of body fat, there may or may not be a transient state of progesterone dominance due to balance from estrone. So, as far as balancing estrogen is concerned, it depends on what your starting point is and if you are trying to prevent a hormonally sensitive cancer or its recurrence.

Progesterone

Most people think of progesterone as the friendly gentle "balancing hormone" for estrogen in the female menstrual cycle and gynecologic health. However, it can be a potent mitogen which can stimulate abnormal cell growth. Just as the case with estrogen, how it acts at the cellular level depends on upon the presence or absence of progesterone receptors. Normally hormonal attachment to receptors activates cellular pathways, including growth. Counterintuitively, high doses of progesterone may be used to fight endometrial cancer. According to laboratory data, this may also be true in breast cancer and others. It is a complex molecular interaction and thinking simplistically can get you into trouble.

The main danger here is attempting to balance estrogen using the many different types of progesterone creams, available in varying doses, on the market. Again, it does not matter if it is synthetic or natural bio-identical. If you have a progesterone sensitive cancer, this can harm you. Everyone's capacity to absorb progesterone, and other substances, through the skin, is different. To make matters worse, progesterone accumulates in fat cells. So, if you overdo it using skin creams or supplementation, high blood and tissue levels can persist even if you stop because the fat cells will continue to release progesterone for a prolonged period of time. Taking it even one step further, excess progesterone converts to estrogen. So, overdoing it can lead to more estrogen dominance, which is the very thing that you are trying to avoid by artificially adding progesterone.

In the absence of a progesterone sensitive cancer, balancing depends on your starting point and goal, just like estrogen. In premenopausal years, there are many regulating hormones involved. Levels change on a weekly if not daily basis.

So it is not a simple matter to decide what is best and when to try to artificially balance them. Having said that, we're only addressing the direct cancer effect here. Chapter 20 goes into more details about symptoms, like anxiety, when progesterone declines relative to estrogen. From a pure cancer perspective, low progesterone only increases the risk of cancer when it is not counter-balancing estrogen well, not because of low progesterone in and of itself. The safest answer in premenopausal years is to look at ways to reduce estrogen rather than increase progesterone.

In perimenopausal to postmenopausal years, there may be a state of progesterone dominance, but it is relatively short lived. Progesterone does not bind well to SHBG, so trying to increase that through weight loss is not as effective as it is with estrogen. On the other hand, it binds to transcortin and albumin, both of which are synthesized in the liver. Unfortunately albumin levels drop with malnutrition and malignancy. So, a diet that focuses on maintaining protein is important in this way among many other reasons.

Testosterone

Most people think that androgens such as testosterone are only present in the male. However, this is not true, and in fact, men and women normally produce androgens, estrogens, and progesterone in varying quantities. In women, androgens are used in breast cancer treatment but can be paradoxically carcinogenic. It's a very complicated issue in both men and women because of metabolic interconversion between sex steroids. Also, androgens are sometimes prescribed for symptoms such as low sex drive in both genders. So, you should just know that this is not without risk for hormone-sensitive cancers such as breast and prostate. Also, as a related side-note, it's important to remember that breast cancer can occur in men as well.

This, as well as all other hormone therapy, is an exceedingly complex topic. Suffice it to say that minimizing meddling is prudent but, when necessary under physician supervision, androgen therapy for symptoms can be considered. If anything, it is best to try to optimize androgen naturally, and the following steps can help.

As far as diet and supplements go, zinc is an essential co-factor in testosterone synthesis, and your diet is the best source. If you're going to use supplements, more is *not* better because it can interfere with other mineral absorption such as copper and be immune suppressive. Stick to doses less than 40 mg per day.

Likewise, it is important to optimize your Vitamin D level. This is discussed below and in other parts of this book as a crucial supplement for health and anti-cancer status. Finally, limiting sugar and high GI carbs (which increase insulin and lower testosterone), optimizing healthy fats (mainly from plants and fish), and increasing branched chain amino acids from high quality whey protein, round out the recommendations for natural testosterone metabolism support.

Resistance training as well as burst training, discussed elsewhere in this book, are known to naturally optimize testosterone levels. Depending upon your starting point, exercise can either increase or decrease your androgen levels.

Stress increases the hormone cortisol which is discussed in greater detail below. Suffice it to say that cortisol blocks testosterone effect. Stress reduction in heaping quantities, like meditation, yoga, laugh and music therapy are all effective solutions.

One additional natural strategy is to optimize free testosterone bio-availability. We know that androgens bind to SHBG. So if the concern is mainly high levels of androgen, losing fat weight and maintaining lean body mass through diet and exercise can help. This naturally modulates testosterone by raising SHBG and limiting androgen bioavailability to tissues.

Cortisol

Cortisol is produced by your adrenal gland and is your "stress response" hormone. It typically fluctuates from a high level in the morning to much lower levels in the middle of the night. Under normal circumstances, it helps regulate blood sugar, immune function, and inflammatory response. With poor sleep habits, chronic stress and depression this fluctuation goes away and high levels persist. This leads to all the negatives of insulin resistance, muscle wasting, immune suppression and rampant chronic inflammation. You have already learned that this is all pro-carcinogenic and worsens other chronic inflammatory diseases such as cardiovascular disease, diabetes, Alzheimer's and is probably at least partly responsible for chemo-brain.

So, OK, you know cortisol is bad in excess. How do you go about reducing it? The good news is that there are multiple ways you can lessen the effect of this supercharger of bad outcomes.

Magnesium supplementation in combination with aerobic burst training can help reduce cortisol.

Omega-3 fatty acids can slightly reduce cortisol production with a greater effect with larger doses, but that can be dangerous for other reasons. So, keep it in moderation.

Music, laugh, and massage therapy are a good set of options.

Soy-derived phosphatidylserine and black tea can reduce cortisol.

On the other hand, staying away from excess caffeine, and getting a regular good night's sleep of at least seven hours can help.

Beyond that, anything that works for you to relieve stress is helpful. Engage in what you enjoy, as often as you can. Consider yoga, tai chi, and meditation among those options.

Thyroid Hormone

Thyroid hormones triiodothyronine (T3) and thyroxine (T4), are essential in the modulation of normal development, growth, and metabolism. However, thyroid status may influence the development of cancer, its growth, and metastasis. This is still very controversial and has been debated for over a decade. In a laboratory test tube, the main thyroid hormone, L-thyroxine (T), acts as an anti-apoptotic agent at normal physiologic concentrations in numerous experimental cell lines. Also, triiodothyronine (T3) has a proliferative effect on a number of cancer cell lines, especially breast. The best clinical information about this is also found in breast cancer, where we know that the risk is increased if there is a history of thyroid cancer. So, there seems to be an association, but it is not clear how strong this relationship is or what the mechanism might be.

Regarding how to balance your thyroid hormones, there are numerous very important issues. First off, your doctor should determine why your thyroid is overactive (hyperthyroidism) or hypoactive (hypothyroidism). On the underactive side, it may be something simple like insufficient iodine intake. But there are other more serious considerations. Regardless of that, we are mainly concerned with hyperthyroidism in this section. An overactive thyroid may harbor a tumor, some of which can be malignant. If you are on thyroid medications for hypoactive thyroid, you may be taking too much.

So, it is crucial not to try to naturally mask symptoms of hyperthyroidism or adjust anything without working with your physician and getting tested.

Leptin/Ghrelin/Adiponectin

Leptin, adiponectin, and ghrelin have varied and extensive roles in controlling inflammation and metabolism, including a central role in the cancer wasting syndrome called cachexia. They are all involved in glucose homeostasis and insulin sensitivity. Ghrelin, adiponectin, and leptin are all elevated in cachectic patients. However, in obesity, leptin is the only one that is elevated. Ghrelin and adiponectin are both decreased.

Ghrelin is secreted by G cells in the stomach and is an appetite stimulant. Leptin is secreted by fat cells and suppresses appetite while increasing energy use. Adiponectin is also secreted by fat cells and is important in energy metabolism. In addition, this hormonal interplay can be affected by thyroid dysfunction, by sex, by the time of day and time before and after eating.

This is an extremely oversimplified account just mentioned here to raise your awareness of another delicately balanced system that influences key factors in fighting cancer wasting on one hand and cancer-promoting obesity on the other. It would be dangerous to go overboard in one direction or the other, and it depends on where you are in the spectrum of obesity to cancer-related wasting. The best way to balance this system is to hold to a solid anti-cancer anti-inflammatory, low glycemic index diet and engage in a balanced exercise program which includes muscle preservation or building through resistance training.

Insulin

We already touched on the critical and multiple effects insulin has on cancer initiation and promotion. I included this snippet here because it is most definitely a hormone you need to keep in balance. Refer to Chapter 4 for a complete discussion.

Endorphins

Endorphins are "endogenous morphines" produced by your central nervous system and pituitary gland, which primarily function in your body as pain blockers and "feel good" hormones in your brain. They are a little off the beaten path as they are technically neuromodulators, and some have called them neurotransmitters. Their function is quite a bit broader than originally thought. So, for the purpose of this discussion I'll refer to them as hormones that need balancing. Put in a better way; they need optimizing and nurturing.

Endorphins are important for quality of life regarding feeling good and being as optimistic as possible. Besides helping to reduce pain, β-endorphin may specifically activate parasympathetic nervous system control of tumor suppressor genes and help your immune system to destroy and clear cancer cells.

Strategies that may increase endorphins include exercise, pleasurable activities such as sex, laughing in response to good comedy, enjoying music, sniffing lavender or vanilla, taking Ginseng, and eating something spicy that includes capsaicin. Most of these are also obviously stress reducers, so you will get the added cancer-fighting benefit of reducing cortisol.

Endocannabinoids

The human endocannabinoid system is quite complex and is involved in many metabolic processes, including inflammation, immunomodulation and pain control. Endocannabinoids belong to a non-traditional set of biochemicals which act sort of like hormones, much like the endorphins, in that they are chemical messengers. Much like prostaglandins, they are: 1) made in multiple tissues (not in one organ like the ovary or thyroid, among other endocrine organs), 2) are produced only when needed by activation of specific enzymes, 3) not stored in vesicles like most hormones and neurotransmitters, 4) mostly act locally on the cells and tissues nearby, and 5) are quickly degraded when their job of activating CB receptors is completed. This activity is named scientifically as "paracrine" rather than "endocrine," which is a category most hormones belong to.

To exert their effect, cannabinoids need to bind to CB receptors. CB$_1$ receptors are found in high levels in the central nervous system (CNS), but also are located in many other tissues. CB$_2$ receptors are mainly found on cells of the immune system but are also located in the intestine, brain, and peripheral nervous system. The goal is always homeostasis or metabolic balance and may be one physical explanation for a mind-body bridge. The two best-known endocannabinoids are anandamide (AEA) and 2-arachidonoylglycerol (2-AG).

In the brain and in the intestine, endocannabinoids increase with fasting and cause hunger and also increase the hormone Ghrelin, which is an appetite stimulant. Active CB1 receptors in the liver are likely also responsible in part for fatty liver. In fatty tissues, CB1 receptors go way up when you get fatter. This sets of a vicious negative cycle of storing more fat the more obese you get. Obesity, as you have already learned, leads to lower adiponectin and to insulin resistance, inflammation and a great environment for cancer to grow. In animals, you can experiment and block CB1 receptors but medications for this are not available in humans nor are there natural ways to do this other than losing fat weight. If you lose weight, you decrease the number of CB1 receptors and lower LDL-cholesterol, triglycerides, and glucose. This creates an anti-cancer environment.

External cannabinoids, most commonly marijuana, are phytocannabinoids (phyto means plant) and are commonly recommended in the treatment of chemotherapy side effects, including neuropathic pain, loss of appetite, nausea, and vomiting. But animal lab studies have also shown that the endocannabinoid system can induce apoptosis, inhibit cancer cell proliferation, and inhibit angiogenesis and metastasis. Other than small case reports there is no sound clinical proof of these direct anti-cancer effects in humans. But there probably is something to this because additional laboratory studies suggest that endocannabinoid signaling is different between normal and cancer cells. Also, remember that the cannabinoid effect on the immune system may be positive or negative.

So what's the upshot? Yes, it is true that the endocannabinoids may have an anti-cancer effect, but it is also true that too many CB1 receptors lead to increasing obesity and a pro-cancer environment. With balance, in theory, it is possible that you can get the good effects of endocannabinoids but that you can limit the harmful effects if you lose weight and have fewer CB1 receptors to create the pro-cancer environment. This is all theoretical but speaks to the need for balance, as in many other things in life.

Studies suggest that an imbalance in the endocannabinoid system and its interaction with sex steroid hormone balance may also promote cancer. Thus the endocannabinoid system might be a good target to help control initiation and progression of prostate, breast, and endometrial cancers. These are all hormonally sensitive tumors, so other cancers which are at least partly regulated by sex steroid hormones may follow.

However, as with everything in life, there are still other cautions. There have been laboratory studies in breast cancer cells lines which suggest that in those cancers where cannabinoid receptors are weak or absent the primary psychoactive cannabinoid (tetrahydrocannabinol or THC) may actually promote cancer. Epidemiologic studies do not support this concern, but nevertheless overindulging with cannabis preparations that contain THC may be counterproductive. This is another example of needing to use discretion and to consider the precautionary principle.

Cholecalciferol

Otherwise known as vitamin D3, cholecalciferol is one of five forms of vitamin D. Active vitamin D3 (1,25-dihydroxyvitamin D3) has a hormonal activity throughout your body. Unfortunately, there is a 30% deficiency rate even in those who live in the sun-belt. Sunscreens also largely interfere with skin synthesis of Vitamin D. This is a huge problem because we know that Vitamin D receptors are widespread in the human body, affecting many functions as a hormone. Vitamin D also influences over 3000 genes. Most importantly, we know that people who have lower levels have a much higher risk of cancer. What we don't know is whether or not increasing Vitamin D levels after a diagnosis of cancer improves prognosis. But the downside to optimizing it is small.

Supplementation is crucial. The Institute of Medicine's recommendations are far too low according to most experts. The good news is that you can have levels measured. In most laboratories, 30 nanograms per milliliter (ng/nl) is the rock bottom within the "normal range." But if levels are lower than 40 or 50 ng/ml, supplementation with 2000 to 4000 IU/day may be required. Test it, supplement it, re-test it and adjust as needed. There is a risk of liver toxicity, but that is at much higher levels. So in the case of Vitamin D, balancing usually means optimizing your blood level by ensuring optimal intake. Finally, to minimize the risk of calcium depositing in your arteries, take Vitamin K2 along with Vitamin D. The optimal ratio is not well worked out but is around 100 micrograms for every 1000 IU Vitamin D. For more information, please review Chapter 14 on supplementation.

Final Thoughts On Balancing Hormones

Part of mainstream therapy against cancers that are sensitive to sex hormones is to increase or reduce hormone production, increase hormones artificially by administering them or to block them using very specific medications. Most often tumor cells from a biopsy will be tested for presence or absence of hormone receptors, which are like little molecular locks on the cell surface or within the cells. If these receptors or locks are absent, the hormones, which are like little keys, have nowhere to plug themselves into to exert their effect. The goal here is not to balance anything. It is to eliminate a hormone or use massive quantities of it to kill or suppress cancer cells specifically. While natural approaches, including diet, exercise and herbals can certainly affect hormones in your body, it is a less precise and longer term strategy. Most importantly, communicate with your oncologist if a practitioner is working on "balancing" your hormones. In some cases it may be helpful, in some cases useless and in the worst case scenario, it can hurt you by interfering with a specific hormonal therapy.

CHAPTER 7
EPIGENETICS, NUTRIGENOMICS
& CANCER STEM CELLS

Talk To Your Genes

It is not the genes you are born with but *largely* what you do with them or allow your environment or habits to do to them. Is that a surprise to you? After all, we are repeatedly told that it's just bad luck and that you get cancer because you must have been born with bad genes and there's just nothing you can do about it. But, there are an overwhelming number of environmental factors that can contribute to cancer, and we have known that for a very long time. The only question that is debated is how many cancers are mainly genetic and how many are primarily environmental? The truth is in between. Even the most conservative estimates are that 30% of all cancers are environmental, which includes diet, toxins, and lifestyle choices. We also know that somewhere between 10% and 20% of cancers are primarily genetic. So, what's in between? There's 50-60% that is missing! This means that most likely, more cancers are affected by your environment than we previously thought, and that puts it at a whopping 80-90% that you can influence.

The following image depicts the balance between genetics and epigenetics. It's not a true balance in that there is more epigenetic than genetic influence on cancer, but you get the idea. Both are important. Differentially methylated regions (DMRs) are associated with a number of diseases including cancer. These are stretches of DNA that have different DNA methylation patterns compared to other areas, and this influences which genes are expressed or not expressed. Genomic imprinting is an epigenetic phenomenon where certain gene alleles are silenced and not expressed. An imprinted gene means you inherit only one working copy (allele) of the gene from mom or dad. So, depending on the gene, one or the other copy is epigenetically silenced. Silencing usually happens due to the methylation, which we are about to cover. Loss of imprinting (LOI) is seen in a number of cancers and in critical genes such as IGF2 or insulin growth factor 2, which we have covered already. With increased expression due to LOI of IGF2, there is tumorigenesis. The last part of the simplified diagram below is CTCF-binding factor which is a transcriptional repressor protein. The CTCF gene which encodes this protein thus plays a significant role in repressing the IGF2 gene, for example. I hope this is painting the very complex picture of epigenetics vs. genetics role in cancer development and progression, but you do not have to understand the extremely complicated details to benefit from this concept.

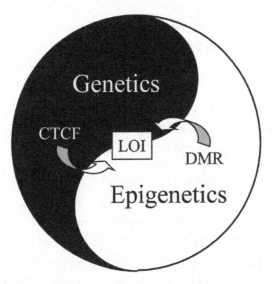

From Proceedings of the National Academy of Sciences (PNAS) http://www.pnas.org [Public domain], via Wikimedia Commons

It turns out that the toxins in your environment, the food you eat, what you drink, the air you breathe, your mood and stress levels, all constantly "talk" with your genes through molecular interactions on the genetic code surface. The 21st century science that is devoted to studying this is called epigenetics, which literally means "on top of genes." Favorable environmental factors can either suppress "bad genes" or enhance "good gene" expression. Epigenetics is formally defined as "the study of heritable changes in gene expression or cellular phenotype caused by mechanisms other than changes in the underlying DNA sequence." How can we do this through natural approaches? We'll get to that in a second. First we have to touch on some basic genetics.

The genetic code that you inherit from your parents and ancestors before them follows a so-called Mendelian pattern. What genes your offspring will have is quite predictable by looking at your family tree. Some genes are dominant, and some are recessive, which means some are more likely to be hidden or not "expressed" in any given generation. Because you inherit two copies (alleles) of every gene (one from mom and one from dad), it also influences which genes result in your phenotype or basically how you look. It's a very complex topic, and it is far beyond the scope of this book to cover genetics. Suffice it to say that some cancers, a vast minority, are inherited in a Mendelian genetic manner. For example, the mutated BRCA genes that are related mainly to breast, ovarian and prostate cancer are inherited this way. When you are born with defects in these genes, the chances of developing one of these cancers during your lifetime skyrockets. However, even when you inherit one of these cancer-prone gene alterations, this does not guarantee that you will come down with cancer. Some folks still dodge that bad gene bullet. Why? Interaction with your environment and lifestyle choices still has something to do with it, and that is at least partly under the influence of epigenetic factors.

So, the genes you are born with are a major factor in some forms of cancer. But in the end, cancer develops because some "bad genes" (tumor promoter genes) are turned on in addition to the "good genes" (the normal BRCA tumor suppressor genes) being altered, turned off or missing. Again, not everyone who is positive for BRCA mutation gets cancer. Beyond this, some people seem to overall have more bullet-proof genes than others. Some can smoke packs per day, eat junk and drink to oblivion and yet live to be a hundred. This is the exception. Most of us are not that lucky, and there is individual and ethnic variation as to how "cancer-proof" we are.

It's also very interesting that you can inherit epigenetic DNA changes or marks, which can influence one or more alleles (i.e. copies of genes). However, they are inherited in a non-predictable non-Mendelian fashion from cell to cell and possibly from parent to offspring. Epigenetic changes are also acquired throughout your life, and some are reversible. We will cover what these epigenetic changes are and how you can influence them. But first, here is an example of epigenetic influence to drive the point home. Identical twins are born with essentially the same genes, yet they "grow apart." Their incidence of high cholesterol, hypertension, Alzheimer's and cancer are quite different. In other words, they largely steer their body towards health or disease by their lifestyle choices.

The main point about discussing both genetics and epigenetics is that purely genetic cancers that you can't affect at all are far less common than those which occur because of an interaction of environment and your genes. You see, it is not just "one thing," not just one gene that is responsible for cancer in the vast majority of people. It is an unfortunate series of events with multiple "hits" or damaging attacks on some of your genes that finally make some cells go bad and become cancerous. The number of "hits" that any individual can sustain before cancer develops is also related to how well their DNA repair genes are functioning. These "hits" (e.g. from toxins and bad lifestyle choices) may be reduced in number and magnitude at any point in your life by making modifications in your diet, better lifestyle choices and avoidance of toxic substances.

Even if you are cancer prone because of the genes you have inherited, nutrients can affect the genetic switches to silence bad genes and otherwise optimize the good genes. Although these are very new sciences compared to anatomy, physiology, biochemistry, or even genetics, they are the scientific glue that connects natural substances and approaches to health. You are what you eat, breathe, consume, and are exposed to. And, lest you think this takes decades for an effect, science says it is quite a bit more rapid. In some cases, it can be almost instantaneous in reversing the damage that has been done. So any lifestyle choices you make today can carry an almost immediate effect in many cases. Could this favorable change lie within you? You simply can't afford to not explore this strategy to wellness.

Epigenetic Modifications

So, what exactly are epigenetic modifications and how do they occur? The three best-studied mechanisms are DNA methylation, histone modification and small non-coding RNA such as micro-RNAs (miRNA). Don't worry; we're not going deep on this. It's an exceedingly complex topic but again highlights how complicated preventing and beating cancer is when you really start studying it. We're mainly going to focus on how you can influence these processes. But to tell the

difference between marketing hyped useless anti-cancer strategies and the real
deal, you need to know the basics.   *GLUE = PACKING*

As the following image illustrates, <u>DNA methylation is the first mechanism that
activates or deactivates gene expression.</u> It is simply the addition of a methyl
molecule to a specific area of DNA (position 5 of the pyrimidine ring of cyto-
sine in a cytosine-guanine or CG base pair). Hypomethylation (i.e. not enough
methyl groups) causes the DNA chromatin to be less densely packaged so that
the DNA can be transcribed. Conversely, hyper-methylation (i.e. too many
methyl groups) can make these areas dense, not transcribable and therefore silenced. These hypermethylated areas are usually found in so-called <u>CpG islands.
In cancer,</u> more tumor suppressor genes are hyper-methylated (i.e. silenced), and
tumor promoter genes are hypo-methylated (i.e. made active). Globally, human
DNA becomes more hypomethylated with age and in cancer cells, especially in
metastatic tumors. However, this can vary widely from organ to organ.

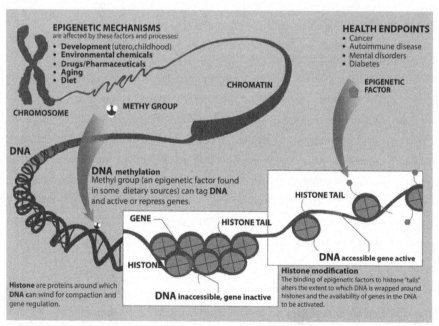

Modified from National Institutes of Health (http://commonfund.nih.gov/epigenomics/figure.aspx) [Public domain], via
Wikimedia Commons

Histone modifications are the second mechanism available, and much is known
about how it works, but less is known about how nutrition may affect it. In a
nutshell, histones are proteins (H2A, H2B, H3, and H4) around which DNA

is wound (kind of like a knitting ball) to make it more compact so that it can fit inside a nucleus. This piece of DNA which is 147 base pairs in length is wound twice around the histones and is called a nucleosome. Nucleosomes are strung together by DNA segments that are about 20-80 base pairs in length. Multiple biochemical processes called mono-, di-, and tri-methylation, acetylation, ubiquitylation, phosphorylation, and ribosylation, of these histones can alter how tightly wrapped the DNA is and how exposed it is for genes in that area to be active or suppressed. What makes it more challenging is that multiple histone modifications appear to be necessary to change gene expression. This makes it very hard to study effects of specific nutrients.

The last main type of modification is due to small non-coding miRNA, piRNA, siRNA and small nucleolar RNA. RNA is normally the intermediary between DNA in genes and the proteins they code for. So, DNA is "transcribed" into RNA and RNA is in turn "translated" into the myriad of proteins we need to sustain life. But small non-coding RNAs are not translated into proteins. These help regulate 30-60% of genes through inhibition of protein translation and various other complex mechanisms.

The above mechanisms usually interact, and all three are often found to be in action within cancer cells. So, what can we do to affect these epigenetic processes?

Before moving to proactive nutrient epigenetics, let's get toxins out of the way. Toxins can either be directly genotoxic (i.e. directly affect and damage genes) or work through the epigenetic modifications we're about to cover. The bottom line is very easy to state: avoid toxins like the plague! A short exposure to even a highly toxic material might not do anything to you other than make you feel a little sick. But long-term and repeated exposures to lower levels of less toxic materials can make all the difference between getting cancer or not. Now, as I repeatedly mention in this book, you can't avoid all of the estimated 65,000 toxins that many of us are exposed to during a year. But you can certainly try as much as you can. Refer to Chapters 14 and 15 to learn more about avoiding or minimizing exposure to both internal and external toxins.

Nutrigenomics And Nutrigenetics

Turning to a more proactive topic, there are two related scientific disciplines that devote attention to how nutrients and genes interact and how diets should be individualized. First, how food talks with your genes is being studied within a broad subject science called nutri*genomics*. So, for example, polyunsaturated fatty acids (PUFA) in fish oil suppress fatty acid synthase gene expression. We know of many direct epigenetic effects on genes like this, but many are yet to be discovered and characterized as to what they really mean. Nutri*genetics* is a highly related field which studies how different people respond to the same diet or specific nutrients differently, based on their genetic makeup. For example, the same diet can lead to different levels of cholesterol and different degrees of blood pressure problems due to genetic variability between individuals. Even more simply put, what's good regarding nutrient mix for one person may not be the best for another. Some may do better with more carbs than with proteins for example. In others, it might be the direct opposite. Nutrigenetics and nutrigenomics are complementary and often confused in terms of usage. Both will become more critical in ferreting out what nutrients will help beat cancer in any given individual.

There are some people hyping and marketing diets and supplements that are supposedly specific to you as an individual, your blood type, your star sign or whatever. There have been some exciting advances over the past ten years but the science for this is still not quite there yet to make major and unique anti-cancer diet recommendations for specific individuals. Here is an example of what is possible. Individual genetic alterations, called single nucleotide variations (SNV) or single nucleotide polymorphisms (SNP), can determine if you are at risk for heart attacks from caffeine. This is great because if you have a specific SNP (CYP1A2) you can alter your caffeine intake and reduce your risk of a heart attack. Unfortunately, this is not well worked out yet for cancer risk and actionable interventions.

So, nutrigenetics and nutrigenomics will both have a huge impact as we go on because this will eventually become very personalized. However, today it is still in its infancy. Anyone selling you anything beyond that is making it up as they go along. Or they are making recommendations based on theory or lab studies and not fact based on human studies, or even animal studies. Having said that, this area is exciting and rapidly evolving.

Even though it is not 100% precise, we know that there are some nutritional components that inhibit the development of cancer on the basis of nutri*genomics*, which is more akin to epigenetics in principle. These components include sulforaphane and isothiocyanates from cruciferous vegetables, folate from leafy green vegetables, grain cereals, caffeic acid from coffee, plums and kiwi, polyphenols such as EGCG from green tea, resveratrol, genistein, lignans from linseed, omega-3 PUFAs, α-linoleic acid, zinc, selenium, vitamin E, among a large and growing list. Unfortunately, the effects may be different in different individuals and can be organ specific, which can also present a challenge.

Which nutrients you need may also be related to the timing and dose when you consume them. The best-known example of that is in normal colon cells, where higher folate levels suppress cancer formation. But if you go too high, it can promote cancer growth. Also, if colorectal cancer is already present, higher folate levels can promote cancer growth. So, keep in mind that there is a risk and benefit to everything. As I keep mentioning over and over in this book, the risk side is probably minimized if you focus on whole foods to get your nutrients rather than higher doses often found in supplements.

The following are some of the best known nutrigenomic interactions. Keep in mind that these are mostly based on lab studies and not on human trials. Also, as mentioned previously, these are not accurately targeted strategies because in some cases methylation of genes results in suppression of tumor promoters and in other situations can result in activation.

All this information substantiates how these nutrients seem to have an anticancer effect in physiologic doses found in a prudent diet. But as you will see, it is not all straightforward and doing things that seem healthy on your own or under the supervision of a less knowledgeable cancer nutrition professional may be counterproductive to your survivorship. I have to stress, again and again; this cautionary advice is especially true if you are experimenting with taking higher, more pharmaceutical level or "orthomolecular," doses of "natural" supplements. Be very careful.

Folate is a vitamin (B9), which means you have to obtain it from diet or supplements and your body converts it to 5,10-methylenetetrahydrofolate (MTHF) which is a methyl donor. It converts homocysteine to methionine, which in addition to choline, donates methyl groups to form S-adenosyl-methionine (SAM). In turn, SAM is an important DNA methylating agent, which is a key epigenetic mechanism of action. Natural whole food sources of folate include leafy vegetables, beans, lentils, asparagus, and avocado.

EGCG from green tea is a potent polyphenol known to decrease the risk of colorectal, breast, esophageal, ovarian, pancreatic, hepatocellular, and prostate cancer. It exerts its epigenetic effects through suppressing methylation of tumor suppressor gene promoters and may have an effect through favorable histone modification as well.

Resveratrol has been shown to affect miRNA in cancer cells but not normal cells, reduce methylation of a tumor suppressor genes and modify histone acetylation. While more may or may not be better, resveratrol appears to be non-toxic at higher doses and is rapidly metabolized. Having said that, there is a concern that very high doses may be carcinogenic through an unknown mechanism.

Caffeic acid is a dietary polyphenol from the coffee bean. It affects SAM bioavailability which, as mentioned already, is a universal methyl donor.

Soy isoflavones genistein and daidzein have a direct effect on estrogen receptors by virtue of being phytoestrogens. Whether or not this is protective against hormone sensitive cancer like breast or prostate is hotly debated, and there is evidence for both sides. When you dig down to epigenetic influences the picture gets muddier because of the different effects of hypo – and hyper-methylation in various suppressor and promoter genes. The picture is mixed and, if you have a hormone-sensitive cancer, your oncologist may or may not want you taking soy phytoestrogens for this combination of reasons.

Sulforaphane and *glucosinolates* are isothiocyanates that are abundant in cruciferous vegetables like cauliflower, broccoli and brussel sprouts. These are the quintessential anti-cancer veggies! They have an inhibitory effect on histone acetylation and are demethylators of some cancer suppressor genes, meaning they can activate "good" genes. Sulforaphanes, in combination with green tea EGCG, can also activate estrogen receptor promoters which can enhance the activity of Tamoxifen in breast cancer hormonal blocking treatment. These are just two examples of the reasons why eating cruciferous vegetables is essential.

Lycopene is an antioxidant carotenoid found in tomatoes and in even higher levels within tomato paste. In combination with animal and epidemiologic evidence, there seems to be a benefit in at least prostate, breast, and lung cancer. This benefit it as least partly related to epigenetic effects and involves activating tumor suppressor and DNA repair genes.

Mineral micronutrients such as selenium and zinc can also have an epigenetic effect. Selenium is known to reduce prostate cancer but its preventative role in other cancers is controversial. Nevertheless, selenium is found in various quantities in many vegetables, depending upon how much selenium is in the soil that the vegetables are grown in. So, you are likely consuming this mineral as well as zinc, which is found in highest levels in pumpkin seeds, sesame seeds, lentils, garbanzo beans, quinoa, and cashews. This is another case where balance is everything. Too much selenium or zinc can be counterproductive, and the body does not need very much. So, taking higher dose supplements is generally not a great idea. There are exceptions for specific circumstances. Regarding its epigenetic effect, selenium inhibits histone deacetylases, which likely helps prevent abnormal histone methylation.

Cancer Stem Cells

Epigenetic mechanisms affect normal cells and cancer cells, but perhaps the most important part of this whole discussion is the epigenetic effect on silencing cancer stems cells and putting them into a dormant state. You have seen many references to cancer stem cells in this book already. These are the generally slow growing cells in your body that have gone bad and whose only purpose is to create rapidly dividing cancer cells which form primary and metastatic tumors. There is more and more research to support the existence of these in all cancers. They are relatively resistant to chemotherapy and radiation and can circulate in the blood and lymphatic systems. Unless you are lucky to have had them completely removed surgically (e.g. hysterectomy, prostatectomy, mastectomy or lumpectomy), or unless you control them or differentiate them (i.e. loss of "stemness") as best as possible through epigenetics, this is likely a major reason why your cancer might recur.

While there is still some debate about the existence of cancer stem cells, overall and in specific cancer types, research is ongoing to try to target these cells using monoclonal antibodies, cell signaling interruption, epigenetic biological agents, and other strategies. Meanwhile, there is no question that natural epigenetic silencing is a real and low-risk option, albeit not very targeted nor clinically proven. In other words, we know it exists from laboratory studies but do now know how much of what will silence which genes. Keep in mind the warnings about too much and wrong time or place effects we just discussed. Remember, diet, and lifestyle modification prevail over higher dose synthetic supplements in most cases and will give you 80% of what you need with generally low risk.

Nutritional and lifestyle modification effect on cancer is not all epigenetic in nature, but in the following positive examples epigenetics and nutrigenomics are likely to be at least partly responsible for the anti-cancer effect. In a recent study, patients with prostate cancer recurrence after radiation or surgery either got a placebo or took pomegranate seeds, broccoli, green tea and turmeric capsules (whole food supplements in physiologic doses so they could compare the outcome). Those that received the nutrients had their prostate-specific antigen (PSA) levels rise only 14.7% vs. 78.5% for the placebo group. Also, the PSA levels remained stable in 46% of the supplement group vs. only 14% in the placebo group. In another study involving a review of breast cancer patients who were BRCA mutation positive, those who consumed a wide variety of fruits and veggies per week had a 73% reduction in developing breast cancer.

SECTION II
CANCER TREATMENT & SUPPORT CUREOLOGY

Chapter 8
Beyond Basic Diagnostic Testing

Once cancer is diagnosed, or even as part of a suspected cancer evaluation, various blood tests and scans are used. These may be used to determine if a cancer is present or if it has spread.

In addition to the standard testing that is used, such as tumor-specific blood biomarkers, CT scans, PET scans, MRI, ultrasound and the like, the following are additional markers that might be of help when assessing your body's anti-cancer status in the integrative cancer care model. Standard medical insurance will not cover many of these because they have not been proven to help in prevention or in following treatment results during cancer therapy. Most of these focus on the state of *you* as opposed to the state of cancer in your body, so it is not part of the mainstream model. Most integrative tests address the risk factors for cancer and cancer growth. This includes blood sugar levels, inflammation, overall immune system health, and nutritional status.

Some of these are proven to be useful, some are based on plausible theory, but all are worth considering. Starting with mainstream tests that are not always obtained, like serum albumin, you can get a better basic idea of what your overall nutritional status is. Some give you another dimension by assessing what your body's cancer-proof status is, or lack thereof. Other tests help by determining what chemotherapy may work for you specifically, as an individual. Still, others assess known molecular pathways that are related to cancer and suggest epigenetic switches you may be able to favorably influence. This is a developing area, and we are not far from testing that will be highly specific to individuals overall, rather than generic tests like white blood cells and hemoglobin levels.

Keep in mind that everyone is different. Ask your oncologist or integrative practitioner about these and if they fit in your case. The rest of this chapter addresses how you can use these tests to monitor your body's status and efforts to reduce insulin resistance, improve nutritional status, enhance immunity, reduce inflammation, increase intrinsic antioxidant activity and the like.

Oxidative Stress Biomarkers

The following tests may help determine the state of oxidative stress and capacity for methylation in your body. There are other blood tests for this, but the following can give you a start: methionine, S-adenosylmethionine (SAM), S-adenosylhomocysteine (SAH), adenosine, homocysteine, cystathionine, cysteine, and oxidized and reduced glutathione. Not all are necessary, but some may be better markers than others, and this is highly individual. The one most likely to be available in standard labs is homocysteine.

The methylenetetrahydrofolate reductase (MTHFR) gene codes for an enzyme which is crucial in the metabolism of proteins and the conversion of homocysteine to methionine. This is directly related to DNA methylation, synthesis, and repair. Alterations in the gene, called single nucleotide polymorphisms (SNP), can contribute to many medical conditions, including heart disease and certain types of cancer, most notably colorectal cancer. Unfortunately, variants are very common but keep in mind these are not mutations. They are just variations, some of which lead to abnormal function.

The good news is that if homocysteine levels are low and red blood cell folate is normal, you do not likely have a significant variant. If there are abnormalities in folate metabolism, these gene SNP variants can be tested for. Routine testing is not accepted by the medical community because the clinical implications are unclear. Keep in mind that most oncologists are not following the integrative model of determining and improving your body's oxidative stress management. Direct to public testing is available these days at 23andMe.com for around a $100.

The Oxidata® Test via Oxidata.com is a urine test which measures the amount of circulating free radicals in your body by assessing malondialdehyde (MDA). The urine test is better than similar blood tests and is simple to use. It is essentially an inexpensive at home colorimetric test, which means you look at the color of the urine in a reagent filled test tube after adding a small amount of urine to it using a dropper. It is not meant to give you and exact number (quantitative), but rather to give you an idea of where you are in the spectrum of free radicals in your body (qualitative). The idea is to test initially, then improve your anti-cancer nutritional and lifestyle modifications and test monthly for progress.

More sophisticated testing of DNA oxidation, such as the 8-oxoG test, are coming but not readily available. Nutrient modification of ongoing DNA damage, with verifiable and measurable testing, is going to be a reality in the very near future.

Inflammatory Biomarkers

Chronic inflammation is now accepted to lead, or at least be associated with, biochemical processes which contribute to the onset and progression of cancer. So, measuring biomarkers of inflammation can give you an idea where you stand in cancer-proofing yourself as much as possible. There is a slew of markers that can be theoretically measured, but few are available in most clinical labs for routine use. Most are for research use only.

The most available test is called C-reactive protein (CRP) or a new modification that is a little more sensitive called highly sensitive C-reactive protein (hs-CRP). Either can give you a solid idea of where you stand, but if available the hs-CRP is a little more telling. The problem is that it may be too sensitive because most of us have some background inflammatory conditions. For example, arthritis or irritable bowel may cause this test to be elevated. The idea behind this testing is to see where you are at baseline, modify your lifestyle and nutrition and re-test. If you are testing at too sensitive a level, you may see discouraging results. It is almost impossible, and not advisable, to remove all inflammation from your body. Remember, you can't micro-manage Mother Nature, and some inflammatory processes are required for healing. You are looking for the big picture by lowering obviously higher levels of chronic inflammation in your body.

Other inflammatory markers that are relatively available in clinical labs are TNF-alpha and IL-6. However, these are going to be a lot more expensive and may not be approved for use in this manner. That's OK as the CRP or hs-CRP will likely give you what you need to know.

In a related manner, since we are aware diabetes and pre-diabetes is an inflammatory state which predisposes to cancer, measuring the long-term status of your blood glucose is a proxy inflammatory marker. This is called hemoglobin

A1c (HbA1c) and is now accepted as a diabetes screen. It can usually be readily ordered, as a blood test, in any clinical laboratory. If you don't have good insurance or for some reason this test is not available, even daily testing of urine sugar (colored sticks), which can be obtained from many pharmacies, can give you an indication of your potential for diabetes. This is not the recommended test, compared to HbA1c. But if your urine sugar is high, you should seek medical attention.

Immune Status

A myriad of immune modulating status tests is available for research purposes. However, as a routine in cancer care, it is not common for an oncologist to order any. Nor are they readily available in most clinical labs. Very specific tests are available if immune deficiency or autoimmune disease is suspected, and this varies from children to adults.

In the extreme, if severe immune deficiency is suspected, a human immune deficiency virus (HIV) test panel can be ordered. There are also groups of tests that are related to this, such as CD4+ (helper) CD8+ (suppressor) lymphocyte status and more. A decrease in CD4+ lymphocytes and a CD4+/CD8+ ratio of less than 1.5 means that there is substantial immune impairment and susceptibility to infection is high. But other than striving for the normal range of twice as many helper than suppressor lymphocytes, there is no strict cutoff as to the risk of cancer.

However, in the integrative model we are interested in potentially subtle but definite immune suppressive factors in your life. How can this be measured? The answer is complicated and there is no universally accepted set of cancer-specific markers to follow in general. This is especially true if your immune system is clinically in reasonably good shape. For example, if you don't get sick very often- that is already a good sign and marker of immune health.

The immune system is exceedingly complex and "bad" molecules, cytokines or cells can act in a "good" way in certain situations and vice versa. So, there are few absolutes. Your immune system is in a delicate balance, but obviously can be thrown off and disease like cancer sets in. This does not mean that there are big switches that should always be turned off and others turned on. It's about the timing, specificity and degree of specific effects.

Having said that, there is a way to test the overall general status of your immune system comprehensively. A blood panel can test for the amount and ratio of T cells, B cells, and NK cells you have. The T cells can be separated into T helper 1 and T helper 2 cells, and more. The argument for getting this type of testing is to determine if you're in reasonably good shape or to send an alert that you may have a lot of work to do to improve your immune status. However, it is not detailed enough to give you an idea of exactly *what* you can do. Several chapters in this book focus on doing everything you can to ensure your immune system is optimized. You should do this regardless of what these tests show. This is why they are not really required. This type of testing is also a little different compared to your HbA1c status or even your inflammatory hsCRP status, where you can significantly impact the result. You can't usually see a major effect on the types of immune status tests available to us today, short of the many research-intensive tests alluded to. The state of the art is just not clinically there yet, but coming soon.

Chemotherapy Effectiveness Assays

A tremendous problem with selecting chemotherapy agents is that cancer cells can either be immediately resistant or become so over a period of time. At some point, all chemotherapy agents stop working.

Many strategies have been used to try to predict what will work. These have included drug sensitivity and resistance testing in test tubes, immunohistochemical (IHC) and identification of proteins that are associated with resistance. In addition to these issues we know that resistance is related to: 1) the ability of cells to detoxify, 2) to repair themselves, 3) gene activation which produce protective pathways, 4) whether or not blood supply is good to the tumor so that the agents can get there, and more factors that are really not testable. Cancer cells use too many pathways to protect themselves from chemotherapy to overcome them all. Ideal tests would look at all of these pathways, but this is still not possible because the human body is far more complex than what can be simulated in a laboratory test tube.

Having said that, a recent extensive review or meta-analysis of scientific publications over the past 40 years showed that resistance to chemotherapy can be predicted correctly in 80 to 100% of cases. Sensitivity, on the other hand, could only be predicted with an accuracy of 50–80%. This means that the prediction of resistance could help in individualizing treatment. In the past, uncovering that tumors were resistant to multiple chemotherapy drugs presented an uncomfortable situation where oncologists would awkwardly offer therapies that were not obviously going to work. But today, with ever increasing options, it can help to know what might not work while formulating a personalized cancer treatment plan.

There are additional tests that help personalize oncologic care today very effectively. If you have breast cancer, then treatment recommendations beyond surgery should be based on the OncoType DX®, which analyzes 21 different genes and stratifies recurrence risk based on the results. It is the new standard of practice and prevents over and under treatment very well. Newer similar test offerings for colon and prostate cancer from the same company are also available.

Testing for specific abnormal variants of genes, such as the BRCA gene, is available and should be used for breast, ovarian, prostate, colon, uterine, and a growing list of other cancers. In some cases, it helps with prognosis, and in some cases, it opens treatment options that only work when these abnormal variations are present (e.g. PARP inhibitor biologicals in breast and ovarian cancer).

On the other hand, so-called "next generation sequencing" (NGS) testing panels for multiple abnormalities faces some difficulties. We know we can find all sorts of genetic abnormalities and aberrant metabolic cellular pathways. The question is what to do with them. The testing has so far outpaced the treatment options that are specific to the findings, so many of these are "non-actionable." This has led to overtreatment in some cases and a sensation of hopeless despair in others when multiple abnormalities are found. They can be ordered and in some centers it is routine. Just be wary of the limitations.

Another set of panels are available through Caris Life Sciences®, Foundation Medicine® and others, which perform tumor profiling as well as offering NGS. These also strive to personalize care through matching of tumor molecular pathways with a database of clinically available and current research treatments. These offerings are very high tech but also suffer from not being ready for prime time because the data is robust but not conclusive in many areas. However, while it may not dictate what treatment is best for straightforward cancer treatment, it can open avenues of "out of the box" thinking for treatments not normally used in any given cancer type.

The other problem is that all of these tests are extraordinarily expensive, from $5000 to $15,000 and up, and not always covered by insurance. Having said that it is something to discuss with your oncologist.

Nutritional Assays

A relatively standard test that is used to check for protein deficiency is serum albumin and pre-albumin. There are others, but this is readily available in clinical labs. It is often used around the time of surgery to predict healing and infection risk and can be ordered any time to monitor this aspect of the status of your nutrition. Keep in mind that protein makes up a lot of your immune system, so this is an important number to stay on top of.

The other cancer-related nutritional assay that is becoming more common is a vitamin D blood level. This is now readily available and, as described in other areas of this book, is important to know because it seems to be a good prognosticator. It is also something that you can easily influence by changing your intake. Keeping in the safe range of 40-50ng/ml is probably ideal. Others recommend higher levels, but there is no evidence that this is better and there may be a risk of toxicity and side effects.

Many other micronutrient values can be specifically tested. These include trace elements and vitamins. For example, if you are fatigued, vitamin B12 is a reasonable test to consider although simply taking B12 may answer the question. Most often micronutrient tests are ordered when there is a clinical problem or deficiency suspected, such as iron or folate deficiency anemia. Also, tests can be run if toxicity is suspected (e.g. copper, lead, mercury). Some practitioners advise blanket testing in these areas but there is no scientific evidence that this can help you defeat cancer.

As already mentioned, there are assays out there that hype personalized nutrition and the ability to match you to specific nutrients based on your blood type and things like that. Outside of a nutrigenetic research program, they may as well be matching you with your astrological star sign. The science is simply not there yet for recommending a completely personalized anti-cancer diet. I am not referring

to diets for certain disorders such as diabetes, hypertension, hyperlipidemia, irritable bowel, gluten allergies and the like. I am talking about any assays which
purport to match you with an ideal personalized overall diet, especially an ideal
anti-cancer diet. Don't waste your money and follow the recommendations in
this book, which will get to at least 80% of the way to your survivorship goals.
The other 20% will come in time as the science of nutrigenetics advances. Today,
we can find a lot of genomic alterations but most are not actionable. This will
likely change rapidly. As it does, nutrigenomic or nutrigenetic analysis and directly related recommendations will become very prevalent.

CHAPTER 9
MAINSTREAM TREATMENT KEYS

Cancer Cureology focuses mostly on the natural support aspects of integrative oncology, but please understand that mainstream diagnostic techniques and therapy are vital to your success. This introduction is meant to explain why.

Legitimate international research and treatment efforts by tens of thousands of scientists and doctors show that all countries include some variation of mainstream therapy in treating cancer. The degree to which natural complementary treatments are also used varies, but no legitimate oncologists anywhere in the world completely ignore mainstream treatment.

Herbals and botanicals are used more in other countries, most often in addition to mainstream therapy. But keep in mind that most herbals are simply unrefined pharmaceuticals. They may help, and they can definitely harm, but in contradistinction to pharmaceuticals, there is less known about the effectiveness and safety. So, you take a much bigger gamble with your life. Only you can answer if it is worth going against common wisdom and reams of scientific literature. Finally, this depends on when in your cancer journey you are considering alternatives. Is it up front when you have legitimate documented curative or meaningful life-prolonging options available? Or is it down the line when nothing mainstream seems to be of benefit anymore, including experimental research drugs? Timing and wise, informed choice is everything!

The other big question that always comes up is: "Does surgery, radiation, and chemotherapy work or does it really just cut, burn and poison without results?" There are misquoted research articles out there which imply that mainstream therapy is useless, only causes cancer and pours fuel on the fire. A famous article from Australia incorrectly asserts that chemotherapy only works in 2% of people. This study lumped multiple cancers together, which obscures results, and it omitted cancers that are highly treatable. It even included cancers for which chemotherapy is not indicated. In short, it was a very poorly designed study. There is another timeworn article that claimed 80% of oncologists would not take chemotherapy if they came down with cancer. There are tens of thousands of other articles in the scientific literature which prove that chemotherapy "works" to either cure or meaningfully extend quality of life in many if not most cancers.

Regarding oncologists "refusing chemotherapy if they had cancer," this article was related to a question asked of them about an unproven and quite toxic chemo-therapy for lung cancer over 25 years ago. That was then, and this is now. So, the assertion that today's oncologists would not take what they dish out in general is completely false. Newer published studies prove this. Knowing what they know, oncologists may be picky about what situation they would expose themselves to chemotherapy, and justifiably so. But in quite a few cancers up to 98% say they would accept chemo. Every situation is different and personal choice is the key, after understanding the prognosis, risk, and benefit. As far as surgery, it is insane to imply that it does not work, especially in early stage cancer. There are hundreds of thousands, if not millions, of cured individuals that say different. Again, even a limited quick review of the medical literature proves that point. The moral of the story is not to listen to quack "shock-jocks" who misquote results and cite statistics that are misleading or incorrect. There is a huge role for mainstream therapy in your fight against cancer, and it leads to cures in many and prolonga-tion of quality-filled life for many more.

We can't possibly cover all of the mainstream treatment options for different cancers because they differ. Why do they differ? Because, contrary to what radical conspiracy aficionados say, we know a LOT about cancer. We understand the different types and what works best to eliminate or control specific cancers for as long as possible. There are millions of medical research papers that are published on the topic, and the advances are increasing every single day. No, we have not won the "war on cancer." This is largely because since President Nixon declared that war, we have learned tons more about the fact that cancers are all different. In other words, it is not one disease like we used to think. So, it is extremely unlikely that we will *ever* have a magic bullet cure for all cancers. Rather, each type of cancer has interested researchers looking into the best treatment options. In that respect, we are winning, and people are living longer or being cured in many more cases. But much more work needs to be done and is being done every single day.

Just to briefly touch on the mainstream treatment options, why they are used and where we are going with them I hope the following gives you a grasp of the basics. For details about the best mainstream options for your cancer ask your oncologist if any "NCCN Guidelines" for your case exist. These are a compendium of the best evidence-based guidelines for cancer care from the National Comprehensive Cancer Network. The major cancers are all represented in this resource which is updated often based on the newest research.

Your oncologists are interested in seeing you either be cured, if at all possible, or at least in helping you control your cancer if it is a particularly aggressive type. That is what they are trained to do, and they devoted their lives to it because of that shared goal. They use the best tools possible and any "alternative" derogatory reference to "cutting, poisoning and burning" is simply a slap in the face of those doctors trying to help cancer patients worldwide. Having said that, face it, there are crooks in every walk of life. It is highly unfortunate that doctors are not excluded. However, at least 99% are very dedicated to your success in beating cancer. Let's look at the reality of these mainstream tools.

Surgery

Surgery is mainly used to remove a cancerous organ when all pre-operative scans and indications seem to say that your cancer appears to be early and localized to the organ it originated from. There are some exceptions to this, like ovarian cancer, where we know that surgery and chemo work so well together that it is worth the surgical risk to remove multiple areas involved by cancer.

As recently as ten years ago, many surgeries required a big incision or disfiguring removal of tissues and organs. While this may still be required in individual situations, we have moved very far towards "minimally invasive" surgeries which offer smaller surgeries, smaller incisions which are sometimes less than half an inch, organ sparing surgeries and the like. The results, for example, are breast cancer patients who have minimal if any visible body image changes, women with cervical cancer whose uterus is spared so they can bear children and many other success stories. The technology of surgical intervention is simply amazing and allows same-day surgery and very rapid recovery in many cases.

The reason surgery is often curative in early stages of cancer is not only that the rapidly dividing wild cancer cells that make up a "tumor" are removed, but the cancer stem cells are also removed with the tumor. Sometimes these stem cells and actively dividing cancer cells escape microscopically undetected and are called micrometastases. When this happens, an apparently early cancer recurs, either nearby or in other organs, despite the surgeon saying "we got it all." There is no way to know if these micrometastases have occurred before surgery and some cancers spread earlier than others. But if all scans look good, surgery can be very curative in many types of cancer. If your oncologic surgeons think they can remove an apparently early cancer, it is well worth the risk in most situations. In some cases, surgery is used in advanced cases as well, but then it is usually used as a helper to radiation or chemotherapy in a combined treatment plan. This is not as likely to be curative in most cases, but each situation is different.

Radiation

Radiation therapy is usually used to treat cancers that may have grown beyond the organ of origin but seem to be confined to the general area of the organ. An example might be uterine or prostate cancer that has spread to the nearby lymph nodes. When I initially trained 30 years ago, we used to use Cobalt radiation which was very difficult to focus. For this reason, many patients suffered either internal organ damage or horrendous skin complications. Today is an entirely different story. Compared to what I just mentioned the state of the art in radiation therapy is Star Trek level, or very futuristic.

Cobalt has been replaced by very focused linear accelerator radiation technologies that can spare normal tissues with precision. For example, for certain brain cancers, an invisible and tightly focused radiation beam can be used with scalpel-like precision. In other areas, similar technologies are available. In many cases, large areas require radiation for "local and regional control." But even in those situations, the side effects are usually limited due to vastly superior and ever-improving technologies. Radiation therapy is not perfect, and complications do occur, but advances keep steadily coming. It is pejorative and even insane to use the term "burn" in the same sentence as modern radiation in the vast majority of cases.

The reason radiation may be curative, or at least reduce the chances that cancer will come back locally, is similar to surgery. If all the actively dividing cancer cells and the cancer stem cells are eradicated in the radiation field (i.e. the area that is radiated, which often includes the organ as well as the lymph nodes in the area to which cancers spread), then there may be a cure. Unfortunately, some cancer cell types, and possibly the stem cells within, are much more resistant to radiation damage than others. The chances that radiation will work differs between cancers, so a risk vs. benefit discussion with the radiation oncologist is critical. Also, just like with surgery, cancer may have micro-metastasized undetected and spread beyond the treatment field. Radiation is useless outside the area that is being radiated.

Unfortunately, even though modern radiation is far better, it is still toxic to normal tissues. In addition to the risk of complications, there is an increased risk of developing a secondary (often different type) cancer in the area that was radiated. In most cases, the relative risk at 40 Gray (an average conventional radiation dose) of developing a second solid cancer in the radiated area is 5–10 times higher than the risk in people who have never undergone radiation therapy or those who received very small doses. Often radiation is given not for a cure but to slow cancer down when the chances of cure are not high. In these situations, the risk of another cancer many years down the line are outweighed by the benefit of treatment. But, if radiation is being given with a high probability of cure, it is important to consider the risks in later life. In some situations there are other options, but in some, there are not. This requires a risk vs. benefit discussion with your radiation oncologist.

Chemotherapy

Chemotherapy is usually used when we know cancer has spread or metastasized widely to many areas of the body. It is recommended when there is a high risk that cancer has spread microscopically but too small to be detected by any scans yet. This is because chemotherapy is usually injected by vein and travels to most if not all parts of the body to fight cancer. Unfortunately, most chemotherapy agents are pro-oxidant toxins that are designed scientifically to kill more cancer cells than normal cells. Usually, they kill rapidly growing cells by generally interfering with cell replication at the cell DNA level. It is not as good at eliminating slow growing cancer stem cells which may remain when all the tumors visible on scans are gone.

We are also not yet at the stage where only cancer cells are killed, and for that reason, people suffer side effects like hair loss, intestinal upset and nerve damage among others. As I repeatedly mention in this book, it's kind of a "brute force" attack against cancer that has collateral damage to normal cells. Each chemo drug has a different profile of side effects and varying degrees of collateral damage. Having said that, the drugs that are used today are much better designed and dosed to minimize side effects. The additional medications used to help with symptoms like nausea are very very effective.

The scientific community and doctors have a lot of work left to come up with more curative drugs that have even fewer side effects. However, the contention that more people are killed by chemotherapy than helped is a brutal and insane accusation. No, it is not ideal by any means, but yes it is an effective treatment that has saved or meaningfully prolonged quality filled years of life in many patients. For some cancers, we have chemo agents that are very effective and/or curative, but for others the results are not very good. This requires a heart to heart deep discussion with your oncologist to assess whether or not chemotherapy is right for any given situation. If you can't get that, then get a second opinion or as many opinions as you need to get an answer you feel comfortable with.

Keep in mind that oncologists are highly trained in cancer treatment, but they are just people. In today's helter-skelter medical practice world, most doctors are pulled very thin to take care of as many people as possible. It's an unfortunate situation which has ruined doctor-patient relationships where they are critical for success. Also keep in mind that people are people. Some communicate better than others and are more compassionate that others. This includes doctors, even if one would think that doctors should be more compassionate to be in the profession in the first place. Find and connect with the best doctor for your needs.

Why does chemotherapy work, or not work? Compared to surgery and radiation, chemotherapy is designed to go to all areas of your body, usually through your circulatory system or through direct contact in some cases (e.g. intraperitoneal chemotherapy for some abdominal cancers, like ovarian, or intrathecal chemotherapy for brain cancer). The reason it needs to be given multiple times is related to something called the "log cell kill" or "fractional kill" hypothesis. Each time the chemo is given, it kills a certain fraction of cancer cells. Unfortunately, between chemo cycles, some of the cancer can regrow. This makes it more complicated because the cancer cells can adapt and become resistant to the drugs being given. However, we can't give chemo continuously in most situations because it would kill people. Your body's normal cells need time to recover between chemo cycles. If you were a Petri dish in a lab where cancer cells are grown, a high enough dose of chemo will kill the cancer 100% of the time. But you are not a Petri dish. So, the idea is to kill as many cells as possible while minimizing the side effects. It has to be aggressive and remain on schedule to keep killing the percentage of cells until ideally all the cancer cells are gone.

We are only beginning to understand why some cancers are more resistant to chemo than others and what we can do about it. Meanwhile, there are measures to take by combining drugs to hit cancer from different angles, using different doses and more. Unfortunately, this is way beyond this basic introduction.

You can rest assured that the doses and combinations of chemotherapy drugs have been tested very extensively through multiple clinical trials in the vast majority of cases. Your oncologist does not guess at the proper, most effective, least toxic dose and combination. Doses are adjusted for body size, kidney and liver function and more. Anything beyond this, like alternative "insulin potentiation low dose chemotherapy" (IPTLD), is unproven and can be very dangerous and/or ineffective. But we'll cover more on this later in Chapter 17.

The final big problem is that cancer stem cells, from which cancer cells are thought to arise, are not as rapidly dividing and are more resistant to chemo. Research is underway to find ways to attack cancer stem cells specifically, but until then lifestyle modification is the best weapon we have. That is largely what this book is about. According to this expanding theory, if you can't eradicate cancer stem cells, cancer will occur and recur.

Regarding chemotherapy being a cause of the cancer it is designed to treat, there is, unfortunately, something to this. Just like the case with radiation, the reason to use chemo in your particular case is important to consider. If you are highly likely to increase your cure, then it may be worth the risk if there are no other proven options. If cure is not an option due to advanced cancer but the chemo is likely to give you months or years of good quality life then it may be worth the risk of possibly getting another cancer many years down the road. Why? Because in this situation the intent is to control the cancer you are fighting now, not a theoretical one in the future, and the likelihood of surviving many years is low.

What exactly is the risk of getting another cancer? That is hard to say with accuracy because new drugs are developed all the time and different doses are given over a variable length of time. So, it is different for each cancer and chemo type. It is true that forty plus years ago some early drugs that were used for chemo commonly caused leukemias in patients many years later. These drugs were given for several years rather than the more limited time frames today. Most of these are not used very much, if at all, anymore. Today's chemo drugs are still basically poisons, but they are not given as long. It bears repeating that this is the reason for a risk vs. benefit discussion with your oncologist because each situation is different.

As far as chemo possibly causing cancer to grow, there is a greater consideration than worrying about what might happen years later. Recent research shows that in some cancers chemotherapy can cause normal cells, called fibroblasts, which live near the cancerous tumor to produce proteins like WNT16B which promotes cancer cells to grow. This happens over time. As these protein concentrations climb, they may contribute to chemotherapy resistance and tumor growth. So, this may be a reason not to use more chemotherapy than absolutely necessary to produce a remission. This concept flies in the face of a trend today called "maintenance chemotherapy" where lower dose chemo is continued for many months or years after the cancer appears to be gone. There is scientific evidence to support considering maintenance chemo or biological agent therapy in specific cancers. However, the benefit is usually measurable in a few months of extra life, and the risk of cancer promotion is now apparently a downside to this type of strategy. Research is underway, and the most prudent plan is to discuss such concepts with your oncologist.

Here is where an integrative mindset opens avenues that are not well developed in mainstream medicine yet. The concept of maintenance therapy to extended remission is not universally available or recommended. But a proactive natural approach to reducing your risk of recurrence is also a "maintenance" strategy and may be much more long lasting. While this is unproven, the downsides are very low and will at least benefit your quality of life. That is partly what this book is about. Given the lack of overwhelming benefit for maintenance chemo in most cancers, this is a plausible low-risk alternative.

Personalized Medicine

We stand at a crossroads with a very exciting future that will rapidly unfold over the next five to ten years and accelerate even faster after that. The non-specific chemotherapy drugs used today kill normal cells as well as cancer cells, which is responsible for side effects. This brute force attack against cancer cells will soon be replaced by agents that specifically target only cancer cells, including cancer stem cells, or help the body beat cancer by harnessing your immune system. We are only scratching the surface here, and the current targeted therapies are not much kinder or gentler than chemotherapy. They interrupt molecular processes in both cancer cells and normal cells, which can lead to side effects. However, in the future, these targeted therapies will become less toxic as we hone in on cancer cell molecular processes and avoid harming normal cells. This is not as easy as it might sound, but we are well on the way to replacing brute force therapies like chemo with these targeted approaches that reflect the molecular biology of the individual patient.

Breast cancer is probably the best model for personalization at the moment. Personalization does not mean that each patient will get an entirely different tailored treatment. Perhaps in the future, it will mean that. But for now, personalization means using the best combination of therapies for groups of patients who test for similar factors. This is already way better than simply giving the same chemo to all patients with a given cancer. Here are just a few examples in today's breast cancer treatment world. Using a 16 gene signature test, Oncotype DX® can help determine if chemotherapy would be helpful for certain types of breast cancer or not. Another test, MammaPrint®, can assist in determining if an apparent early stage breast cancer patient might have metastatic disease, using a 70-gene expression profile. These, and other assays, now help guide recommendations for treatment using chemotherapy, hormones or targeted monoclonal antibody therapy using Herceptin® (trastuzumab) when HER2/neu gene amplification is discovered. These high-tech analyses avoid unnecessary treatment and increase the chances that the best treatment combination is used for each individual situation.

Hormone receptor analysis from tumor biopsies can help determine if hormone therapy would be useful for breast, uterine, ovarian and prostate cancer. Hormones for cancer treatment only work if there are "receptors" on the cell surface that recognize and allow the hormones to attach. If there are no receptors, the hormone therapy won't work. For each of these cancers, the exact type of hormone or hormone blocker varies.

We have an ever increasing group of cancer-fighting agents that are called "biologicals." These are substances that attack cancer cell metabolic pathways specifically or interfere with cancer cell requirements, such as blood vessel formation required for access to the nutrients cancer needs to grow and spread. One example is the trastuzumab monoclonal antibody we just mentioned. Another example is Avastin® (bevacizumab) which has been used in fighting a number of malignancies and mainly works by interfering with blood vessel formation (angiogenesis), starving cancer cells. This was originally the idea behind shark cartilage, but that did not pan out as an effective therapy. Many others are entering the market and are cancer type specific. So I will not delve deeper into this other than to once again suggest that this is a topic of conversation with your oncologist.

Back in the 1960's and 1970's there was some excitement regarding immunotherapy for various cancers but did not work out very well at the time. Since then we have learned an enormous amount and treatments related to antibodies and other immunologic manipulation is back with a vengeance. Various targeted "monoclonal" antibodies are used in the biologicals mentioned above, but the story is much more complicated than that. In fact, it is advancing so rapidly that anything I could write here would be outdated by next week. It bears repeating that while generically "boosting" and optimizing your immune system has some merits, the complexity of the immune system is staggering. It is not that simple to naturally get your immune system to reliably eliminate cancer once millions and billions of cells are present in a cancerous tumor. Having said that, action on your part to optimize your immunity is a goal of integrative oncology, which is why an entire chapter in this book (Chapter 5) is dedicated to exploring your natural options on that front.

Future Research

The future in mainstream therapy, beyond what we just covered, is likely in direct gene manipulation, immune recognition, and stem cell research. Although some of these options may become available sooner than you might expect, this is largely still bench laboratory research. When these treatments enter clinical trials, and some are already out there (e.g. TILs), they are worthy of consideration. I will leave it at that since this book is not focused on this topic.

CHAPTER 10
NUTRITION CORE

Other than being a good idea to "eat right," why is nutrition at the center of fighting and defeating cancer? It's because science is evolving rapidly towards knowing exactly how nutrients affect biochemical pathways which prevent and potentially target cancer directly. As we come to understand the molecular and genetic aspects of cancer on a more granular level, we learn how to interrupt bad signals and boost the right ones. This can be done with new biological agents in the research pipeline and with nutrients. Again, except at the miracle level, doing everything right with diet and lifestyle choices will still not prevent all cancers. Unfortunately, as oncologists, we all see fitness fanatics who have developed cancer. Likewise, except perhaps in a miraculous instance here and there, nutrition by itself will not cure any individual of cancer. However, you can go a very long way towards primary prevention. You can also support your body in your fight against cancer. Although not proven, you may also help with a direct anti-cancer effect, and in doing everything you can to prevent recurrence by affecting cancer stem cells. All of this is possible using 21st century nutrition knowledge.

The following is repeated in this book multiple times, so you really latch on to the concept. According to the National Cancer Institute, roughly 1/3 of all cancer deaths may be ascribed to our diets and bad lifestyle choices. If one includes chronic exposure to toxins, this number is very likely MUCH higher. Only about 10% of all cancers are purely genetic in origin over which you have much less control. In 90% of cases, YOU are very much in control of your destiny through the sciences of epigenetics, nutrigenomics and nutrigenetics. We've already covered what these are, so in this chapter we're getting at more practical recommendations, starting with the nutritional anti-cancer core.

You do not need to understand the intricacies of these very complex sciences involving gene-nutrient and gene-environment interaction. You simply need to know that it is a subject of intense research and what you eat and expose yourself to directly "talks" to your genes and other processes at the molecular level. This area of epigenetics, nutrigenetics, and nutrigenomics was covered in Chapter 7.

Anti-cancer diets aren't very elaborate and should not be expensive or confusing. There are also a lot of superfoods and spices that may help in the fight against cancer, and you can concoct what works for you by following the basics and then modify to your personal taste. There is a lot to choose from, and there is no proof that one is far better than another. So, that should take some stress away. We'll cover some more details and benefits of specific foods and diets, but first, we need to get a few popular burning questions out of the way.

Does The Sugar I Eat Feed Cancer?

Yes and no. It is true that cancer's preferred food is sugar. In fact cancer's *most* preferred sugar is fructose, which is what is naturally found in fruits and vegetables. It is also almost impossible to remove ALL sugar and carbohydrates (which are broken down to simple sugar) from your diet. Even if you did, your body needs glucose to survive. So the liver becomes more efficient in converting the protein you eat into glucose.

So yes, the final main food for cancer is *all* forms of sugar, but no you shouldn't and really could not cut all sugar out. Having said that, some diets like the ketogenic diet at least tries to minimize the amount of circulating glucose in your body by severely restricting both carbohydrates and proteins, and focusing on fat intake (preferably plant fats). It is in clinical trials for several forms of cancer but is very difficult to sustain in the long run due to side effects and complications. We will cover it in more detail later.

The most prudent thing to do is to avoid an excess of sugar intake, particularly refined sugar (because of additives), and focus on berry type fruits for their benefits in antioxidant value. By itself, sugar is sugar, and there is no completely "healthy" sugar. The junk that is quoted about cancer only using dextrorotatory refined sugars and the safety of natural levorotatory sugars is just that, junk. The proof is that the most sensitive PET scanners use tracer labeled fructose, otherwise known as levulose or levorotatory sugar, because cancer cells avidly take up fructose. Standard PET scans use fluorodeoxyglucose (FDG), which can be dextrorotatory or levorotatory.

A few quick tips. The most common sugar we are all exposed to is high fructose corn syrup. Stay away. If you have a sweet tooth, use stevia root. This is a natural non-sugar substance that gives you all the sweetness you desire without any of the downsides.

Should I Alkalinize My Diet?

It is true that the Standard American Diet, aptly shortened to SAD, results in a small net acid load produced in your body every day. We are talking about milli-molar minuscule changes which do not result in any significant pH change in your blood or tissues. It is also true that in experimental situations (i.e. Petri dishes in the lab) cancer does better in an acidic environment than an alkaline environment. On the other hand, one of the most effective short term anti-cancer diets is the ketogenic diet, and it is quite acidic. So, the answer is not that simple.

What is not true is that you can significantly impact the environment your cancer lives in within your body by drinking expensive "alkaline water." Your body is not stupid. By the time anything you ingest gets to a cancerous tumor, it has been metabolized and buffered a hundred times over because your body is an incredible machine designed to maintain homeostasis and limit dangerous change. Also, the toxic chemicals produced by cancerous tumors and as part of the inflammatory immune response are overwhelming and acidic. Anything you take in by mouth that is alkaline can be easily overpowered by the time it is metabolized and reaches cancer cells. So, it's not a simple proposition of simply dousing acidic cancer with supposedly life-saving alkaline water. That's just too simpleton and does not work that way.

Having said the above, it is prudent to eat food that is not inflammatory and acidic in nature because chronic exposure to even small amounts of acid may influence genetic expression and cellular metabolism efficiencies. It is the difference between tending toward an alkaline balance in your diet for prevention purposes vs. expensive and aggressive alkalinization attempts as part of ineffective treatment. This is unproven but falls under the Precautionary Principle discussed elsewhere in this book. Veggies can range in their degree of alkaline content. By choosing wisely, you can have quite an alkaline diet without spending a lot of money on hyped alkalinizing water.

Should I Avoid All Meat?

There is a lot of compelling scientific evidence that strictly plant-based whole food diets are as anti-cancer as you can get. But if you are not already in vegetarian mode, it is hard to go completely vegan. So, the likelihood of far worse outcomes from eating some meat in moderation is low. Remember, even though the world's Blue Zones (where people tend to live longer quality lives) are mostly in vegetarian or vegan mode, not all of them are. The final answer will come from nutrigenetics when we determine the individualized nutrient impact on disease. Meanwhile, it may be prudent if you are going to consume meats, to avoid red meats. At least make sure they are from grass fed free range sources. This is not based on absolute data but rather on the precautionary principle which is invoked a number of times in this book.

Also avoid high temperature grilled, charred and blackened preparations. The more char you see, the more it means there are cancer-causing Heterocyclic amines (HCAs) and polycyclic aromatic hydrocarbons (PAHs) being produced. There are no precautionary regulations that address this, so you are on your own to watch out for yourself. I know this goes against the urge to eat those beautiful barbecued steaks and burgers, but this is the scientific reality. To be fair, the evidence is pretty strong in animals but whether or not these chemicals cause cancer in humans is not conclusive. However, given these are potent carcinogens, it is prudent to err on the side of caution. These cooking precautions go for fish and poultry as well, but not for veggies. When you grill veggies or even char them, they do not form these same dangerous chemicals.

The other problem with meats, farmed fish, and poultry, is that they are full of growth hormones and antibiotics which are passed on to you. These can act as xenohormones, can be endocrine disruptors, serve as carcinogens, and can affect your gut flora microbiome negatively. This is not the case with fresh caught wild fish but is certainly true of some farm raised fish. It is hard to ascertain which farms use antibiotics and hormones and which ones don't. The levels of Polychlorinated Biphenyl (PCB) can also be low, but they are measurable and sometimes up to eight times higher than that found in wild caught fish. On the other hand, mercury levels will be lower in farm raised than in wild-caught fish. So, there is no perfect answer.

If you absolutely can't break away from red meat in your diet, at least try to minimize it by consuming grass-fed rather than grain-fed beef. You will find about 100 milligrams of omega 3 fatty acids in a 100-gram steak (about 3.5 ounces) from grass fed steer. This is better than almost zero in grain feed beef, which also contains a lot of pro-inflammatory omega 6 fatty acids. However, keep in mind that wild salmon contains about 2.5 grams or twenty-five times more omega 3 fatty acids per 100 gram cut of fish. Even the lowest sources of omega 3, sardines and oysters, contain ten to fifteen times the amount found in the very best grass-fed steak. So, of all animal protein "meats" wild caught fish is arguably the best.

Ideally, all of your animal protein should come from fish. Not long ago, farm raised fish were completely raised on corn and did not contain much in the way of beneficial omega 3 fatty acids at all. Today, most farm-raised fish have more omega 3 but also have very high levels of pro-inflammatory omega 6 fatty acids. Cold water wild caught fatty fish such as cod, salmon, herring, and sardines contain high levels of omega 3 fatty acids. Extracts of these have been used to prevent and treat multiple chronic inflammatory diseases including cardiovascular problems such as coronary heart disease, high blood pressure, and stroke. There are many other inflammatory and non-inflammatory diseases on the list, but the evidence is strongest in the area of cardiovascular health.

In general, eating fish three to four times per week leads to most of the benefits while limiting risk. But if you can't stand fish, then taking supplements may be your only solution. We'll cover more about the risks and benefits of fish oil and omega-3 fatty acid supplementation in a bit.

Should I Avoid Dairy?

Dairy products are a very complex group of foods and composition varies by region and origin because of livestock raising practices and more. For example, casein [the main protein in cow's milk], has been vilified as a carcinogen primarily from experiments related to the China Study by Professor Campbell. However, it is plausible that other components of milk are the culprit. So, while this has become a very heated debate, it may or may not be true.

Overall, making a determination of dairy product association with cancer risk is tough. For most cancers, the data are inconsistent or lacking. For some, like bladder and colorectal cancer, there seems to be a protective effect. On the other hand, high calcium, which may be the result of consuming a lot of dairy products increases prostate cancer risk. Dairy products also contain rumen-derived metabolites and fermented milk products which may have a favorable effect on the human gut microbiome, which in turn influences the immune system. However, if the source contains antibiotics or hormones, which is the result of livestock raising practices, this is a very plausible but incompletely proven cause for concern. Studies suggest that cultured milk, yogurt, and low-fat dairy products might be the preferred choices if you're going to consume dairy.

What About Whey Protein?

This topic comes up often because whey is often added to smoothies and promoted in muscle building. It is true that maintaining lean body mass (i.e. your muscle mass) is also important in fighting cancer. All proteins are made up of about 20 different amino acids. Nine of these are "essential," meaning your body cannot produce them, and you have to consume them.

Maintaining protein is no problem when you eat red meat. But that should be largely off the table in an anti-cancer diet. So, we are left with white meat, poultry and fish for animal protein and of course vegetable protein. All of these can give you sufficient protein, although you have to make sure you have the right combination of veggies to ensure intake of all nine essential amino acids for making protein if you are vegan. A vegan diet may contain "adequate" protein for routine life, but the catabolic muscle wasting cancer state is anything but routine. Having said that, it is popular to consume whey for extra protein as long as you can eat dairy, based on medical, philosophical and religious reasons (there are kosher formulations available). Why? For one thing, it is very easy to mix into smoothies, but let's look into the critically important details.

Whey protein contains higher levels of leucine (an essential amino acid that also signals genes for muscle building), is highly bioavailable and incorporates into muscle arguably better than many other sources. You need only consume a few ounces of whey to equal the amount of leucine in roughly a pound of chicken or 12 eggs, never mind lesser protein foods. So far, so good.

An important side note is that building or even maintaining muscle mass means the optimal use of the protein you take in. This primarily happens if you take in protein soon before and after exercise. In other words, sitting on a couch and eating protein will not lead to improving your lean body muscle mass, no matter what your source of protein is. Using your muscle is what maintains or builds it, assuming you give it the proper building blocks of amino acids and protein. This does not have to be a muscle beach or gym level program, and we cover exercise in more detail in Chapter 16. In general, it has to be something far more than sitting around with intermittent low-energy exercise.

Here's the rub about whey protein. Most commercially available whey products are cheap for a reason. They are poor quality and can harm you more than help you, especially if you are looking for an anti-cancer effect. Too often whey is processed from highly pasteurized milk using use acid and heat, which destroy protein and make it putrid and in an un-natural form (D form optical isomers). To make the whey more palatable and mixable in smoothies, manufacturers often add a ton of chemicals such as flavoring agents, surfactants (same as used in soap), GMO soy and sweeteners. This means that if you do not purchase high-quality whey, you may be exposing yourself to an acidifying toxic waste dump.

So, how do you find the good stuff? It's not easy. You'll have to read the fine print and look for manufacturers that do the following. Ideally, the source should be organic and grass-fed (means the cows are rich in healthy fats and their milk is more immuno-supportive), and minimally processed. Minimal processing means no use of heat or acid. If processed properly, the whey should be soluble in water and taste creamy and full. Buy whey protein concentrate, not isolate which is almost all acid processed. There should be no sweeteners, or if present, stevia root is best.

One of the best sources of whey is that derived from raw milk cheese. But during chemo, this may be a dangerous proposition since non-pasteurized dairy can become spoiled with potentially toxic bacteria. After chemo, concerns about contamination remain, but they become less critical compared to periods of very low white blood cell counts during chemo.

Is Fiber Anti-cancer?

Multiple research studies reaffirm what nutritionists have stated for years: consuming lots of high-fiber foods is a fantastic way to protect your health. That may sound like a steep claim, and really basic. But according to investigators conducting the biggest-ever study into the relationship between diet and cancer, this is factually true. Many other studies support this contention, and it is due to multiple factors.

It is true that some researchers feel the jury is still out on fiber's role as a cancer fighter, and we are not just talking about colon cancer. However, even if you are skeptical about the anti-cancer effect, it would be a shame to die of a heart attack or stroke after having beaten cancer. Given the many advantages of high-fiber foods like whole grains, fruits, and veggies, the arguments for contributing more fiber to your diet are overpowering. A high-fiber diet may cut levels of blood cholesterol, help keep up regularity, and avert gastrointestinal conditions like diverticulitis. Both soluble and insoluble fiber offer health benefits.

Contrary to their processed counterparts, like white rice or white bread, whole-grain foods hold their original fiber, the nutrient-rich bran and germ, and the starchy endosperm. That may sound academic, but from a nutritional point of view, it makes a huge difference.

Processing whole grains to produce a refined grain takes away most of their nutrient and fiber content. Individuals erroneously believe that adding synthetic micronutrients to white flour for "enrichment" purposes counterbalances the many useful nutrients lost during processing. It's true that a few synthetic vitamins and minerals are added to white flour, but this does not even come close to reestablishing all the lost nutrients.

Whole wheat, for instance, contains calcium, iron, magnesium, phosphorus, sodium, zinc, copper, manganese, selenium, vitamin C, thiamin, riboflavin, niacin, pantothenate, vitamin B6, folate, and vitamin E. That's a lot of nutrient power which is stripped out in processed flour.

The body converts all carbohydrates into glucose. But it breaks down processed or refined grains much faster than intact or whole grains. The speedy breakdown of processed carbs (high Glycemic Index), which causes wide sways in blood glucose, may trigger hunger cravings, cause the release of stress hormones, and contribute to the buildup of arterial plaques.

Basic whole grains include brown rice, barley, millet, oats, buckwheat, rye, and whole wheat. All are good but differ in nutrient content and amount of fiber. Don't forget about fruits and veggies for fiber content. You may also want to try out some traditional Native American grains such as quinoa ("keen-wa") or amaranth, found in health-food stores. Healthy whole-grain recipes are simple to find on the web. But savoring these highly nutritious foods may require patience. Whole grains commonly take longer to cook than refined grains. It's worth the wait!

What Is An Anti-Inflammatory Diet?

We know that cancer is a pro-inflammatory state. In other words, it thrives in inflammatory conditions and part of how it comes about in the first place is related to inflammatory biochemical pathways that are triggered in the body. How are these inflammatory pathways triggered? The answer is very complicated, so we can only scratch the surface in this book. However, one strong reason is that our Western diet contains a gross imbalance of Omega 3 (anti-inflammatory) to Omega 6 (pro-inflammatory) fatty acids. We need *both* as building blocks for various metabolic processes, but thousands of years ago the ratio was 2:1 of Omega-6 to Omega-3 fatty acids. By the early to mid-1900's with more and more processed foods, the ratio went to 4:1 and now it is a staggering 25:1 in favor of pro-inflammatory Omega 6. Omega 3,6 and 9, all of which you need, comes from fish oil and flaxseed in our diet. Here is a list of foods that are high in Omega-3 fatty acids you should consider as well as a list of omega-6 containing foods you should avoid.

Anti-inflammatory Omega-3	Pro-inflammatory Omega-6
Anchovies	Bacon
Avocados	Butter
Bluefish	Cheese
Brazil Nuts	Corn Oil
Canola Oil	Donuts
Flax Seed Oil	French Fries

Anti-inflammatory Omega-3	Pro-inflammatory Omega-6
Green Leafy Vegetables	Ice Cream
Herring	Lamb Chops
Lean Meats	Margarine
Mackerel	Mayonnaise
Olive Oil	Onion Rings
Salmon	Potato Chips
Sardines	Processed Foods
Trout	Steak
Tuna	Sunflower Oil
Walnuts	Whipped Cream
Whitefish	Whole Milk

Flaxseed avoids the mercury contamination problem found in wild-caught saltwater fish. However, it is not as complete because it only contains alpha-linolenic acid (ALA), which may be an inferior source for several reasons. Omega 3 fatty acids eicosapentaenoic acid (EPA) and docosahexaenoic acid (DHA) are initially made by algae and other microorganisms found in our oceans. These are consumed and metabolized further by fish, after which they become our primary source of omega 3 fatty acids. Vegetarians only consume ALA and no EPA or DHA. ALA is converted to EPA and DHA in our bodies, but poorly. Blood EPA and DHA omega 3 concentrations in vegetarians and vegans are lower than in omnivores (non-vegetarians). Whether or not this makes any difference in overall and cardiac health is very debatable. Vegetarians already have a reduced risk of cardiac events. But when we are discussing cancer and have a goal of higher omega 3 tissue levels, this may not play well.

The best sources for omega 3 remain cold water fish (farmed fish are getting much better as well) or Krill (a shrimp-like organism), but there is now the added concern about mercury and radiation contamination. Krill, being on the lower end of the food chain, has less time to accumulate mercury contamination before harvesting and is superior in this regard. There are other similar sources, such as the New Zealand Green Lipped Mussel.

So, choose where the omega source comes from wisely in planning your diet. Sometimes, supplement forms are purer in this regard compared to natural sources and can be one of the exceptions to the whole food over supplements rule. Non-fish-oil DHA and EPA are becoming available, but this is a semi-synthetic solution and is much more expensive. Finally, beware of flaxseed supplement labels which boast much higher omega 3 amount (typically 7 grams) than those found in fish oil supplements (typically 1 gram). Remember that all this ALA in the flaxseed has to be converted to EPA and DHA and 7 grams can yield about 700 milligrams of these omega fatty acids. This is higher than the 300 milligrams of DHA and EPA you get in a typical 1 gram fish oil capsule. But fish oil capsules do not require a 7 to 1 ratio to deliver a good amount of DHA and EPA. So, watching the amounts on the label is important as a 1 gram or even 5 grams flaxseed oil supplement is inferior to a 1 gram fish oil capsule.

Eat Less? Calorie Restriction And Free Radicals

As mentioned, cancer and other diseases are at least partly caused by free-radical damage to your cells. Free radicals are unstable molecules which are produced as part of normal metabolism in your body all day long. You can do two things about this. First, a calorie restricted diet can reduce the number of free radicals that are formed. These are hard diets to adhere to but can lead to significant benefits regarding longevity and potentially preventing disease, including cancer. However, one has to be very careful not to suffer the consequences of malnutrition and severe vitamin deficiencies. So, there is a trick to this in order to be done safely. A safe recommendation would be to look at the number of calories you are consuming per day and reduce that number by 20% or so. Just to be clear, this is a proven effect in mice but research is in progress in humans. Nonetheless, it is low risk. Also, to the extent that it at least reduces the ill effects of obesity, calorie restriction is something to consider but only if you are in a baseline nutritional balance. In other words, doing anything like this during cancer treatment can be dangerous. Reserve it for potentially helping to prevent recurrence after treatment.

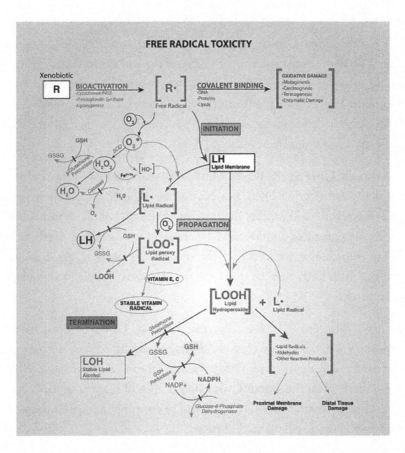

By Dan Cojocari (Own work) [CC BY-SA 4.0 (http://creativecommons.org/licenses/by-sa/4.0/)], via Wikimedia Commons

Even if you can't prevent all free radicals from forming, you can help your body quench them by having a substantial amount of anti-oxidants in your diet. These are usually in the form of fruits and vegetables, with vegetables being favored because their sugar content is lower. There are specific types of vegetables as mentioned in this book which are better than others (e.g. cruciferous vegetables) and there is a lot more to this story than can be covered here. Also, anti-oxidants can become harmful *pro*-oxidants when taken in the wrong dosage or mix and *cause* cancer. So, to emphasize, more is not better when taking supplements in high pharmacologic or orthomolecular doses. Focus on diet! It's hard to overdose on veggies, and a veggie-focused diet will tend towards calorie restriction.

What's The Best General Anti-Cancer Diet?

Even if you throw out all your supplements and focus on whole food, it's hard to keep track of all the anti-cancer superfoods out there in isolation and which ones to choose to create a "diet." Which combination diet is "better"? The reality is we do not yet know which foodstuffs overall are best for any given individual, so that makes this a loaded question. That day is coming soon through the sciences of nutrigenetics and nutrigenomics.

The best-studied diet on the planet which has anti-cancer and other health benefits is the Mediterranean Diet. You can't go wrong here, especially if you lean towards the plant-based aspects of this diet. A strictly whole food plant-based diet is also documented to have anti-cancer properties but not nearly as many clinical or epidemiologic studies back this up. Having said that, based on increasing evidence, it is likely that the more you steer towards a whole food plant-based diet, the better.

Finally, as a rule, aim for a low Glycemic Index or Glycemic Load food mix. This means lower amounts of simple sugars, especially refined sugars but also natural sugars such are fructose. With a Mediterranean Diet, leaning towards low glycemic whole plant-based foods, you will get 80% of the way to the "best diet" for you. Mix in some superfoods that we will be covering in the next chapter, and you will find yourself miles ahead of most.

More radical anti-inflammatory cancer-fighting diets exist, such as the ketogenic diet. However, these are in clinical trials, not proven and are notoriously harder to follow with substantial side effects. Many others, such as the "alkaline diet" as the sole anti-cancer strategy, are more confabulation than fact and proffered by those who don't understand how the human body works. Most offer precious little over what has been mentioned so far. We cover more about specialized diets later in this book.

Let's move on to the components of a basic anti-cancer, anti-inflammatory, antioxidant diet.

Veggies

Which veggies should you pick? Cruciferous vegetables like broccoli, cauliflower, kale, Brussels sprouts and cabbage contain two major and very potent antioxidants, lutein and zeaxanthin. These veggies also contain sulforaphane, which has direct and powerful anti-cancer activity. Most fresh veggies contain additional antioxidants, vitamins, and minerals, like selenium and zinc, which likely also contribute to an anti-cancer effect. A guiding principle is to make sure your diet contains a "rainbow of colors." These colors represent the presence of a very broad variety of cancer-fighting nutrients.

Fruits

All fruits have something to contribute and balance is everything. But some are better than others when it comes to cancer prevention and anti-cancer support. Some fruits, as well as vegetables, also contain very high levels of sugars. Natural or not, sugar is the preferred food for cancer. So, look at the glycemic index and glycemic load to balance the benefits of anti-oxidants, anti-inflammatory effects and epigenetic influences on genes.

For the glycemic index, a value of 100 is set to pure glucose and standardizes the rest of the table. Anything above 100 causes your blood sugar and insulin levels to spike higher and faster. Anything below 100 causes them to go up less after meals. The glycemic load helps adjust for portion sizes and is calculated as follows. Glycemic index x grams of carbohydrates / 100 = glycemic load. This is merely an example list. There are many to choose from online.

Carrots 101	Wheat bread, white 101	Bagel, white 103
Watermelon 103	Swede (rutabaga) 103	Cheerios 106
French fries 107	Donut 108	Waffles 109
Total 109	Broad beans (fava beans) 113	Pretzels 116
Rice Krispies 117	Cornflakes 119	Potato, baked 121
Glucose 137	Parsnips 139	Glucose tablets 146
Maltose 150	Cream of wheat 100	Melba toast 100
Chana dal 12	Yogurt, artificially sweet, low fat 20	Soya beans 25
Rice Bran 27	Cherries 32	Fructose 32
Peas, dried 32	Barley, pearled 36	Grapefruit 36
Milk, full fat 39	Kidney beans 42	Black beans 43

Apricots, dried 44	Milk, skim 46	Fettuccine 46
Lima beans, baby, frozen 46	Chickpeas (garbanzo beans) 47	Rye 48
Pear, fresh 53	Whole grain Spaghetti 53	Apple 54
Haricot/Navy beans 54	Plum 55	Pinto beans 55
Millet 101	Apple juice 58	Black-eyed beans 59
All-bran 60	Peach, fresh 60	Orange 63
Macaroni 64	Linguine 65	Lactose 65
Grapes 66	Pineapple juice 66	Bulgur 68
Rice, parboiled 68	Peas, green 68	Grapefruit juice 69
Pumpernickel 71	Ice cream, low fat 71	Orange juice 74
Special K 77	Banana 77	Sweet potato 77
Oat Bran 78	Buckwheat 78	Sweet corn 78
Rice, brown 79	Popcorn 79	Apricots, fresh 82
Honey 83	Rice, white 83	Split pea soup 86
Oatmeal 87	Ice cream 87	Raisins 91
Beets 91	Sucrose (table sugar) 92	Couscous 93
Pineapple 94	Grapenuts 96	Stoned Wheat Thins 96
Cornmeal 98	Wheat bread, wholegrain 99	Shredded Wheat 99

Berries are a solid way to go as far as fruits are concerned, and to some extent, it's a matter of taste. Some berries have higher antioxidant content than others, and you could use the Oxygen Radical Absorbance Capacity (ORAC) scale to help you pick. This, and other reference scales attempt to measure the total antioxidant capacity of different foods in a test tube. The higher the number, the better. It's not perfect, but it can help you pick those that you like that have high values. The ORAC is most often used to look up fruits, but you can also look at ORAC values for vegetables and spices in making your selection of those foods. You may be surprised to learn that the ORAC value of spices, herbs, and certain nuts is a lot higher than that of fruits. It can exceed values of several hundred thousand. You can find multiple lists online for over three hundred different whole foods and nutrients.

Food Type	Serving Size	Antioxidant Capacity per serving
Small Red Bean	½ cup dried	13727
Wild blueberry	1 cup	13427
Red kidney bean	½ cup dried	13529
Pinto bean	1 cup	11864
Blueberry	1 cup	9019
Cranberry	1 cup	8983
Artichoke hearts	1 cup cooked	7904
Blackberry	1 cup	7701
Prune	½ cup	7291
Raspberry	1 cup	6058
Strawberry	1 cup	5938
Red apple	1	5900
Granny Smith	1	5381
Pecan	1 ounce	5095
Sweet cherry	1 cup	4873
Black plum	1	4844
Russet potato	1 cooked	4649
Black bean	½ cup dried	4181
Plum	1	4118
Gala apple	1	3903

Table is from USDA and is in public domain

Some melons, such as cantaloupe, have been shown to be protective against breast cancer in epidemiologic studies. Laboratory, but not human studies, have also demonstrated that bitter lemon extracts are particularly active against multiple cancer cell lines. The mechanisms of action are epigenetic as well as through insulin growth factor pathways.

Citrus fruits, such as oranges, mandarins, lemons and limes, contain abundant levels of antioxidant flavonoids and vitamin C. Certain flavonoids, such as nobiletin, are particularly active as anti-angiogenic factors. Not to be left out, pectin is also anti-angiogenic, may help prevent tumor progression and metastasis and induce apoptosis. Finally, when you consume fruits don't throw away the rind! It does not always taste good, but figure out a way to incorporate it into your diet. Citrus rind contains D-limonene which is a potent apoptotic in lab and animal studies involving various cancer cell lines. Finally, a word of caution about citrus. As another reminder not to overdo anything, several large epidemiologic studies involving over 100,000 people suggest that eating citrus more than twice per week increases the risk of melanoma. Worse, the more you eat, the higher the risk. This study is epidemiologic, which means it can suggest but not prove association. Nevertheless, there is a strong suggestion that overdoing citrus may be a bad idea.

Apples are particularly rich in quercetin, which is the most commonly consumed flavonoid. It is a potent antioxidant and has anti-inflammatory properties as well. It also works at the epigenetic level modulating the p53 tumor suppressor gene, as well as at the cell signal transduction level by influencing tyrosine kinase. In other words, it has multiple anti-cancer effects, but almost all of this data is from laboratory and animal studies.

Papaya fruit contains papain, which is a proteolytic enzyme that has been shown to have anti-cancer effects in the laboratory. Proteolytic enzymes are thought to be immunomodulatory and antiangiogenic.

Pineapple, similar to papaya, contains another proteolytic enzyme called bromelain. It works much the same way. Also, bromelain may reduce inflammation and swelling after surgery, but this is not proven. One word of caution is in order. Bromelain is anti-thrombotic and can lead to excess bleeding when taken with anticoagulation medications such as warfarin.

Peaches, apricots, plums, cherries and nectarines belong to a class called "stone fruits" because of their large central seed. They all contain vitamin C and anti-oxidant polyphenols that have anti-proliferative effects in the laboratory model against multiple cancer cells lines. While some of these have been hyped to be strongly anti-cancer (e.g. amygdalin or Laetrile from apricot seeds), the data seems to be weakest here compared to other fruits. Nevertheless, adding these into your diet for flavor and potential benefits is very reasonable.

Overall, a healthy mixture of fruits is critical to your health. Aim for several servings of fruit per day, focusing more on vegetables than fruits in your diet. The exact ratio is not definable scientifically, and this is only mentioned because of the concern of excess fructose intake. Keep in mind; vegetables also contain fructose. In most cases, they contain less than fruit.

Nuts

Nuts are full of antioxidants, which can also suppress the growth of cancer cells. These are highly under-rated. Consider walnuts, almonds, and brazil nuts. However, be careful of nut allergies, which are relatively common. If you're not used to eating nuts, try a tiny sample first or put a small sample on your skin.

Teas

Research confirms that various teas have cancer-fighting powers. While all teas are good for the body, green tea and white tea are made from unfermented tea leaves. Consequently, they have a higher density of antioxidants than black teas, which are more processed. The antioxidants in tea are known as polyphenols. Epigallocatechin Gallate (EGCG) is the most effective cancer chemopreventive polyphenol in tea. Based on studies, three to five cups per day are recommended.

Polyphenols

Other than EGCG, many other polyphenols are essential to the battle against free radicals. They are found in many foods, mainly fruit and vegetables, green tea, black tea, red wine, coffee, chocolate, olives, and extra virgin olive oil. Many herbs and spices, nuts and algae also are high in these beneficial micro-nutrients. A very specific anti-cancer polyphenol you may have heard of is quercetin, which is found in fruit, vegetables, cereals, leguminous plants, tea, and wine.

Specific Immune Boosting Gems

As noted in the immunology and immunotherapy sections of this book, naturally "boosting" the immune system to help it fight cancer better is a very complex and incompletely proven strategy. The most that can be said is that you should optimize your immune system as best as possible by removing immunosuppressive influences and adding nutrients that your system requires to function optimally. There is quite a bit you can do in this regard that is simple and inexpensive. Again, don't be fooled into thinking that some expensive concoctions are better than others in your fight against cancer. This should smack of quack if it is really outlandish in promises. This is especially true if the supposed actions of a marketed concoction can be replicated for far less cost with more benefit through diet and superfoods.

According to some studies, garlic contains alum compounds that seem to "support" the immune system. Another well documented general immune boosting food source is mushrooms and one of the main active ingredients called Polysaccharide-K (PSK). There are many to choose from, but some can be hard to find. Maitake and Shitake are perhaps the best studied and easiest to come by. But even the lowly white mushroom found in all supermarkets can be beneficial, compared to no mushrooms at all. Astragalus stands out as an herb with immune-boosting potential.

The degree of immune support that can be achieved by consuming these nutrient groups is scientifically controversial, BUT there is very little downside. Therefore, from a risk vs. benefit perspective, they are recommended strongly. Remember not to go overboard. The synergies between various dietary nutrients are important and that works well. However, if you overdo a supplement or herbal in pharmacologic doses, you run the risk of immunosuppression.

Adaptogens

The concept of foods containing adaptogenic substances is relatively recent, first described by a Russian pharmacologist N.V. Lazarev in 1947. Adaptogens are defined as natural metabolic regulators or biological response modifiers which increase the ability to adapt to environmental factors and to avoid damage from such factors. While the concept is still controversial, even the Food and Drug Administration accepts this as a functional claim for certain herbs. Basically, these are a group of substances that can be considered as "balancing agents" or stress busters and immune system facilitators. Top contenders are arguably Ashwagandha, Rhodiola, Siberian and Red Ginseng, and Maca, although Reishi and Maitake mushrooms are often part of the conversation. This is a very vague area of investigation, so numerous nutrient sources have been proposed, but none stand head and shoulders above the rest.

Spices

Turmeric, which is a member of the ginger family, helps battle cancer. Hot chile peppers and jalapenos contain capsaicin, which is thought to be a cancer-fighting agent. Rosemary, which is a flavorful spice, might also help in the battle against cancer. The best way to use these superfood spices is to make your food taste better rather than buying capsules full of extracts. There simply is not enough data to pick one over another, and certainly not enough to recommend mega-doses. So, food to taste is the order of the day.

Avoiding Gluten

Gluten is a natural protein found in wheat and other grains that helps the dough rise in the process of cooking. There is an association between celiac disease, which is an increasingly prevalent autoimmune disease related to gluten allergy, and gastrointestinal cancer. Specifically, there is an association with lymphoma and the rare small bowel adenocarcinoma. Interestingly, the risk of lung and breast cancer seems to be decreased. There is not enough data to explain why. However, in general, the incidence of self-described gluten allergy and intolerance seems to be increasing.

First, if you think you have a gluten allergy get tested for celiac disease. Do not simply cut out all gluten containing food because it is popular to do so. Fewer that 1% of people actually have celiac disease. The downside is that gluten is a major source of protein and avoidance of whole grains can be counter-productive. Gluten free products are expensive and can be high is calories.

Having said that, it is true that many people test negative for celiac disease who still experience resolution of symptoms with a gluten elimination diet. So something may be going on with "gluten sensitivity" or intolerance. In many cases, this can simply be a wheat allergy specifically. In those situations, you can still benefit from other whole grains.

Combining that with the growing acceptance of the "leaky gut" concept, which is aggravated by inflammatory foods, suggests that it is prudent to avoid gluten if you are sensitive to it, along with other pro-inflammatory foods. From an anti-cancer perspective, the focus should be on avoiding inflammatory bowel symptoms while not cutting out too many beneficial nutrients.

Juicing

The advice here is simple, don't juice! There is a better way. Say what? Certainly, fruits and veggies are extremely important for many reasons, but here are the concerns. First of all, if you BUY bottled juices, they are full of additives, sugars, sweeteners, corn syrup and more. Even the high pulp bottled juices are suspect. This is a definite no – no for any health benefit, let alone fighting cancer.

If you have a good juicer, there is still a problem. Remember that fruits have a lot of fructose in them. This is less of a problem in most vegetables. However, even if you have the world's best juicer, it is going to leave some or all of the pulp behind. The pulp is crucial because fiber has health benefits and contains tightly bound beneficial nutrients. You are leaving a significant part of the nutritional value behind if you leave out the pulp. As far as sugar is concerned, if you eat an orange, the fiber contained in the pulp will reduce the sugar and insulin spike that will soon follow. Neither of these effects are good for you. If you drink a glass of fresh squeezed OJ, you don't get that benefit because the fiber that retards the sugar absorption is missing. So, either set your high-end juicer to conserve all the pulp, if you can, or buy a high-speed blender which is usually cheaper and way better for you because it retains all the pulp. You can dilute it with some water to make a thick shake more drinkable.

If you juice but take the pulp in later as a snack that is still not good. This is because Mother Nature designed micronutrients in fruits and vegetables to work together, at the same time. By separating them, you lose these interactions. Also, that sugar and insulin spike prevention that was just mentioned is lost.

There are, of course, others who argue for juicing and not blending. Think about it this way. If Mother Nature wanted us, humans, to drink juice rather than eat fruit and veggies, she would have evolved things that way. By juicing you're meddling and trying to make that case that humans are smarter than Mother Nature.

Food Safety Tips

During chemotherapy, you may get recommendations to avoid a lot of things like veggies and salads and other foods that seem to be good for you. Most of the time the concern is a risk of infection while your white blood cell counts are low. These concerns are important, but the truth is you don't need to avoid whole foods with critical nutrients. You just need to take some precautions.

First of all, the primary interface with the outside world when it comes to food is your intestinal barrier. This needs to be healthy to avoid harmful bacteria getting across and potentially making you sick. To do this, make sure you are taking probiotics and prebiotics as discussed in Chapter 5. This helps limit the damage to the barrier which chemo, inflammation and cancer itself can cause.

Beyond keeping your intestine in the best shape possible, you need to handle foods with extra care. Here is a list of tips.

For cooking:

1. Before handling and preparing foods that you will be consuming wash your hands with warm, soapy water. Then wash them again before you eat.

2. Keep your foods refrigerated at a temperature below 40° F.

3. Don't eat food that has been sitting around for a while, especially if there is mayonnaise or dairy involved

4. Be careful how you thaw food. Do not thaw it at room temperature and make sure if any water accumulates in the process, keep that separate in a drip pan under the thawing food.

5. Do not re-freeze frozen foods.

6. Make sure you refrigerate perishable food soon after you're done buying, preparing or eating it, preferably within an hour.

7. Wash fruits and vegetables well. Do this under running water and not in a container. You do not need to use soap. But if any have crevasses or irregularities, make sure you scrub them with a brush to remove any dirt or soil.

8. Leafy veggies should be washed or rinsed under running water, one leaf at a time. Make sure any dirt or soil has been washed off. Do this even if the salads or veggies have been marked as pre-washed.

9. Do not consume raw vegetable sprouts (e.g. alfalfa, radish, broccoli, mung bean). These carry a high risk of *Salmonella* and *E. coli* contamination. Dispose of any fruits and vegetables that have visible slime or mold.

10. Avoid foods that have been prepared or cut in the grocery store because their areas can be contaminated.

11. Clean off the tops of canned foods with soap and water before you open them.

12. When cooking, use different utensils, pottery, bowls, cutting boards, etc. than those you will be serving or eating with. Until the food is cooked it may harbor bacteria which may stay on the cooking utensils or plates and bowls.

13. Dispose of eggs with cracked shells

14. Do not eat raw fish preparations like sushi, sashimi or ceviche because of the risk of parasites.

15. Err on the side of caution. If it looks, smells or feels bad, throw it out.

16. When you cook, make sure it is thorough enough for meat and fish (160° F) and poultry (180° F). Use a thermometer which is accurate. If you are not sure, you can put the thermometer in boiling water where it should read 212° F. If you must use a microwave, then verify that the food is properly exposed or rotated enough to be evenly cooked.

For shopping:

1. Pick the freshest products you can find based on the posted "sell-by" and "use-by" dates. Certainly, don't buy anything out of date.

2. Check the integrity of the packaging, whether it is plastic, metal or paper. Make sure everything is sealed properly and not overtly damaged.

3. Pick veggies and fruits that are not damaged or old and bruised.

4. Avoid tofu packed in water

5. Avoid unpasteurized foods, including dairy and juices. This may be a contentious point for some natural foodies, but during chemotherapy, it is crucial to avoid contamination with potentially very virulent bacteria.

6. Avoid eating at fast food, delis, sandwich and bakery shops where food is prepared on site. While this may be appealing, you have no idea what their cleaning habits are or when the person who prepares food last washed their hands or changed gloves.

7. Do not eat from mass food dispensers of products like ice cream softies and yogurt

8. Refrigerate perishables immediately.

For Dining Out:

1. Avoid crowded establishments or go early or late

2. Avoid self-serve dispensers for condiments. Ask for single serving packets instead.

3. Do not eat from high-risk food sources such a salad bars, delis, portable food truck kitchens

4. Avoid any raw food when dining out.

5. Inspect the utensils and make sure they are clean and set on a napkin or placemat rather than on a table that may not have been washed.

6. If you take leftovers home ask for the container and package it yourself rather than sending it back to the kitchen where it can be mishandled and contaminated.

Some of the above may seem like overkill, but you just can't be too careful. Use common sense to avoid eating contaminated food.

CHAPTER 11
MORE ANTI-CANCER SUPER FOODS

As you might already be noticing, there are "superfood" qualities to many foods. As we just covered, even the essential anti-cancer diet contains many of these by default. There are many foods today specifically sporting a so-called "super foods" designation, but the problem is that who calls them superfoods varies. This chapter draws attention to an additional select few that impact cancer.

These top superfoods include tomatoes, olive oil, green and white tea, garlic, and apples. There are undoubtedly others, and in certain individual cases you specifically might require some superfoods over others, but those listed here stand out as top performers in the general advanced anti-cancer diet.

Tomatoes

Lycopene is the main ingredient for discussion in tomatoes. It is a bright red carotene and carotenoid pigment and is a phytochemical found in tomatoes and other red fruits and vegetables, such as red carrots, watermelons, and papayas. Although lycopene is chemically a carotene, it has no vitamin A activity.

Lycopene is technically not an essential (meaning you could live without eating it) nutrient for humans but is commonly found in the diet, mainly from dishes prepared from tomatoes. Of interest, the best-concentrated source of lycopene seems to be from tomato paste, not fresh tomatoes.

Research has shown an inverse correlation between consumption of tomatoes and cancer risk, particularly prostate cancer. More research is needed, but the preliminary evidence and scientific reasons for this claim are striking and here's why.

Lycopene may be *the* most powerful carotenoid quencher of toxic singlet oxygen.

It is 100 times more efficient in test tube studies of singlet-oxygen quenching action than vitamin E, which is known to be a potent anti-oxidant. Why is this important? Singlet oxygen is not a free radical per se, but it can chemically transfer energy and act as a catalyst for free radical formation. Of course, free radicals are known to cause cellular oxidative damage. Where prolonged oxidative damage occurs, cancer results.

Given its strong antioxidant properties, substantial scientific and clinical research has been devoted to a possible correlation between lycopene consumption and general health. Research suggests some benefit for cardiovascular disease, cancer, diabetes, osteoporosis, and even male infertility. Evidence for lycopene's anti-cancer benefit is strongest for cancers of the lung, stomach, and prostate gland. While lycopene hasn't been explicitly associated with cervical cancer prevention, it can enhance the body's ability to battle infection. Thus it may be useful in clearing relentless HPV infections.

What is some of the science behind this? In lung tissue, lycopene is valuable in protecting lymphocytes from nitrous dioxide damage, which is found in lung cancer. In the stomach, lycopene may help decrease the impact of the oxidative load from H.pylori infections which can reduce ulcerative disease and cancer. It may reduce the risk of many cancers by activating special cancer preventive enzymes such as phase II detoxification enzymes, which remove harmful carcinogens from cells. Lycopene is also known to suppress insulin-like growth factor-1 (IGF-1) which is a major regulator of breast and endometrial cancer cell growth. There may be a similar effect on colon cancer. Superfoods affect multiple biochemical cascades and targets. That's what makes them "super." Lycopene is an example of a "uber" super-food.

While many veggies are more nourishing raw or whole, lycopene is found in greater concentrations in tomato sauce, tomato paste, and tomato juice. So setting aside small cans of tomato juice at work or in the frig can help avert the need to turn to unhealthy snacks while preventing or fighting cancer.

Olive Oil

Olives, obviously the source of olive oil, come from the family Oleaceae. It's one of the main components of the famed Mediterranean Diet and has been used to treat many inflammatory conditions, including arthritis, migraines, cancer, and cardiovascular disease. It has also been recommended in the management of diabetes mellitus (the common form of diabetes), treatment of gallstones in conjunction with apple juice, various infections (viral, bacterial and protozoan), and intestinal disturbances. When applied to the skin, it has been a popular treatment for stretch marks after pregnancy. The list is quite extensive, but you get the idea. It has been used for just about everything, although the evidence that it works for all these conditions is very variable.

The active ingredients are mono-unsaturated (MUFA) fatty acids: oleic, palmitic and linoleic acid, as well as other important ingredients called oleocanthal and oleuropein.

Based on a lot of available research making olive oil part of your diet will likely help prevent cardiovascular disease and possibly some cancers, notably breast and colon cancer. If you already have mild diabetes or blood pressure problems, olive oil may help keep blood glucose and blood pressure under control. Olive oil will help regulate bowel movements by acting as a mild laxative.

Dietary intake of olive oil from 20-50 grams per day (typically 2-4 tablespoons) has been the reported range in studies which examined prevention or treatment of cardiovascular disease and blood pressure control. Higher doses have been reported but not recommended since there is no evidence that more is better.

A few words of caution are in order. As an orally ingested oil, used in various cooking dishes in dietary amounts, it has been used to safely provide 10-20% of daily calories (that is only two tablespoons). Used on the skin, it can produce allergic reactions, so it does have allergic potential in some people. If you are taking medications or natural supplements for the purpose of decreasing blood sugar (diabetes) or improving blood pressure control, be careful since olive oil can increase the effect causing your blood sugar or blood pressure to go too low.

Acting as anti-inflammatory agents, the phenols present in olive oil are natural antioxidants. They also dilate blood vessels and prevent platelets from aggregating. These effects reduce the formation of arterial atherosclerosis or plaque formation and otherwise contribute to the health of the internal arterial lining, called the endothelium.

Olive oil also helps other nutrient balance which helps curb inflammation in your body. It increases omega-3 fatty acid levels, which are also anti-inflammatory. While doing this, it also reduces the pro-inflammatory omega-6 fatty acid levels. The additional anti-inflammatory effect is due to the presence of oleocanthal which is a COX-1 and COX-2 inhibitor. Inhibiting the COX 1 and 2 enzymes impedes the production of the chemical messengers (such as prostaglandins) that mediate inflammation.

The oleuropein component is both an anti-inflammatory and a natural antibiotic, which can affect a large number of bacteria. The benefit from that is unclear clinically, but natural antibiotics help in defending your body against opportunistic infections during cancer treatment.

White And Green Tea

We've already touched on the anti-cancer benefits of tea. Here we go more in depth. White tea leaves belong to the family Theaceae and have been sipped as a tea, chewed as candy, applied as a poultice or as a topical to treat a wide variety of inflammatory conditions. Other common teas not made from specific herbs, including green tea, generally come from the same bush, the Camilla Sinensis. They all contain similar ingredients but undergo variable amounts of processing. White tea comes from immature leaves, is processed the least, and is known for a much higher antioxidant potential, at least partly explaining its wide range of uses. Although green tea has been studied the most, based on higher levels of virtually the same active ingredients, the effects of white tea may be amplified.

The main active ingredients are the polyphenols: catechin flavonols, theanine, gallic acid, theobromine. Also there is caffeine and phytoestrogens (plant estrogens). Catechin is a strong blocker of the pro-cancer pro-inflammatory substance NF-kappa B.

The most effective documented use has been topical application of an ointment or poultice to genital warts. This is due to the main catechin which is active in the extract, epigallocatechin gallate (EGCG). Again, the data is for green tea and is FDA approved for this use, but the active ingredients are even higher in white tea.

Drinking the tea likely has an effect on reducing various forms of cancer, including ovarian, cervical, bladder, pancreatic, esophageal, prostate, and possibly lung.

Information about breast cancer is not conclusive. It may also prevent pre-cancers of the uterine cervix and mouth (similar tissues in these areas), as well as improve oral hygiene overall by reducing gingivitis, an inflammatory condition.

For oral consumption, 4-5 cups per day have been studied, and tea preparation is generally 2-2.5 grams (approx 1.5 teaspoons) of tea leaves for every 6 ounces of water, steeped for 10-25 minutes in less than boiling water. This limits deactivation of ingredients and reduces harshness in taste. For a cooler refreshing drink, you can consider whipping up a batch of sun tea, which means a prolonged natural steeping preparation of iced tea.

Can there be problems with something as simple as tea? Well, allergic reactions do occur and can be severe. However, the usual limiting factor is the amount of caffeine, which can start climbing after 4-5 cups. Caffeine can cause agitation, blood pressure changes, and can cause dehydration because it is a diuretic. It can also react with a slew of prescription and non-prescription medications. The good news is that caffeine content of white tea is lower to begin with, in the range of only 15mg per serving. During pregnancy and breastfeeding, caffeine intake is controversial but less than 200mg per day has not been reported to be harmful.

Interaction with herbals and drugs which affect platelets can increase the risk of bleeding. In general, caffeinated substances can interfere with blood glucose control, so diabetics beware. When applied to the skin and genital area, as is done for genital warts (not cancer) blistering and swelling can occur. This is usually quickly reversible.

Many polyphenols are active ingredients in green and white tea, and as a group is responsible for the health and anti-cancer benefits. The ingredients are 1) anti-mutagens (anti-cancer), 2) anti-angiogenic (prevent abnormal blood vessel formation), which is a mainstream anticancer strategy, and 3) potent anti-inflammatory substances (including COX-1 and COX-2 inhibition) and other biochemical pathways. The higher the polyphenol level, the greater the anticipated benefit. Polyphenols are also anti-bacterial, which is partly why they help with gingivitis prevention and treatment. So, other than the caffeine warning, you can enjoy quite a bit of tea within any specific health limitations.

Garlic

Garlic belongs to the family of Alliaceae, to which onion also belongs. People have used the garlic bulb to treat a huge list of disorders, most of which are inflammatory in nature. Both oral intake and application to the skin have been recommended. The main active ingredients are allicin and ajoene.

Best studied is the effect of garlic on cardiovascular health. Oral garlic doses of 300-1000 mg/day have been shown to reduce arterial wall hardening (which helps prevent blood pressure problems) and can also lower blood pressure when hypertension is already an issue. Although more controversial, some studies indicate that it may also favorably affect your overall lipid levels and lower cholesterol. Less well studied, there is a potential cancer prevention benefit and possible prostate health support.

When applied topically there is a risk of blisters and scarring. However, a 0.6% ajoene gel is effective against various fungal infections, including jock itch (Tinea cruris), ringworm (Tinea corporis), and athlete's foot (Tinea pedis). This is mentioned because fungal skin infections do occur during cancer therapy, and this might be an option to consider if you don't wish to use prescription medication for that.

Oral intake in the range of 300-1000mg/day has been studied. The problem is that raw garlic may differ from the various formulations of supplements out there. Beware that odor free preparations may not contain Allicin and its derivatives, which are the active ingredients. So again, consider just staying with natural whole food intake.

Allergic reactions are common and can be severe. Also, if you start taking garlic in larger doses, expect some intestinal disturbances due to direct irritation and effect on the bacteria normally found in the intestinal tract. In addition, garlic can affect platelet function, which can increase the risk of bleeding internally or during surgery. You should discontinue use of garlic at least two weeks before any planned surgery and tell your oncologist if you are taking substantial amounts while on chemotherapy. During pregnancy and breastfeeding, in addition to the warnings noted, doses higher than normal dietary intake may be dangerous based on a few reports.

Interactions with other supplements or herbals and prescription or over-the-counter synthetic drugs are pretty extensive. In particular, any herbals, supplements or drugs which can affect bleeding should not be taken at the same time. Typical examples are Coumadin® (warfarin), heparin, aspirin, ibuprofen, ginkgo or vitamin E. Garlic can also affect the liver and metabolism of many other drugs, including oral contraceptives, isoniazid or INH (used for tuberculosis treatment), and antiviral drugs, including those used for the treatment of HIV. So, as I keep emphasizing, more is not usually better and can be dangerous.

As far as cardiovascular health and cancer prevention is concerned, the active ingredient Allicin and its metabolites help protect the inner lining of arteries (endothelium) by acting as an antioxidant. Ajoene has been shown to cause apoptosis (cell death) in various tumor cells when studied in test tubes as well as stimulation of the immune system in several ways (humoral/antibody as well as cell-mediated). The clinical effect is not as apparent, but there is plausible fundamental research which shows how it might work and it is low risk with moderate intake.

Finally, allicin and ajoene can also help fight off several types of bacteria and viruses, including the dreaded MRSA or methicillin-resistant Staphylococcus aureus bacteria and herpesvirus. So, this might be of help if stress related herpes breaks out during treatment, or an infection occurs or for prevention of all of these.

Apples

Apples are a member of the Rosaceae family and are available pretty much globally. No significant studies have been done to try to discriminate details between different types of apples. People have used apples to treat everything from intestinal disturbances and gallstones to cancer. The most active anti-cancer ingredient is quercetin. But an additional component, pectin, may be of help for chemo related intestinal disturbances.

For intestinal disturbances such as diarrhea or constipation, pectin is the active substance and the amount you need depends on upon how much of a problem you have. Don't overdo it as you might end up with the opposite problem, too loose or too constipated. So you have to adjust intake to get the desired effect.

Pectin makes up a lot of an apple's pulp bulk. When it absorbs water, it swells even more. By doing that, it can form bulky stool that is not too firm or watery, making bowel movements regular. Phloretin is a natural antibiotic and might have some effect on normalization of bacterial flora in the large intestine.

Other than possible allergies, there is no evidence for harm when eating the fruit of apples in dietary amounts. On the other hand, eating apple seeds can be dangerous and very toxic, or even lethal, due to hydrogen cyanide. How much? Well, best to stay away altogether, but reports have noted about a cupful of seeds as being lethal. Finally, apple juice can reduce absorption of certain medications, notably fexofenadine (Allegra®).

Conclusion On Superfoods

This was just a lightning quick review of a few very useful cancer-fighting superfoods. There are many others, and the trick is definitely to use them in moderation and mixing for variety. Ideally, they should be utilized in the "right" combination and preferably related to your specific circumstances and cancer type. Unfortunately, the science is not that tight yet on this topic. So, adding superfoods to taste, variation and moderation are just fine and is likely a better plan than you have now. Don't overthink this. Just do it and start with what we covered here.

Remember a base antioxidant anti-inflammatory diet will get you 80% of the way there. For supercharging your fight, selectively adding superfoods to taste can fill in the rest. The good news is that unlike the potential interaction and overdose danger with supplements, you can mix and match food at will with few exceptions. There is no way to overdose on whole food nutrients. So, for example, if you find something interesting based on new research, add at will.

At http://CancerCureology.com, here are others that we cover in greater detail and depth: genistein in soy products, choline in eggs, more mushrooms, artichokes, pomegranate, black raspberry, black cumin seed and much more. As I mention many times in this book, Mother Nature's pharmacy is quite a bit larger than the one you will find at your corner drug store. This book and CancerCureology.com only scratch the surface, but we try to get to those topics that will help you the most.

Chapter 12
Alcohol: The Good, Bad, and Ugly

Scientific evidence consistently and strongly indicates that consumption of alcoholic beverages is a risk factor for cancer. On the other hand, you've probably heard that wine is supposed to be protective. Why the confusion?

I included this chapter because many people enjoy some recreational alcohol and, given the stress of having cancer and other life's pressures, what is the appropriate thing to do?

Bad Alcohol

There is no question that drinking alcoholic beverages increases the risk of mouth & throat cancer (larynx and pharynx), esophageal cancer, intestine cancer (colon and rectum), liver cancer and breast cancer. That's the bad news up front. Also, escaping behind alcohol is not a good coping strategy. With that out of the way, let's explore what you need to know.

It is probably the actual alcohol molecule itself (ethanol) which is the main culprit, and even small amounts of alcoholic beverages increase risk, but the more you drink, the higher the risk. This holds true for all types of drinks but obviously the higher amounts found in hard liquor may be the biggest danger, assuming you drink it straight and a lot of it. So, avoid binge drinking and multiple drinks each day.

How does alcohol raise cancer risk? It can cause direct damage to cells in the mouth and intestinal tract, acting as a pro-inflammatory irritant. It can help other toxic chemicals get into cells, like the toxins from cigarette smoke. It can lower folate levels which is a documented risk for breast and colon cancer. Finally, it can raise estrogen levels, thereby increasing ovarian, endometrial and breast cancer risk, among others. There are other theories, but with these warnings let's move on to the good news.

Wine

What about wine? How might that be different? Red wine is a rich source of biologically active phytochemicals, which are beneficial biochemicals found in plants. Particular compounds called polyphenols found in red wine—such as catechins and resveratrol—are thought to have antioxidant and anti-cancer properties. They are found in the skin and seeds of grapes. When wine is made, the alcohol produced by the fermentation process dissolves the polyphenols contained in the skin and seeds. Red wine contains more polyphenols than white wine because the making of white wine requires the removal of the skin after the grapes are crushed. The phenols in red wine include catechin, gallic acid, and epicatechin.

Resveratrol

What about resveratrol in particular? Resveratrol is a type of antioxidant polyphenol called a phytoalexin, a class of compounds produced as part of a plant's defense system against disease. It is manufactured by the plant in response to an invading fungus, stress, injury, infection, or ultraviolet irradiation. Red wine contains high levels of resveratrol, as do grapes, raspberries, mulberries, peanuts, and some other harder to find plants.

Resveratrol has been shown to reduce tumor incidence in animals by affecting one or more stages of cancer development, such as initiation and promotion. It has also been shown to inhibit the growth of many types of cancer cells in culture. Evidence also exists that resveratrol can reduce inflammation and reduces activation of pro-cancer NF-kappa B. Remember, this is a very important protein produced by tumor cells and the body's immune system when it is under attack. This protein affects cancer cell growth and metastasis. Also, resveratrol has some beneficial epigenetic effects on tumor suppressor genes.

Research studies published in the International Journal of Cancer show that drinking a glass of red wine a day may cut a man's risk of prostate cancer in half and that the protective effect appears to be strongest against the most aggressive forms of the disease. Men who consumed four or more 4-ounce glasses of red wine per week have a 60 percent lower incidence of the more aggressive types of prostate cancer. This is supported by lab evidence that resveratrol reduces tumorigenesis in prostate cancer cells lines by several mechanisms including mTOR and SIRT1.

Similar beneficial effects have been seen in gynecologic cancers, but recent studies are also troubling. Based on results from the 88,084 women in the Nurses Health Study, women were at significantly higher risk of developing breast cancer if they consumed one standard drink (15 grams of alcohol, or 118 milliliters of wine or 355 milliliters of beer) a day, regardless of whether or not they were smokers. This was markedly different for men who only increased their risk with light drinking if they also smoked. The problem is that resveratrol has some estrogen-like effects and can up-regulate development of estrogen and androgen receptors. This means it can increase the number of receptors. The more receptors there are, the more circulating hormones may increase tumor growth. It can also increase angiogenesis and reduce apoptosis, which is clearly not anti-cancer. So, anyone with a hormonally sensitive cancer should be careful. Avoid excess.

Overall, studies of the association between red wine consumption and cancer in humans are rather early. Although use of large amounts of alcoholic beverages may increase the risk of some cancers, there is growing evidence that the health benefits of red wine are related to its non-alcoholic components. So, lower alcohol content red wine in moderation is the key. Read the label. You will see alcohol content in red wine ranges from 12-16%. Also, although hard to find, quality alcohol-free red wine contains the same amount of polyphenols and resveratrol in particular.

If you don't like to drink alcohol or want to eliminate the possible ethanol risk or don't like the taste of wine, you can consume resveratrol supplements. Once again, more is not better. Even a small supplemental dose of 10-20mg is equivalent to many bottles or even cases of wine. So don't get carried away! There are studies which document *pro*-cancer effects at higher doses. Also, resveratrol can activate or inhibit the liver detoxing cytochrome p450 system, which means it can interfere with numerous drugs, including safe dosing of chemotherapy agents.

Red Wine Varietals

It turns out that not all red wines are the same regarding potential health benefits. In addition to containing different amounts of alcohol, the amount of resveratrol also varies. The winner is Pinot Noir which is grown in cool, rainy climates. Boutique wineries also beat out large wineries because the larger ones who want their wines more drinkable faster add chemicals to do so. Madirans, Cabernets, Syrahs, and Merlots are high in procyanidins, which are potent antioxidants. Overall, dry red wines like Cabernets have higher levels of beneficial flavonoids than sweeter wines like Zinfandel. So, vary these during the week to your taste to garner all the potential health benefits, but err on the side of caution regarding the total amount per week.

CHAPTER 13
SUPPLEMENTS & BOTANICALS

Antioxidant Warning

There are many advantages to antioxidants in terms of prevention of disease, including cancer. Who benefits the most from supplement antioxidants will be determined as nutrigenetics evolves and gives us the answer. For now, it is generally accepted that antioxidants are a good thing. They act by neutralizing reactive oxygen species (ROS) and reducing free radical damage to DNA. This is assumed to help prevent cancer. The modifying caveat to that, which is mentioned many times in this book, is that whole food antioxidants are likely to benefit you more at the least possible risk. However, even supplementary antioxidants are likely to produce more benefit than harm in most people for primary cancer prevention. This is not always true, and some primary prevention clinical trials were aborted when the risk seemed higher in those receiving antioxidants. An example was a study done involving male smokers who received antioxidants in the Alpha-Tocopherol, Beta-Carotene Cancer Prevention Study (ATBC). Those who consumed the antioxidants had a higher incidence of lung cancer than those who received a placebo.

Once you have a diagnosis of cancer, multiple disturbing new studies in mice suggest that antioxidants may actually be harmful. It's true that mice are not the same as humans, but we use laboratory and animal research data to help guide us in the absence of clinical data, for both effectiveness and harm. Also, when several studies show the same thing one should be appropriately cautious and apply the Precautionary Principle and not overdo it.

Studies in mice using melanoma and lung cancer models showed that antioxidant supplementation might promote cancer growth and metastasis. These studies were performed in Sweden and Texas. In the study involving lung cancer, the antioxidants N-acetylcysteine (NAC) or vitamin E accelerated cancer progression. At the molecular level, they reduced DNA damage from ROS inside cancer cells and interfered with the tumor suppressor gene p53. In one study involving melanoma in mice, the number of lymph node metastases nearly doubled. On a molecular level, antioxidants reduced oxidative stress and DNA damage specifically in the metastatic cancer cells but not in healthy cells. In the other mouse melanoma model antioxidants allowed more metastasizing cells to survive. This means that it is possible that reducing oxidative stress through antioxidants benefits cancer cells more than normal cells.

The possible pro-cancer anti-oxidant effect is extremely concerning and means you should think twice about taking fistfuls of high dose antioxidant supplements after a cancer diagnosis. Further research will hopefully shed more light on this. For now, it seems safe and prudent to use antioxidants for primary prevention. Whether or not this applies to prevention of recurrence likely depends on whether or not all actively dividing cells have been eliminated with surgery, chemo or biologicals and radiation. It is anyone's guess if you have straggling metastatic stem cells remaining or not and impossible to tell using today's scans and blood tests. So, this calls for a risk vs. benefit discussion with your oncologist. Finally, it is far more likely than not that a prudent antioxidant whole food diet is safer than high dose supplementation.

Legal Overview

While the word "natural" carries a well-intentioned and warm feeling, "natural" does not necessarily equal safe regarding supplements. Unfortunately, there is a popular statement in circulation that supplements and herbals have never killed anyone and that drugs do. While it is absolutely true that drugs and drug interactions and "mistakes" in drug administration definitely kill people, the truth is that no one really knows how many bad effects there are from supplement and herbal use. Other than voluntary reporting, no one is watching, at least not to the degree that prescription medications are monitored. This is due to a law that was passed in 1994 regarding FDA regulation of supplements.

The FDA regulates dietary supplements under a different set of regulations than those covering "conventional" foods and drug products (prescription and over-the-counter medications). Even before release, new drugs are scrutinized with an eagle eye at multiple levels by drug companies and the FDA, but not every harm is caught during clinical trials. Drugs found to be dangerous after release (e.g. Vioxx®) get pulled from the market, albeit sometimes later than we all would have hoped. However, under the Dietary Supplement Health and Education Act of 1994 (DSHEA), it is only the dietary supplement manufacturer that is responsible for ensuring that a dietary supplement is safe before it is marketed, not the FDA. The FDA is responsible for taking action against any unsafe dietary supplement product after it reaches the market. This occurs only if and when the FDA finds out about problems. Also, manufacturers do not need to register their products with FDA nor get FDA approval before producing dietary supplements. Manufacturers must make sure that product label information is truthful and not misleading. Everyone is mad at the FDA, but do you see a potential conflict of interest here with manufacturers? If they know that there is a problem with their product; they are on the honor system. If unscrupulous, they can hide problems with their product until and if they are caught.

FDA's post-marketing responsibilities include monitoring safety. This includes monitoring voluntary dietary supplement adverse event reporting and product information evaluation. It also includes evaluation of misrepresentation on labels, inserts, and literature about what the supplement does. If a supplement is represented to act as a drug, it is pulled from the market and legal action is taken.

Regarding monitoring for adverse events, the key word here is "voluntary" adverse event reporting, which can mean "don't ask don't tell" on the manufacturers' part. Because of this, it is crucial to deal with reputable manufacturers. Otherwise, two things that you need to keep in mind: 1) no one is watching, and 2) buyer beware. Hopefully, anticipated changes to the laws will make it safer while not overly restricting access to supplements that people might choose.

Finally, many imported herbal concoctions are contaminated by animal excrement, dead critters and bugs and other not so nice additives. Beware where you obtain these products from and only use them with an experienced herbal professional. Bona fide experts can be hard to find, but someone who has completed coursework at an accredited Oriental School of Medicine en route to acupuncture certification often also has expertise in this area. Accreditation is problematic in itself because there are a lot of diploma mills out there as we discussed earlier in this book. So, performing due diligence is critical to your health. The best resource available to the public for free is http://mskcc.org/AboutHerbs. They even have a smartphone app for those who want to keep this information handy.

Dietary Nutrients vs. Supplements

One of the main core messages in this book is that whole foods beat supplements, whether synthetic or "natural," one hundred percent of the time for baseline anti-cancer requirements. However, we have also repeatedly said that there are some targeted exceptions to this rule or situations where a little more of something may be beneficial. That is what this chapter focuses on. It is not meant to be a reference for all possible anti-cancer supplement effects. Rather, it points out the particular benefits of very few specific supplements. Beyond this discussion, Chapter 19 gives you some more information on supplement and botanical solutions for specific treatment and cancer-related symptoms.

Far too many patients come to me saying, "I have a lousy diet. Can't I just buy a bunch of supplements that they say fight cancer?" Here's my answer and it is not just based on my opinion. It's based on scientific facts.

Read the next paragraph carefully, and then *read it again*, before going shopping for a gazillion supplements that will usually not help you and might even harm you. We have touched on some rather common foods which fight cancer or otherwise support your body. Do they all act the same way more or less? Although there is some overlap in function of various natural biochemicals in food, the beneficial activity comes in several forms and may be largely due to synergy between nutrients.

Various nutrients can interact and enhance different parts of the immune system, can act as detoxifiers, can help squelch free radicals before they damage your cell membranes and DNA/genes, and they can even have a direct anti-cancer effect. The latter three functions can reduce cancer promoting "hits" we discussed earlier. And that is just the beginning. In fact, the exact details of how beneficial nutrients interact optimally for health benefit are still largely unknown. Mother Nature may have laid it out for us over eons, but we haven't discovered it all yet. Therefore, walking around the health food store aisles and randomly grabbing what looks good, or Googling up the "best" anti-cancer supplements, or listening to random practitioners pitch anti-cancer supplements is simply gambling and trying to outsmart Mother Nature.

Why did I ask you to read the above paragraph twice? What I am strongly suggesting is that the main anti-cancer answer for today is still "whole foods," largely plant based, and not fistfuls of supplement pills made up of various synthetic concoctions. Artificial mixing of supplements in doses that are usually just made up for no particular reason cannot replicate Mother Nature's cancer-fighting arsenal. Mother Nature has reasons for nutrient combinations that humans have not even thought about, let alone figured out yet. Also keep in mind that supplements are artificially created using various manufacturing and synthesizing practices. This means they can contain harmful or at least non-useful fillers. Furthermore, supplements are often stored in crates and warehouses for some period of time, exposed to the elements in some cases; then they sit on store shelves for another unknown period of time. All the while, they don't usually go "bad," but can be losing potency. Sure, they all sport an expiration date, but that is based on pure guesswork.

Even so-called "whole food" supplement pills are created using some kind of proprietary enzymatic or heat process to extract nutrients from the whole food sources. In doing so, there is a good chance that some of the best nutrients are left behind.

Stop and think about it. They are trying to outsmart Mother Nature's plan in this complicated nutrient-nutrient symphony orchestra synergy. Outsmarting Mother Nature simply cannot be done with today's knowledge. There are a few exceptions where focused supplements might be of benefit, and we'll address these shortly.

To clarify, many nutrients help prevent cancer or support health in general but the best way to get these nutrients is through diet, not processed supplements. Also, although it may seem logical to think that more of something good is better, in this case, it is not and can be dangerous. In other words, if you take in a nutrient at a dose that far exceeds what you can get in a diet this becomes a "pharmaceutical" dose, like a drug. This can be ineffective at the very least and at most can be dangerous or carcinogenic.

If you absolutely positively just won't modify your diet to a healthy one, then, by all means, you should go to the store and buy a lot of very expensive pills and powders to fill in your nutrient gaps. This is far inferior to whole food but is possibly better than nothing. I say "possibly" because you will never know if you are getting what the bottle says you are getting. For all the reasons outlined above, it is simply an inferior approach to supporting your body and defeating cancer. Just be careful.

The exceptions to this diet over supplements rule are primarily vitamin D, calcium, melatonin and possibly omega fatty acids if you don't like fish or are concerned about Mercury. Also, if you don't eat fermented foods, probiotics and prebiotics round out the supplement recommendations. There are other targeted exceptions discussed in more detail as we move on. You will find them to be very personalized. They require close collaboration with a health professional rather than opting for a supplement store shopping adventure based on generic internet or book advice.

An additional circumstance that requires particular attention is the time around surgery. There are dangers and benefits of certain supplements and botanicals and we'll cover that in this chapter as well.

Vitamin D

Vitamin D is a highly recommended supplement because it is unlikely that you can get enough from the sun, even if you live in a sunbelt region. We know that people with higher blood levels of vitamin D are less prone to developing colorectal and breast cancer, possibly prostate, and likely many others. They may also have better outcomes after a diagnosis of cancer. However, we do *not* know if increasing vitamin D levels after a diagnosis improve survival or how it affects most cancers. So, the upside is unclear but achieving a mid-normal blood level is prudent and low risk with reasonable doses. Fortunately, you don't have to guess. Blood tests are readily available. The usual "normal" range of greater than 30 ng/mL may be too low for purposes of optimal health, especially in the face of cancer. Getting to 100 ng/ml or higher risks toxicity, mainly from elevated calcium. While there is no consensus, levels in the range of 50 ng/ml may be the best target.

Ask your oncologist about your Vitamin D level because this is potentially far more important than balancing copper levels or some other esoteric recommendations. Also, keep in mind that Vitamin D is essential for more than cancer prevention and support. It's healthy for your bones and possibly general immune regulation. Let's explore this further because it is one of the biggest exceptions to obtaining all your nutrients, vitamins and minerals from your diet.

Vitamin D exists in several metabolic forms, and the most bioactive form is calcitriol, which mainly controls calcium and phosphate levels. However, as far as supplements are concerned, it is extremely important to seek cholecalciferol (D3) and not ergocalciferol (D2). D3 is far more effective in converting to calcitriol and is more potent.

Most people think they can get enough vitamin D from sun stimulated skin synthesis. This is certainly the most natural way to get your daily required amount. Unfortunately, up to 30% of those who live in the sun-belt are deficient. So, if you are not in the sunbelt your risk of having low levels is even higher. There are also some downsides to sun overexposure, like skin cancer, including potentially life-threatening melanoma.

Related to the multiple "hit" cancer development theory which we discussed, you have to get multiple sunburns to get into trouble with skin cancer. But there's more to preventing sunburn and skin cancer than a lot of individuals recognize, and many sunscreens, unfortunately, contain a lot of potentially toxic chemicals.

If you are going to try to get all your vitamin D from sunlight, you need to know what is good about sun rays and what is bad. Ultraviolet rays, or UV rays, can induce skin cancer, sunburn, and untimely wrinkling of the skin. Ultraviolet rays can be further categorized as UVA and UVB rays. UVB rays are the ones that induce sunburn but also stimulate the most D3 production. These rays are more potent the closer you are to the sun, such as during the summertime, if you are at a higher elevation, and if you live closer to the equator. UVA rays induce untimely wrinkling of the skin and are present in the same potency no matter where you live. In other words, they can cut through cloud cover easily and reflect from many surfaces like water and sand. They can also penetrate thin T-shirts. The result is that you can get burned even when you think you're protected with clothing and a hat.

Vitamin D is a prohormone which promotes healthy growth and remodeling of bone. But it does so much more! Vitamin D affects neuromuscular function, reduces inflammation, and influences the action of many genes that regulate the proliferation, differentiation and apoptosis (normal programmed cell death) of cells. In other words, it works to help cells regulate themselves not to become unruly wild cancer cells. The good news is that it is stored in our body, as long as we make enough in our skin or consume enough as a supplement.

We do not synthesize vitamin D in the dark or with inadequate sun exposure, and there are no ideal guidelines for a "healthy amount" of sun exposure due to the risk of skin damage and skin cancer. So, what is the ideal situation? Some suggest 15-30 minutes of early morning or late afternoon sun when its rays are less intense. But this is highly individual and it's just a guesstimate.

Sunburn is prevented by blanking out mainly the UVB rays of the sun with any sunscreen lotion SPF 15 or greater. You are more likely to avoid sunburn by avoiding the sun's most blistering rays during the summer and before 10:00 am and after 4:00 pm, and reducing exposure time to the sun near the equator and at higher altitudes.

However, for skin cancer prevention and premature wrinkles, there's more to the equation. You need a sunscreen with both UVA and UVB protection or broad spectrum protection. The problem is that some sunscreens contain toxins, which can be counterproductive. To some extent, wearing a hat and some clothes offer some protection, but again we don't know how much sun we need exactly for creation of any specific amount of vitamin D in any given individual. So, you do need to expose some skin. How can you do this safely?

If you pick up most sunscreens, you will find a lot of chemical names. Most have been associated with toxic effects in the long run. However, two stand out as being safe: Titanium Dioxide & Zinc Oxide. If you find a sunscreen with these ingredients plus supportive skin friendly materials like aloe and vitamin E, you have found a winner. Keep in mind one more crucial point. Sunscreens, although prudent for reducing skin cancer, can cut vitamin D production in your skin by 95%.

As a final precaution, some chemotherapy drugs sensitize the skin to burning quickly. Please watch out! You can get a wicked sunburn while on chemo. Check with your doctor.

Fortified foods, like dairy products, generally don't contain enough vitamin D. Plant sources provide the inferior D2 form. Additional animal sources include fish and egg yolks, but these provide lower levels as well. So, if you can't get enough D3 through exposure to sunlight, supplementation is the alternative. The standard recommended daily dose is 400 to 800 IU per day. That may be fine for individuals who get a lot of sunlight, but grossly inadequate for most. It is true that there is no scientifically established optimal anti-cancer dose, and studies that have shown benefit have ranged from as little as 50IU to 4000IU per day or greater. Remember, toxicity is possible, and there is a suggestion that high doses may increase the risk of pancreatic cancer. This goes along with the admonition about antioxidants at the beginning of this chapter. Moderation is key and more is not necessarily better. However, up to 4000 IU per day is often recommended, at least in the short term.

There are a few precautions you should consider. If you take thiazide diuretics, your calcium levels may increase and cause problems like kidney stones. So, monitoring your intake of calcium is also important. If you take aluminum hydroxide as an antacid, vitamin D can increase absorption of aluminum from food, air and water and your blood levels may rise. Over time, this can be toxic and felt to be a contributor to the development of Alzheimer's.

Fish Oil, Flaxseed Oil And Omegas

We have already touched on this regarding dietary intake. To refresh, the human body cannot produce the main ingredients of fish oil, which are the anti-inflammatory omega-3 fatty acids: docosahexaenoic Acid (DHA) and eicosapentaenoic acid (EPA). We also can't convert pro-inflammatory omega-6 fatty acids (common in Western diets) back to omega-3.

Although plants produce omega-3 fatty acids, they are not quite as beneficial as those derived from fish oil for cardiovascular effects. That is interesting because fish do not actually produce omega-3 fatty acids. They accumulate them by eating algae or feeding on fish lower on the food chain. But the inter-conversion of omega-3 fatty acids in fish seems to create an effect that is measurably different from omega-3 fatty acids derived directly from plant sources, such as flaxseed. For anti-cancer effects, it is not clear if fish derived or plant derived omega-3 is better.

Fish oil intake appears to accelerate healthy weight loss and maximize lean body mass. Maintaining lean body mass, which is indicative of body protein levels, is crucial for fighting cancer. This is because there is good evidence that patients who have muscle wasting, as experienced in cancer, can slow this process down or even reverse it by taking fish oil. This could be related to both a physical effect and an antidepressant effect. To increase muscle mass, the dose has to be in the higher 5-10 grams/day range.

While many of the beneficial effects of omega-3 fatty acids are dose dependent (meaning more might be better to a point), there seems to be an upper limit in the 40-50g/day range at which point the benefits disappear, and stroke becomes a significant risk. Even at a MUCH lower dose of 3g/day bleeding becomes a risk. This can be made worse if you are taking Coumadin or other medications or herbs that thin the blood. Fatal bleeding internally has been reported, so please be careful with this. Trying to get a benefit while increasing your risk of very severe complications is very questionable.

The primary high-benefit omega-3 fatty acids found in fish oil are docosahexaenoic Acid (DHA) and eicosapentaenoic acid (EPA), both of which are potent anti-inflammatory agents and antithrombotic, meaning they thin the blood. The other is alpha-linolenic acid (ALA) and is important but not as important as DHA and EPA. On the other hand, ALA can be converted to DHA and EPA within our bodies and ALA is very much available in high doses from plant sources like flaxseeds. The problem is that conversion from plant based ALA to DHA in humans is not very efficient, even in healthy people. So, if you are vegan you can get some "fish oil" benefit without eating fish, but you might want to consider supplements to get DHA directly into your body.

In addition to many cardiovascular effects, DHA and EPA suppress multiple inflammatory cytokines, including tumor necrosis factor (TNF) and interleukin alpha. These are only the main effects. There is an arm length's more published biochemical data on the comprehensive benefits and risks of omega-3 fatty acids. But the main message is clear. Whether by plant intake or by eating fish, or supplementation, fish oil is an essential cancer-fighting nutrient.

Probiotics, Prebiotics And Synbiotics

Although estimates vary, it appears that there are at least as many microbial cells on or in your body as your cells. This includes what is on your skin, in your intestine, inside the vagina and so on. The roughly 39 trillion microbial cells are sharing your body space and are collectively known as the microbiome. Why are they there?

The Human Microbiome Project (HMP) was launched in 2008 and is trying to answer the question of what this all means. However, what we know is that these bacteria must be kept in a proper balance to maintain health. This includes not only intestinal, vaginal and skin health. It also impacts your immune system as a whole, helps with autoimmune disease modulation, and much more. Although seemingly far-fetched, your microbiome may be in communication with your mind. People with depression, anxiety, and autism have different types of predominant microbiota. Going even further, the findings of psychoneuroimmunology, microbiome research, immune surveillance and immune modulation activity overlap. In essence, you are not alone in your body, but the study of how and why this is important is in its infancy.

The definition and concept of probiotic supplementation have changed quite a bit over the last 40 years as well. We used to think that our intestinal bacteria or microbiota do not change very much, if at all, after the first three years of life under ordinary conditions. Cancer, chemotherapy, radiation, taking in a lot of toxins or even standard antibiotics are certainly not typical conditions. But even under typical conditions, dietary choices can alter your microbiome rather rapidly to accommodate for your vegetarian vs. omnivorous lifestyle. It is not simply "you are what you eat." Your microbiome's health is also based on what you eat, so that it can optimally help digest what you take in. With chemo and radiation, these microbiome changes are accelerated in the opposite or negative direction.

The new concept is that live microorganisms are not the only things that can benefit you, and the goal is not to simply replace harmful bacteria but to feed the "good" bacteria and their beneficial functions. So, providing "good" bacteria with prebiotics, which are nutrients for "good" bacteria, can help in many ways. Synbiotics are supplemental formulations than contain both probiotics and prebiotics.

So now that we have covered what probiotics and prebiotics are, how do they help? First of all, the typical conditions that are required for intestinal bacteria to be in balance are not always "typical" for everyone. Many factors can lead to a long-term shortage of "good" bacteria, which include chronic stress, poor diet and exercise habits, fatigue or frequent exposure to antibiotics, let alone chemotherapy and radiation. Therefore, the "supplementation" for your microbiome may be more important than ever to counteract these factors and the resulting intestinal bacterial imbalance.

In addition to helping keep the pathogenic disease-promoting bacteria away, probiotics can enhance the gut associated lymphatic function and reduce inflammation which decreases the migration of toxins and allergens across the intestinal mucosa. There are numerous research studies which support the use of probiotics in various conditions and diseases. Although unproven it is fair to consider that they would not hurt prevention either, even though the basic bacterial balance is difficult to alter in otherwise healthy individuals significantly. But since probiotics are safe in adults who have good basic immune function, there is little risk and possible significant benefit to taking them.

One big challenge is to figure out which species and strains (subtypes) of bacteria and probiotics are the best for any individual or any specific disease. Studies have not been done to that level of detail. Therefore, unfortunately, other than some specific disease-related research in the references section it is a scientific "best guess." In general Lactobacilli, Bifidobacteria and certain Bacteroidetes strains are considered beneficial.

Dosing is also unclear. For adults, up to 20 billion colony forming units (CFU) per day have been described in studies. The best chance for success is to take them on an empty stomach. This is when acid, which can destroy a lot of the bacteria, is at its lowest levels. Another unknown is what the duration of treatment should be. It varies depending on the reason for taking probiotics, but repeated doses are clearly required. Developing information suggests that probiotic spores (dormant form of bacteria), which are heat and acid resistant, may be a better way to recolonize the colon. This is because of the first problem, that being acid destruction of probiotic bacteria in the stomach. Finally, don't forget that *pre*-biotic nutrient formulations are also available which help keep the "good" bacteria growing. These are often packaged with probiotics. Here is a good example. Firmicutes bacteria are the sugar eaters, whereas Bacteroidetes thrive on fiber and vegetables. In patients who are obese, the ratio is heavily in favor of Firmicutes. Studies show that to lose weight, and thereby gain other health benefits, tilting the ratio in favor of Bacteroidetes is beneficial. So, you can influence your microbiome a lot by just adopting a healthier diet.

One cautionary note is in order. While probiotics reduce chemo related complications, there are cases that have been reported which suggest you should be careful consuming probiotics during periods when your white blood count is low. This is usually, but not always, mid-cycle between treatments. The cases involved sepsis (severe infection) from probiotic bacteria that are generally considered to be "good" bacteria and not pathogenic. This is a rare occurrence, but the caution here is not to over-do it because bacteria in your gut can get into your circulatory system. Finally, the American Academy of Microbiology reported in 2006 that "at present, the quality of probiotics available to consumers in food products around the world is unreliable." Unfortunately, this has not changed much to date. Your best bet is still dietary sources for both probiotic bacteria as well as the nutrients which support them. But if you buy a synbiotic supplement, which ideally contains spores, go with reputable manufacturers.

Melatonin

Melatonin is a multipronged anti-cancer helper. It may lower toxicity from chemo and reduce neurotoxicity, nephrotoxicity (kidney), myelosuppression, mouth sores and cardiotoxicity. It is also a favorable immune modulator and has direct anti-cancer effects. The downside is that it is a potent antioxidant and your oncologist may have a problem with that during pro-oxidant chemotherapy, so discuss this before starting to take melatonin. To help alleviate this concern, studies show that at least at one year, survival rates are better in many cancers when melatonin is taken. As mentioned already, a starting dose of 2.5 to 5mg should suffice as a sleep aid. Toxicity seems to be very low. Safely tolerated doses as high as 30-50mg per day have been reported in studies. However, if you're not used to it, this dose range can make you very tired and sleepy.

Minerals

Various minerals are necessary for your body to function properly. A handful of these are particularly essential for fighting cancer. In general, we get minerals in our diet from the soil, but obviously, it is not by eating dirt. Minerals are pulled in from the soil by plants, which means dietary intake depends on upon how rich the soil is where our veggies and fruits are grown. Another source is from the animals that eat the plants if you eat animal products. With a proper balanced diet, you should get all you need.

We require two categories of minerals, the macro-minerals (e.g. calcium, potassium, magnesium, phosphorus) and micro-minerals (e.g. iron, selenium, zinc, copper, iodine) that we need only in trace or small amounts. A proper balance is required for optimal health of all of these and more that were not mentioned above. But a few of these are more essential for fighting cancer, and we cover them below. So, if you don't get enough through food sources, supplementation may be helpful. If you're not sure, the levels of quite a few of these can be measured in your blood.

Calcium

This mineral is essential for bone health. You should aim for a total intake of 1500 to 2000 mg per day from all food sources. It has also been associated with a reduction in cancer risk in several types of cancer. The mechanism of anti-cancer action is unknown and likely multifactorial. Higher intakes compared with low intake can lead to a 30-35% risk reduction in colon cancer. A cancer protective effect may also be seen in breast cancer, especially in premenopausal years, and ovarian cancer.

Be careful. More than the required amount can lead to hypercalcemia and all the potentially severe complications associated with that. Also, higher calcium intake may be associated with increased risk of prostate cancer, so men should probably avoid supplements and let dietary sources suffice.

What works in one cancer may not in another. We will learn from nutrigenetics what the best solution is for individuals, but this is simply not known yet. Just make sure you take the recommended amount and don't push beyond that. Dietary intake is mostly from dairy, with relatively low amounts present or available from plants. The best plant sources are leafy greens and soy. Also, higher protein and caffeine intake increases calcium excretion. There are many other dietary factors which affect how much calcium is absorbed, excreted and retained. So, simply counting up how much calcium you are taking in and retaining from your diet can be tricky. This is why supplements are often recommended as it is a more reliable intake. As far as supplements go, some formulations have higher bioavailability than others with calcium citrate being the best, followed by calcium carbonate.

Selenium

Selenium is a key cofactor for antioxidant selenoprotein enzymes which help recycle the antioxidant glutathione, reducing oxidative stress on cells. Higher selenium intake seems to reduce prostate cancer risk, based on several studies but there have been conflicting troublesome reports. Studies are still underway to get to the bottom line. Other studies show that selenium deficiency might substantially increase the risk of multiple other cancers including those of the colon, thyroid, stomach, bladder, lung, esophagus, and liver.

Lab studies have suggested that selenium can sensitize breast cancer cells to doxorubicin, which may allow patients to take a lower effective dose. Interventional clinical studies in non-Hodgkin's lymphoma and head and neck cancer were shown to improve outcomes. So, there is something very significant in this developing story. There are many forms of selenium, but specifically sodium selenite, L-selenomethionine, and selenium-methyl L-selenocysteine have anti-cancer effects and seem to complement each other. Keep in mind that you only need to avoid deficiency and going beyond that is not well grounded in clinical data. Having said that, most studies have used doses in the range of 200 *micro*grams per day.

Magnesium

Magnesium is involved in hundreds of known biochemical processes in your body, one of which is insulin efficiency. It is probably through this mechanism that a major anti-cancer effect is present. Magnesium reduces insulin resistance and has been associated with a 12-25% reduction in colon cancer when consumed in a range of 320 to 350 mg per day. Since we have already covered insulin resistance as being a key factor in cancer genesis and progression, it likely affects other cancers as well. Dietary sources are green leafy vegetables, whole grains, and legumes. But we know that most folks are not getting enough, and magnesium deficiency is really at epidemic proportions in the United States. As another benefit, calcium and magnesium have been shown to reduce chemo-related neuropathy. So, supplementation should be a consideration here if there is a dietary deficiency. More is covered about magnesium in Chapter 19, within the context of symptom management.

Zinc

Zinc is an interesting story. It is a powerful cancer suppressor, yet at high levels zinc is toxic to most human cells. This is also the case for selenium, which again reinforces the concept that more is not always better. But in the prostate gland, special mechanisms have evolved to resist zinc toxicity and allow zinc to prevent initiation of cancer in prostate cells and to limit progression by inducing apoptosis. The beneficial effects are also clinically seen from studies in esophageal, breast and other cancers. Oysters contain more zinc per serving than any other dietary source.

Unfortunately, red meat, poultry, and dairy are the main sources in the American diet, which means if you are cutting these out you need to look for other sources you are not used to. This includes beans, nuts, lobster, crab, and whole grains. Optimal adult supplementation seems to be in the range of 30-65 mg per day, but if more than 50mg are consumed 2mg per day of copper is required to limit copper deficiency. The safest approach is to ensure adequate dietary intake in most cases.

Perioperative Supplements and Herbal Precautions

If you are about to undergo surgery or chemotherapy, there are some very special considerations to keep in mind. Mainly, you may increase bleeding risk and other potentially life threatening dangerous medication interactions (e.g. with anesthesia) may occur. There can be downsides and upsides to some of these. First, let's look at some of the potential dangers. The primary interactions we will be talking about are with medications used around the time of surgery. But keep in mind that some of these medications are also used with chemotherapy. Since a number of these complications are related to bleeding, bear in mind that chemo can reduce your blood clotting activity. So, additional blood thinning can increase the risk of at least bruising and at most catastrophic bleeding.

Echinacea

Echinacea angustifolia, Echinacea pallida, and Echinacea purpurea are the three most common forms of Echinacea botanical products. Most people take it as an immunostimulant for the prevention and treatment of various types of infections, in particular for the common cold. Unfortunately, how it works has not been determined and more recent studies over the past decade say that it does not work as well as originally hyped. This is because Echinacea is composed of many bioactive substances that probably interact, and can vary widely in potency.

Although echinacea is nontoxic and safe for most, its use has been associated with severe allergic reactions and liver toxicity. So if you are allergic to daisies, mums, marigolds, and ragweed you may experience an allergy to echinacea.

Many laboratory and animal studies have shown that echinacea acts as an immunostimulant. But the problem is that use longer than eight weeks may result in immunosuppression and poor wound healing. Immunosuppression is obviously not what you want in the face of cancer.

Ephedra

Ephedra is a central Asian shrub that is more commonly known in Chinese medicine as "ma huang." It is regarded as the world's oldest "medicine," discovered over 5000 years ago. It was a very common ingredient in weight loss and energy boosting products and remains a remedy for respiratory conditions like asthma and bronchitis. But it was banned for use in weight loss products by the FDA in 2004 because of excess cardiac complications and death directly due to its components of ephedrine, norepinephrine, and related metabolites. It's still available internationally at full strength, and online a lower dose ephedrine HCL (8 mg) is still available without a prescription for asthma treatment.

Overall, because of its high potential for cardiovascular complications, ephedra is regarded as one of the most dangerous herbal products, especially for perioperative patients. One of the reasons is that ephedrine is often used for low blood pressure and slow heart rate that can occur during surgery. Having taken ephedra or ephedrine HCL before surgery may increase this effect and overcorrect the blood pressure or heart rate. Ephedra can also interact with some anesthetic agents and cause arrhythmias.

If you are using ephedra or ephedrine HCL, it should be stopped at least 24 hours before surgery. Any heart or blood pressure or neurological conditions is an absolute contraindication to using anything containing ephedra, ephedrine HCL or possible "ephedra-contaminated" supplements.

Garlic

Garlic is also a long studied medicinal herb. It may lower cholesterol, help prevent or reverse atherosclerosis and blood pressure problems, is a natural blood thinner and has anti-cancer properties. These beneficial effects may be related to allicin, ajoene, and other metabolites.

The problem is that the blood-thinning effect, based on dose-dependent inhibition of platelets, can be dangerous when you're facing surgery. Ajoene can also increase the effect of drugs such as indomethacin, dipyridamole, and prostacyclin. The point is that it can interact with agents used around the time of surgery and possibly increase bleeding complications. Allicin can lead to lower blood pressure, which is great except that it might be a problem around the time of surgery. Based on pharmacokinetic studies which reveal how long garlic metabolites stay in circulation, it is best to discontinue use of garlic at least a week before surgery.

Ginkgo

Ginkgo has been used for natural treatment of various conditions from altitude sickness and vertigo, to memory issues like dementia and Alzheimer's. Many people take it for these reasons, mainly as a memory stimulant. It's probably the flavonoids and terpenoids that are responsible for these potentially beneficial but incompletely proven actions.

Ginko can also inhibit platelet-activating factor, which means it can, unfortunately, increase the potential for bleeding around the time of surgery. This is particularly the case if nonsteroidal anti-inflammatories like aspirin or ibuprofen are used at the same time. Lethal complications have been reported. Terpenoids are highly bioavailable and stay in your blood circulation for over a day. So, it is advisable to discontinue its use at least two days before surgery.

Ginseng

There are various forms of ginseng but American and Asian are the most commonly used. It's used by many as a "balancing" adaptogen. The main active ingredients belong to a group of biochemicals called ginsenosides. The potency is variable, and combinations in commercial supplements can vary, which make this a bigger challenge.

As with most of the other herbals discussed so far, it can inhibit platelet aggregation and adds risk for bleeding during surgery. In this case, the effect can persist for weeks like it can after aspirin use. Also it can lower blood glucose, which is a good thing except if it is before surgery. This is because patients are usually asked not to eat anything before surgery to make sure nothing is in the stomach that could come up and cause aspiration and pneumonia. Thus, ginseng use could lead to a dangerously low blood glucose level before surgery.

Elimination of ginsenosides varies from hours to a day or so. It is the risk of irreversible platelet function blockade that is the basis for a recommendation to stop its use seven to ten days before surgery.

Kava

Kava has been used as a sedative and anxiety relief agent, and there is some clinical data to support this. However, since there are over 100 varieties with different effects, the picture is clouded. It's also known as kava kava and the main activity is probably based on kavalactones.

Kava's known psychomotor effects led to the discovery that it is highly likely to interact with anesthetics and sedatives used around the time of surgery. These effects seem to be dose dependent, so the danger around the time of surgery varies depending on how much kava is being consumed. In the worst case scenario, this can risk coma. When used at a higher dose and for longer periods of time it can cause scaly eruptions on the skin. This is not dangerous but could interfere with wound healing.

There was a transient concern about severe liver toxicity based on a European case series published in 2001, but dozens of other studies did not confirm this. Nonetheless, since there are other concerns around the time of surgery who knows what other liver toxic medications may create this picture on an individual basis. Best to be cautious.

Pharmacokinetic studies show that kavalactones are excreted rather quickly in the stool and urine. So, the recommendation is to stop kava use at least 24 hours before surgery.

St. John's Wort

St. John's wort, derived from Hypericum perforatum, can help as a short term solution for mild to moderate depression, but not as a long-term solution. It's also
been used with mixed success for premenstrual syndrome and perimenopausal
hot flashes. The active ingredients are hyperforin and hypericin.

The biggest problem with its use is that it strongly stimulates the cytochrome
p450 liver detox enzymes. This becomes extremely dangerous if you are taking
medications. Obviously many types of medications are used around the time of
surgery and St. John's wort can interfere with dozens of them, creating potentially
life-threatening situations of all kinds. This can get even worse if other herbals are
being used which also stimulate the same liver enzyme pathways.

Based on pharmacokinetics, the half-life of all the metabolites of St. John's wort
ranges from nine to 43 hours. Considering the extreme risk here, it is best to
avoid taking St. John's wort for at least a week before surgery. Also, beyond surgery, make sure you look at the medications you are on and review them with a
pharmacist. You may be markedly reducing the effectiveness of your medications
by taking St. John's wort.

Valerian

Valerian is a commonly used sedative, a remedy for anxiety and a sleep aid. It's
derived from the dried root of Valeriana officinalis, and its main activity is probably from sesquiterpenes. It's dose dependent, so the more you take, the more of
an effect you get.

Around the time of surgery, a lot of sedatives and anesthetics are used, and valerian can amplify their effect. Also, valerian withdrawal has been the cause of
postoperative cardiac complications and delirium.

Pharmacokinetics show that valerian is eliminated in a complicated bimodal way.
This means there are two phases to its elimination from your body. For those you
want the technical information, the half-lives are one and five hours. But keep
in mind the withdrawal complications mentioned above. Either taper and stop
taking valerian several weeks prior to surgery or speak with the anesthesiologist
about it. As long as they know about it, benzodiazepine can be given after surgery

to treat symptoms of withdrawal if they occur. Overall it is simply best to stop using it several weeks before surgery.

Arnica Montana

Before we finally get to what may help you, I added this because Arnica is probably the most commonly recommended naturopathic (undiluted) and homeopathic (highly diluted) remedy for pain. Homeopathy is highly controversial, generally regarded as implausible by the National Center for Complementary and Alternative Medicine (NCCAM), but has growing scientific support for a few specific substances. Arnica is not one of these. It has been *proven* to be about the same as placebo for relieving pain in multiple studies. It simply does not work in either homeopathic or naturopathic mode. Interestingly the difference between the two doses is a factor of about 65,000. If you can't prove effectiveness within that large of a dose range, something is wrong with it.

Arnica has been classified by the FDA as unsafe because of multiple side effects. This includes bleeding after surgery if taken in undiluted naturopathic doses. It is especially dangerous if taken orally because it contains a highly toxic substance called helenalin. Watch out for its other names of Leopard's bane, mountain tobacco, wolf's bane, and mountain arnica.

Willow Bark

Bay willow, black willow, and white willow contain salicin and are natural sources comparable to aspirin. As such it has similar properties and similar side effects which include stomach ulcer risk and bleeding from thinned blood. Plain aspirin is not likely to help you with pain relief from major surgery and willow bark won't either. Also, risk of bleeding is not something you want to increase around the time of surgery. After the danger of bleeding post-operatively decreases, days or weeks down the line, then it becomes an option. Be careful if you are already taking blood thinners like warfarin. However, keep in mind that a plant-based diet contains salicylates from many fruits, vegetable and spices. The highest levels are found in cumin. So, mild postoperative pain may be relieved just by safely consuming these anti-inflammatory nutrients through food.

Potentially Beneficial Perioperative Support

Well, we've covered the dangers and some controversies. But there are also some potentially beneficial supplements that can help you heal faster from surgery and possibly help during chemotherapy and radiation. Every situation is highly personal. So, keep your treating physicians informed about any herbals or supplements that you are taking.

Capsaicin

Any surgical incision, from largest to smallest, can produce pain during healing. Also internally, even if the incisions are small like the case with laparoscopic or robotically assisted minimally invasive surgery, the surgical procedure may be substantial and cause a lot of tissue trauma. A lot of that can produce pain. Usually, you are prescribed pain medications, often narcotics. These may be very effective in controlling pain, but can cause you to be a little loopy and can cause constipation. Is there a natural way to minimize pain as an alternative or to reduce the amount of narcotics you might need?

There is evidence from multiple small studies and reports that capsaicin can help with surgical scar pain. This is the main substance in chili peppers that make them taste "hot." Several topical preparations are available, notably a "high dose" 8% patch. Mainly it has been used for residual pain after a Herpes virus outbreak (post-herpetic neuralgia) but has also been used for surgical pain relief. How it works is unclear, but likely related to the release of "substance P" and its effect on pain receptors.

Modified Citrus Pectin

Surgery done the wrong way may reduce your chances of survival. In colon cancer, the so-called "no-touch isolation technique" has been shown to provide a survival benefit of 6% over conventional technique where the tumor is handled more. It is also likely to be a better technique in pancreatic cancer surgery and liver tumor resection. It would not be surprising it this were proven to be the standard of care in all cancer surgery, but this has not been proven. Nor is it always possible. Why is this an issue? The problem is that surgery itself can increase the risk of metastasis. Research suggests that surgery increases tumor cell adhesion. During and after surgery, binding of cancer cells to blood vessel walls can be increased up to 250%, compared to cancer cells that are not exposed to surgical physiologic conditions. Unknown conditions during surgery and recovery may cause circulating tumor cells CTCs, which are cancer stem cells that have separated from the primary tumor, to attach to blood vessel walls and burrow deeper into their wall. This potentially sets the stage for metastatic tumor growth. Most cancer surgeons do not concern themselves with this, despite growing evidence that this is a truly important and modifiable risk seemingly under their direct control. Why? Because there are no reliable and proven ways to avoid this technically. Having said that, there are some low-risk options to try to reduce tumor cell adhesion.

Citrus pectin is a dietary fiber which can't be absorbed through the intestine. But when it is altered into a modified form it can be. It can then inhibit cancer cell adhesion by binding to cancer cell surface galectin-3 adhesion molecules. This may prevent cancer cells from sticking together and from binding to blood vessel walls. Although this research is mainly from mouse and laboratory models, early human studies are promising as well. It turns out that cimetidine, a heartburn drug, has similar effects. In several colon cancer studies, survival was almost doubled in those patients given cimetidine and felt to be related to this effect of preventing CTC adhesion to blood vessel walls. Improved survival was also seen in renal cell cancer and melanoma. Based on this, a combination preoperative regimen of modified citrus pectin (14g) and cimetidine (800mg) has been suggested. Although plausible, there is no clinical proof that this combination is better than either approach alone or that this strategy is truly clinically effective at all. However, other than some gastrointestinal disturbances and possible allergies, the downside is low. Regardless, do not try this without discussing it with your surgeon.

Honey And Propolis

Manuka honey from New Zealand, gathered from beehives around the Manuka *(Leptospermum scoparium)* bush, is used for the treatment of wounds of various types. It is antibacterial and initiates cytokine cascades which promote wound healing. It turns out that Cameroonian honey may have similar properties. Clinical trials may not prove that it is better than conventional methods, but it is a bona fide natural method to accelerate wound healing. Based on laboratory research, the flavonoids in Manuka honey are indeed anti-inflammatory and antimicrobial.

Bee propolis, which is a resinous mixture of pollen and beeswax, also has wound healing as well as anti-cancer properties. However, this is mostly based on laboratory research. Clinical studies in humans are absent, and there are reasons for concern for allergic reactions and no obvious benefit. Based on inhibiting the liver detox p450 system, dietary intake can also increase the activity of many medications. For example, with a normal dose of warfarin for blood thinning catastrophic bleeding can occur. Also, laboratory studies show that it can be pro-oxidant, mutagenic and cytotoxic to normal cells. So, oral dosing may not be safe.

In summary, oral administration is suspect, but topical application is potentially as efficacious as standard collagenase methods in enhancing wound healing in problematic open wounds. Both methods were deemed to be inconclusive by the independent Cochrane Collaboration, but both are used today in clinical practice. Thus there is a lack of consensus about the best method, but specific types of honey seem to be an option for topical therapy of problem wounds. On a final note, neither treatment is required if the wound is healing well. Collagenase and honey therapy are meant for problem open wounds that come apart after surgery due to infection or other issues.

Bromelain

Preclinical laboratory studies show that bromelain, derived from pineapples, can reduce inflammatory biochemicals like prostaglandin E2 and thromboxane A2 and reduce swelling postoperatively. It is plausible, but the clinical proof is lacking for oral bromelain having a beneficial effect. Also, keep in mind that part of normal surgical wound healing is some degree of limited inflammation. Bromelain can inhibit infection-fighting neutrophils from going to the wound, which may not be a good idea. On the other hand, in burn and complicated wounds, probably based on proteolytic enzyme activity, bromelain has been used topically to help debride wounds.

A direct anti-cancer effect for bromelain has been suggested as well. As you may have gathered from this book, a myriad of natural substances may have an anti-cancer effect but some have more scientific support for it than others. In this case, the suggested proof is only in the laboratory and not from clinical data. Bromelain can directly inhibit tumor cell growth, modulate the immune response, increase apoptosis, interfere with protein kinase cell signaling, and much more. However, so can a lot of substances tested in the laboratory to date. Rather than guessing about possible clinical effects and what the "optimal" bromelain supplement dose is, it is probably best to simply focus on including pineapple in your diet in moderate amounts. This may change with further research, but for now is the most prudent approach for oral use.

Vitamin C

Focusing on recovery from surgery, deficiencies in vitamin C can impair wound healing and high dose intravenous vitamin C has been shown to improve healing from massive burn injuries. Studies that have looked at intermediate doses in multiple wound models have produced conflicting results. It is certainly plausible that vitamin C helps all wounds to heal by facilitating collagen synthesis, but taking vitamin C supplements has not been reliably shown to do so. It is possible that beyond a clear deficiency, Mother Nature has designed it so that more is not better. Also, more can be harmful. We know that vitamin C can lead to kidney stone formation, intestinal cramps, and diarrhea, or more severe complications of hemolytic anemia in those who are deficient in G6PDH enzyme.

The potential anti-cancer effect of high dose intravenous vitamin C is debatable but somewhat plausible and should be subjected to more clinical research. But suffice it to say that high dose oral supplementation does not seem to help anything, is not anti-cancer and can make you feel miserable. Having said that, avoiding deficiency is certainly a goal and dietary sources from citrus fruits, veggies and berries are more than adequate for that. Likewise, a typical multivitamin dose of vitamin C is adequate for preventing overt deficiency as well.

Arginine

Arginine is an amino acid and has been recommended to enhance the immune system, increase athletic performance and accelerate wound healing postoperatively. Amino acids are the building blocks for protein synthesis, but arginine specifically is made by the human body. So it is not an "essential" amino acid per se. Strictly speaking, you will not become deficient by not consuming it in your diet, but it is argued that optimal levels can only be achieved with dietary intake or supplements. Dietary sources include red meat, fish, poultry, dairy and many plant sources such as soybeans, pumpkin seeds, spirulina and peanuts.

Around the time of surgery, arginine can be taken orally, in combination with eicosapentaenoic acid (EPA) from fish oil. This may reduce the risk of postoperative infection and improve wound healing. It can also safely be applied topically to potentially help wound healing, but this remains unproven.

There is a risk of allergic reactions, and combination with some herbs can result in low blood pressure, which is obviously a problem around the time of surgery. Herbs that interact include andrographis, cat's claw, and lycium. Also, it is recommended that you avoid arginine if you take medications for hypertension, heart conditions or erectile dysfunction because they can all reduce blood pressure to dangerous levels when arginine is added.

To better explain, the amino acids arginine and citrulline, taken together, increase nitric oxide in your blood vessels, which can naturally optimize your cardiovascular health. This can naturally help normalize your blood pressure over time. But if you are already on blood pressure medications or are heading into surgery when medications are used to help keep blood pressure in a safe range, blood pressure can fall too much.

Because blood pressure issues may arise, it is recommended to avoid arginine for at least two weeks before surgery. It is best reserved for the postoperative situation, within limits of the warnings we just covered. For topical administration, 4 grams of 12.5% arginine cream applied to the wound several times a day is likely safe. However, never use anything without first discussing this with your surgeon. Wounds differ, and you do not want to accidentally disrupt healing.

Chitosan

Chitosan is produced from chitin, which is a component of the shell of sea crustaceans like shrimp and lobster. It has been sold as a weight loss product because it may bind fat in your diet and not allow some of it to be absorbed. This has not been clinically effective, but what it does do is impair absorption of important nutrients such as fat-soluble vitamins (e.g. D3) and calcium. So, it's a bad idea to take chitosan orally. However, there is scientific evidence that it can promote healing when used topically on wounds.

Research shows that chitosan improves wound healing and hemostasis at the wound by improving the function of fibroblasts, polymorphonuclear leukocytes, and macrophages. It seems that this is independent of the blood clotting cascade per se. These benefits plus its natural antibacterial activity supports its use in postoperative bandages. The only warning is that it should not be used in anyone allergic to shellfish.

Eicosapentaenoic Acid (EPA)

Eicosapentaenoic acid, also known as EPA, is an omega-3 fatty acid found in fish and krill oil. Omega-3 fatty acids have many benefits as is covered in multiple places in this book. In the perioperative period, it is known to reduce infection and promote wound healing, especially when combined with arginine.

Generally, EPA is safe to take orally and even intravenously, but in the operative period it can inhibit platelet aggregation and increase the risk of bleeding. This is especially true if taken with herbals like garlic, ginkgo and ginseng and at higher doses of greater than three grams per day. Rarely there are cross allergies to aspirin, and multiple intestinal side effects have been reported. One troubling but clinically unproven effect in cancer is that EPA can inhibit natural killer (NK) cells and otherwise interfere with immune function.

So, EPA should be discouraged preoperatively and stopped at least ten days before surgery. It is also discouraged in supplement doses during chemotherapy, because of the bleeding risk. After surgery, in combination with arginine, it may help with wound healing as already mentioned. In the long run, this is a case where more is not better due to the potential bleeding and cancer facilitating effects. A typical dose of 5 grams of fish oil contains 72-312 mg of DHA (the other main omega-3 in fish oil) and 169-563 mg of EPA.

Given the risk and the benefit, this is another example of how Mother Nature's solution of consuming whole foods is best. No one on this planet has an Earthly idea what the "ideal" overall omega-3 dose is after considering all of the risks and benefits. Anyone that says different is either ignorant or a liar. So, instead of bickering about what supplement pill to buy, better to consume fish. Or if you really can't stand fish, consider plant sources of omega – 3 fatty acids.

Glutamine

Glutamine is the most common amino acid in the body and is synthesized by cells of most tissues. As such it is a non-essential amino acid, meaning your body makes it, and it is not an absolute dietary requirement under normal circumstances. By the way, it is in the same family as glutamic acid, which is a neurotransmitter but is different. It has been used orally and intravenously for improvement in wound healing because of the increased need for nitrogen in the repair process. In fact about one-third of the nitrogen that metabolically mobilizes to repair wounds comes from glutamine. Also it is depleted during the postoperative period because it is being used up for repair. This impairs white cell function, which increases infection risk.

Glutamine can be administered safely in doses up to 40 grams per day, either orally or intravenously. This assumes no pregnancy, no allergies to monosodium glutamate, no seizure history, and no significant kidney or liver disease. A cautionary note is that glutamine can be a preferred food for cancer, so it is not for prolonged use in the presence of cancer. This is often balanced against the beneficial effects it has, including reduction or prevention of chemotherapy-related neuropathy and intestinal support.

If you take seizure control medications, including carbamazepine, phenobarbital, phenytoin (Dilantin®), primidone (Mysoline®), and valproic acid (Depakene®), discuss utilizing glutamine with your doctor.

Ornithine Ketoglutarate

Ornithine ketoglutarate (OKG) is another non-essential amino acid which is made by the body but has been used to enhance athletic performance and to promote wound healing. It helps prevent glutamine depletion and can amplify muscle protein synthesis. While it's generally considered safe when administered intravenously, there is limited safety data for oral intake. The dose range reported in various studies varies from 350 mg to 30 grams per day. More is not necessarily better. One study which looked at the improvement in protein synthesis after hip replacement showed that 280 mg per day was adequate to limit glutamine depletion.

Ribose

Ribose, also known as d-ribose, has been used for increasing heart and muscle energy, increasing athletic performance and reducing fatigue. Especially around the time of surgery, it has been shown to substantially improve cardiac performance.

Ribose use is considered safe when administered either intravenously or orally over a short-term period, with most of the data being from cardiac surgery patients. Long term use safety and benefits are not clear, nor is an extrapolation to other types of surgery. However, there is a plausible reason to believe it can accelerate postoperative recovery.

Nothing is perfect, and there are some possible side effects that have been reported. These include a reduction in blood sugar, headache, nausea and gastrointestinal disturbances as the main issues. So, it is wise to limit the use preoperatively and discontinue a few weeks before surgery. After surgery, within limits above, it may help recovery.

Essential Oils: Rosemary And Basil

Rosemary and Basil can be used on your food as spices with multiple benefits. Here is a novel additional use to limit infection in the perioperative period or if you happen to find yourself in the hospital or other high-risk areas. Used as essential oils, rosemary and basil have strong infection preventing and fighting properties, even against antibiotic-resistant bacterial strains. You can rub a little on your hands, put a little on your upper lip or even soak a cotton ball and leave it laying at your bedside. Make sure you do not ingest essential oils. They are highly concentrated and may damage your intestinal microbiome. It is totally unclear what a safe oral dose may be. Test essentials on a small portion of your skin for allergies before using them topically. When used externally it's a low risk and potential high upside strategy for preventing infection.

CHAPTER 14
TOXINS: WHERE AND WHAT ARE THEY?

A very common burning question is, should you detox for cancer prevention or support? The answer is a resounding *yes*, but not in the ways that are usually pushed on us by slick marketing. This hype is usually related to weight loss or parasite elimination, rather than specific health benefits. There are too many fear tactics used in telling you that you are full of parasites, viruses, fungi and other varmints. Also, the usual detox "programs" are seasonal or every once in a while or when one wants to lose weight or some other artificially timed reason. These detox schemes often cost money and are essentially worthless because they all try to outsmart Mother Nature. It's not nice to mess with Mother Nature, with the risk of bad complications and even death. The answer is to help your body detox on a daily basis, and that's what we are about to cover in detail.

Before we get into how to detox properly, let's lay the background about the dangers of toxins.

According to the Centers for Disease Control (CDC), we are exposed to 60,000 chemicals on average every year. They are found in the food we eat, what we drink, the air we breathe, what we put on our skin and hair and so on. We are also exposed to over 200 radioactive substances on average per year. You simply cannot get away from them all. So, the trick is to assess your surroundings and limit exposure. Some toxins are relatively harmless in small quantities over a relatively short period, and that is what the Environmental Protection Agency (EPA) bases its exposure recommendations on. What is not accounted for is chronic exposure and the interaction of multiple toxins, which can accelerate development of a disease like cancer. The only one watching out for you is *you* in this regard. So be careful about choosing your personal care products and limit other exposure hiding under your sink, in the closet, in your carpet, and in your garage.

Toxins and pollutants are brought into our homes day-after-day through water, food, dirt, dust and household cleansing products. For instance, phenol is a serious toxin and may be detected in a few disinfectants, antiseptics, and air fresheners. You will be surprised when you discover how many "safe" and "approved" substances are slowly killing you every single day. Some of these substances you slather on your skin, your head, and even bathe your babies in. Some are even supposed to prevent cancer, such as sunscreens. They may be "safe" in that they will not kill you in a day or a week or even a few decades. However, in the long run, cancer and other diseases can be the result. Just like nutrients, toxins "talk" to your genes, except toxins do this in a negative way.

Continued exposure to phenols and other toxins might have injurious effects on our nervous and respiratory systems. It's crucial to educate yourself to enable you to cut down your risk and exposure. When you start to educate yourself about the chemicals and toxins on the labels of the products in your house, you should seek to substitute some of the toxic agents you discover with non-toxic options.

So, job #1 is to take a toxic substance inventory today! See what you're up against in your home and workspace. Remove or distance yourself from the worst offenders as much as possible. Some of these toxins are far worse than others, but determining the extent of the problem is in your best interests.

Before going further, it should be noted that the reason you may not be aware of a lot of proven or potential cancer-causing foods, products, and surrounding toxins is that the scientific evidence for this is not consistent. By that, I mean that in some cases it is proven in humans, but in most cases, it is mainly animal research data that is concerning or epidemiologic data is worrisome. The problem with epidemiologic data is that it does not prove that something causes cancer, it only points to a possible association. It is rare that epidemiologic data alone is so overwhelming that it can "prove" a point by proxy. This is the major problem with The China Study, for example. It strongly suggests that a plant based diet is superior, but does not prove it. While animals and humans are not the same, and epidemiologic data does *not* prove causation in most cases, consider the time-honored saying that "where there is smoke there is usually fire."

Without delving into conspiracies, keep in mind that a very strong profit motive is alive and well in most of the Western world. This means that there are many levels of possible deception or avoidance of changing products until the proof is overwhelming. It costs money to not grow livestock and chickens to as large a size as possible using hormones and antibiotics. There is more product to sell, and it is faster to get to market. It costs money to avoid putting potential toxins into a personal care product when that ingredient is the cheapest one that makes your hair silky and shiny. However, manufacturers are technically in the ethical "OK zone" and legally in the right because there is no absolute proof of harm. The question is, do you personally want to be part of the experiment or do you want to heed the "where there's smoke there's fire" admonition?

Precautionary Principle

In many parts of the world, something called the Precautionary Principle is often applied when there is some doubt of safety. I mention this many times in this book. Unfortunately, this is not a particularly strong movement in the United States. The European Union invokes the precautionary principle "when there are reasonable grounds for concern that potential hazards may affect the environment or human, animal or plant health, and when at the same time the available data preclude a detailed risk evaluation." This means the best available scientific evidence, whatever it may be, is looked at carefully and a recommendation is made on that basis. Do not underestimate the difference between this approach vs. that which exists in the United States where extensive proof is required before any mention is made of possible risk. This is critical to understand and apply liberally to protect yourself, not just from toxins but from literally everything that does not seem quite right.

Toxin Discovery Tools And Tips

Cautiously read the list of components on all labels of your household products to make certain you are not utilizing products that contain toxins. Review the following sites:

http://healthandenvironment.org/tddb

http://ewg.org

Click on the various chemicals you find on the labels of household materials. It will enlighten you greatly. You'll learn about a lot of risky substances, one of them being Silica that's detected in many abrasive cleansers, and about a potent reproductive toxin Toluene (which is found in many nail polishes). There are roughly 65,000 to 80,000 other toxins to choose from. Aren't we lucky? You cannot eliminate all exposure, but you *can* limit it.

Pick your seafood with wisdom to limit the measure of mercury that you absorb. Restrict the amount of canned tuna fish and avoid swordfish, shark, and bluefish. Instead buy salmon, tilapia or Pacific cod. Farm raised will have higher levels of Polychlorinated Biphenyl (PCB) toxins, but wild caught will contain more mercury. Nothing is perfect. Avoid frying food and utilize grilling, broiling or roasting cooking techniques. If possible, buy organic when selecting those fruits and veggies that otherwise have the highest pesticide levels. In all cases, wash your fruits, lettuce, and vegetables thoroughly because the pesticides can linger. This is especially true if you buy produce from other countries where the pesticides are not monitored well. Foods that are more likely to absorb pesticides are apples, peaches, strawberries, nectarines, cherries, lettuce, kale, celery, sweet bell peppers, collard greens, and potatoes. Wash them especially well under warm running water.

I will not get into the topic of GMO (genetically modified organism) foods here, except to say that as a cancer survivor or person at high risk for cancer it may be prudent to avoid them. This is purely based on the precautionary principle and absolutely no solid data. It's very important to realize that GMO was not invented by vilified companies such as Monsanto. The concept of genetic manipulation by splicing together different foods has been around since 12000 BC, but newer technologies have taken us to the edge of the unknown. We are unfortunately the subjects of a long-term experiment. While GMO efforts may arguably benefit humanity in many ways, like providing food where there would otherwise be starvation, we simply do not know the long-term effects on cancer causation. So, if you can identify them, you might want to limit intake of GMO foodstuffs.

All foods are not uniformly labeled, but the voluntary labeling of GMO-Free is gaining ground. Keep in mind that GMO is very pervasive and not just in a few foods. For example, it is estimated that 70% of processed foods contain GMO. Even if you stay away from processed foods, which you should do for other reasons anyway, the following foods are genetically modified in the 90% range: corn, soy, cottonseed, and canola. Do your research before your next shopping trip.

Set up a water filter to prevent the consumption of excess heavy metals (e.g. copper, zinc, selenium, mercury). You can review the performance rating of a lot of top brands of water filters by Googling water filter comparisons, where there are many sites to choose from. Keep in mind that some metals, like copper and zinc, are required for normal bodily functions. So it is the excess that you are trying to avoid for many of these, not complete elimination.

Attempt to minimize the utilization of Teflon or any pan that has a non-stick coating. The Environmental Working Group discovered that this cookware more rapidly reaches temperatures that bring about toxic particles and fumes. You might want to pick stainless steel or cast iron for your cookware, not aluminum which can leach into your food.

Never microwave in plastic. Utilize packaging that's labeled "microwave safe" or utilize glass or ceramic containers. Although the literature is controversial, many health advocacy groups feel that dioxin is brought out in plastic when it is microwaved. Ideally, even if it is a *plastic* labeled microwave safe, you should consider using glassware instead.

Be conservative about utilizing antibacterial soaps. They may contain pesticides that may be absorbed through the skin. Utilize a simple soap with water and scrub hands for twenty seconds.

Attempt to minimize the utilization of herbicides and insecticides. The toxic components can get into our system by skin contact and inhalation. Again, review the database links provided earlier in this chapter.

EM Radiation: Cell Phones

These days we are all wired with electronics, which means our exposure to electromagnetic and microwave radiation is higher than ever before. This is still controversial, but low-level radiation from your phone, in particular, can be dangerous over the years. In fact, the World Health Organization has classified cell phone radiation as a potential carcinogen in humans. We also know that children's brains absorb more radiation than adults do. So, protect your kids even more than yourself.

Whenever possible, do not put the cell phone up against your head. Radiation levels drop off *very* rapidly the further you are from the source. In the case of low-intensity radiation from cell phones even 6-12 inches makes a world of difference. Also, keep in mind that cell phones emit radiation all the time, not just when you are talking. So, try to keep it away from your body or at least body parts such are breasts and testicles that might be more susceptible.

Here are some tips. Use your cell phone speaker more often. Wired headphones and Bluetooth devices can still transmit radiation, but it is far weaker than pressing that phone up to your ear, especially for long conversations. Limit your use of the phone in weak signal areas because the phone works harder to transmit signal in these areas. Radiation shields have actually been shown to increase exposure because the phone is working harder to acquire a signal, so don't waste your money. Although less personal perhaps, consider texting more often rather than talking as this really reduces your exposure and still gets the point across.

Home Routines

Take off your shoes before walking into the house. Pesticides from outdoor dust, lawns and invisible toxins on the ground may be easily tracked from outdoors back into your house and persist there for long periods.

Restrict your use of bleach and utilize lemon juice alternatively for whitening. Just because a few companies are using great "green marketing gimmicks" don't trust the advertising. Read all components on your detergent bottles. Restrict a number of chemicals mixing with your clothes by averting the addition of any softeners into your washer or dryer. Anything you can't pronounce is not likely very good for you in the long run.

If you get any of your clothing cleaned by professional cleaners, let these clothing items remain outside for about eight hours to keep some of the chemicals and odors from returning into your house.

Vacuum with a good filter in place or for even more benefit use a "HEPA filter." A HEPA filter snares tiny particles that other vacuums might re-circulate back into the air of your house. Since there may be multiple allergens in your home, including dust mites, vacuum, and dust on a regular basis.

Personal Products And Cosmetics

Pick personal care products and cosmetics that are created by companies that don't use toxic elements, or at least fewer of them or weaker potential toxins. You can look up products on the web that you either are presently using or research data on products you are considering buying for known or suspected hazards. Although a product might be listed as a low hazard on a site, there's no guarantee that it's safe in the long run, especially if you are susceptible to cancer in the first place. It bears repeating that there are over 60,000 chemical toxins we are exposed to regularly. We have no idea how they interact to increase damage and cancer causation potential. This is completely unknown, and it is crucial to understand that the only one that is watching out for you is you. Remember the precautionary principle.

Keep in mind that although recent laws have improved consumer safety, personal products manufacturers do not have to get FDA approval for everything contained in their new offerings before going to market. So, you may not even be aware of a potentially harmful substance, and they can apologize later if they are caught with potentially harmful ingredients. Pick those manufacturers who have a track record of being as green as possible. You can find these using the links provided at the beginning of this chapter. Again, you can't stay away from all toxins, but you can minimize your exposure.

Before we get into proper detox, let's dive even deeper into toxins, both external and internal.

Major chemical toxin sources include aluminum, arsenic, cadmium, lead, mercury, alcohol and artificially created toxicants such as drugs, herbicides, pesticides, food additives, and preservatives. Most toxins are fat-soluble, which means they dissolve in fat. Bio-accumulation or bio-concentration of toxins can and does occur in fat cells throughout your body. This means not just your love handles or butt, but also all of the internal organs which can have fat in them. That is a lot of room for toxins to hide and cause damage and deterioration over the years. Once in there, you can't eliminate them with a weekend, a weeklong or even a monthlong detox.

Consider that body size and age also makes a difference here. The US Environmental Protection Agency standardizes its recommendations regarding "dangerous" exposure levels. Of course, one can debate the impact of having *any* level of toxins around us, especially those that are man-made. However, that aside, the standards are based on 160 lb middle-aged men. So, children are at higher risk at lower exposures for many physiologic reasons as well as older people whose detox mechanisms are not as effective. Over the past decade, the CDC has published reports on blood and urine levels of over 200 chemicals in a representative sample of US citizens. These 200 are those chemicals that are of most concern. It's sort of like the FBI most wanted criminal list. This list represents only a small sample of the 80,000 or so registered chemicals in the US, but it's a good place to start.

You may have a specific cancer-causing material in your house that is virtually undetectable. It is colorless, odorless, tasteless, highly carcinogenic and is present in over 8 million households (1 of 15 homes) at dangerous toxic levels. This substance is Radon gas. Radon is a radioactive gas which is produced in the earth beneath us and released into the atmosphere in tiny amounts, but when it gets trapped under a house it can concentrate, and higher levels can get into your house through cracks in the foundation. The good news is that your friendly neighborhood hardware store should have a cheap test kit available in the range of $10-15. This may be the best $10-15 you will ever spend. When you get the results, you should know that the US Environmental Protection Agency has set the "safe" level at less than 2 pCi/L. There are fairly inexpensive ways to siphon or pump this toxic gas away from your home.

It is very difficult to give specific advice on what to avoid since the list of toxins is very long and varies depending upon your personal environment. In other words, everyone uses different products, eats different foods and is exposed to different substances in different amounts. So it is not possible to issue a blanket recommendation of "things to avoid." It will be different for every person, but you can examine your personal environment and get rid of the worst offenders, which is mainly those things you consume or get exposed to on a daily basis.

Unfortunately, although information about potential toxins is readily available, "safety standards" take years or even decades to develop. So again, beware that something considered safe today is not necessarily going to be on that list into the future. Regarding food, drink, and personal care products, if you want a global golden rule to live by, here it is. Try to avoid long chemical names that you can't pronounce (with a bunch of letters and numbers) whenever you see them on package inserts.

However, let's keep things in perspective. Even good clean, pure water can be "toxic" if consumed too rapidly and in large amounts. In fact, you could die from the physiologic imbalance that occurs with drinking too much water too fast. This has happened in some unfortunate but well-publicized fraternity hazing incidents across the country. Another example is oxygen, which most people assume is a pure, healthy substance. Some of us even belly up to "Oxygen Bars," often found at airports, for a "quick detox fix." There is a reason why the air we breathe is not pure oxygen. Air is 78% Nitrogen, 21% Oxygen, and the rest is a mix of minor gasses. If you were to breathe PURE Oxygen over an extended period (days to weeks), your lungs would severely scar (fibrosis), and you would die. That is why extremely sick patients in the intensive care unit who have a need for higher oxygen amounts are "weaned" or backed off from high oxygen concentrations as soon as possible. If you are an "Oxygen Bar" aficionado, don't worry. The light masks and nasal prongs found at "Oxygen Bars" do not deliver 100% oxygen anyway. However, pay attention to what chemicals are used to make the oxygen "flavored." Some may be natural, and others may be full of artificial potentially toxic chemicals.

Having said all of this about external toxin dangers, to a large degree our bodies *can* eliminate toxins and deal with various chemicals and acute imbalances fast enough such that they will not cause problems. The problem is that no one knows exactly how much of a problem chronic exposure presents. It is logical to assume that the impact is much greater than generally appreciated. Also, it follows that we can help our body by minimizing exposure. We can minimize the risk that our internal detox systems get periodically or chronically overwhelmed and in this way contribute more to vibrant healthy longevity. The degree of benefit is scientifically unproven and is highly likely to be different from one individual to the next.

Lastly, while trying to live healthily and do good things for your body, please keep in mind that some herbs and supplements can be toxic themselves. This may be due to a number of things including 1) taking too high of a dose, 2) interaction between other herbs and supplements, 3) physiologic conditions which reduce your body's ability to clear the metabolites of herbs and supplements, and 4) due to interaction with prescription or over-the-counter drugs.

Internal Toxins

Now that we have covered the external toxins out there is that it? Is that all we have to worry about? The answer is unfortunately not.

Your body is an extremely active biochemistry lab, and in too many cases it resembles a toxic waste dump. It is a chemical factory with a large amount of byproducts being created every second, all of which has to be monitored for excess production and detoxified. Of course, there is no big visible smokestack spewing toxic smoke into the environment, but internally that is actually what is going on... just without the smoke!

These products and byproducts of thousands of normal and abnormal metabolic processes include blood sugar, ammonia, bilirubin, urea, creatinine, carbon dioxide (CO_2: which affects your acid/base balance), and many more. The key is keeping things in balance for some of these, as we have already covered. For example, balancing your acid and base by complex biochemical reactions in the kidney and lungs requires CO_2 gas. However, in excess amounts it is toxic. Likewise, you clearly need blood sugar to survive and feed normal tissues for energy. Processes called glycosylation and glycation occur when excess sugar (in diabetes and pre-diabetes) over time gets attached to proteins and fats forming advanced glycation end products (AGEs). These are toxic and form part of the reason for vascular damage, blood pressure problems and resulting organ damage (e.g. kidneys and eyes). By similar mechanisms, it is a risk factor for Alzheimer's. AGEs can also be introduced into your body through the process of cooking, which is one reason some health gurus advocate a raw diet.

The key to internal toxin control is to minimize the production of some of these or keeping things balanced in other cases. We will cover how to do that, coming right up.

CHAPTER 15

DETOXIFICATION

Clearly environmental toxins you eat, drink, breathe, touch or are otherwise exposed to have an effect in causing cancer. The debate is about how much of what and for how long. One thing is for sure. Too many anxiety-producing alarmists are missing the point. It's not just "one thing" you need to steer clear of like the residual mercury that might be in your tooth fillings. You have now learned that we have two sources of toxins: (1) external and (2) internal, and in most cases a combination of the two. However, before delving into proper detox let's cover a couple of "no brainers" to get rid of.

No Brainers

Hopefully, most readers of this book are beyond this. But if not, there are two MAIN no-brainers to "Just Say No" to:

- Tobacco (purely external)
- Junk Food (external internal hybrid)

No more hacking coughs, or losing money to "XYZ Tobacco" day in and day out. No more shortness of breath and no more social alienation. It's time to quit smoking and get up off the junk food couch potato lifestyle for good. Seriously. Your life completely depends on upon it, beyond beating cancer.

Limit obesity, metabolic syndrome and cancer by just putting that junk sugar candy fix down. Directly, sugar is the preferred fuel for cancer cells, and high glycemic index processed sugar fixes can only give you death through multiple diseases. Beyond that, sugar leads to obesity and a vicious cycle of internal toxin production.

You might be thinking that smoking and junk food are not in the same league. Nothing could be further from the truth. If you included a loaded gun, you would round out the trio of equally lethal threats.

If you are a smoker or junk food junkie, ask yourself, "Why might I be motivated to give up smoking or my sugar fixes?" This may be to prevent or beat cancer, to be fitter, to provide a better environment for kids, to breathe well, to lose weight, to save income, and the list goes on. If your "Why" isn't firm you won't stand by it. For instance, have you ever set a goal to do something and never adhered to it? I'm sure most individuals have. I know I have.

Why is it that occasionally we adhere to our goal and other times we don't? It's because of the cause behind it. If the cause to give up smoking or dropping the junk food is potent, and you truly believe it, you're much more likely to become a non-smoker and healthy eater.

Put your "Why" list on paper and keep it on you where your cigarettes or junk food commonly are. An illustration could be, "I'm going to become a non-smoker for…". Your causes should be very potent and motivating! Different individuals have different motivations for stopping smoking or junk food. Consequently, it's crucial to write your private reasons. Is " I don't want to get my cancer back and die" motivating enough for you?

When weighing your causes, ensure they're not based on pressure from loved ones/co-workers or acquaintances as this makes you less likely to adhere to your reasons. You have to strongly want to give up smoking or start eating healthy yourself, not base it on others' beliefs and advice.

If you carry cigarettes or have junk food in easy reach, you're more prone to give in just because it's there. It's crucial to discard your cigarettes and lighter and get rid of readily available junk food to guarantee they don't sway you.

Set the money you'd commonly spend on cigarettes or junk food in a jar. This is a very potent technique; many people don't sit down and work out how much they are really spending on bad habits annually. When you virtually see the income saved that you'd normally have spent on this stuff, you are more likely to remain motivated.

It's important to tell your friends and family that you have already quit because that is very potent psychologically. When individuals say "I'm *trying* to give up smoking or junk food" it isn't as potent. When individuals state they are trying to stop that gives them the reason to state, "Well it didn't work, but I attempted it!" This is not good enough!

When we achieve our goals, we're proud even though we don't always acknowledge it. So when you acknowledge you've quit smoking or quit junk food because of your "Why," make certain you're proud of it. Honor yourself with the jar of money you've laid aside!

Your habit may be that you smoke when you wake up, or get in the car, or have a cup of coffee, or after a meal or when you're stressed out. You may be tempted to sneak junk food when you're tired or stressed. Try this! Instead of the smoke or junk food, substitute them with a glass of fresh juice or better yet eat fruit, or another natural treat that you know you like. So when the itches are there, you need to alter your behavior. Anything is good just as long as you're distracted from a smoke or chomping on junk.

The simple reality is this. Please take note. This can save your life! There is something called the 80/20 rule or Pareto Principle. It says that you get 80% of your effect from 20% of your effort in almost anything you do. So, in this case, if you did *everything* else in this book and did NOT stop smoking or eating junk food, you lose! These two simple steps of no-brainer quitting outweigh *everything* else you can do. Conversely, even if the *only* thing you did is quit cigarettes and/or junk food, you would get 80% of your result in optimizing health and minimizing cancer. I would certainly suggest you do the rest, but this would be a tremendous start!

Second Hand Smoke

Keep in mind that inhaling second-hand smoke from those smoking around you means exposure to a lot of toxins and carcinogens. How much exposure is the critical tipping point remains unknown. Second-hand smoke not only increases lung cancer risk but may also increase breast cancer risk according to recent research. More likely the effects stretch to other cancers, but the proof is not yet available. So, you have a choice. You can either wait for the proof or prudently avoid second-hand smoke as much as possible.

Daily Detoxification

Beyond these obvious "no brainers" you can limit but can't completely avoid exposure to most toxins. Is there anything else you can do? Can you limit the toxins' effects on you? You bet! Your body processes and clears toxins through literally millions of metabolic processes and the organs involved include the lungs, skin, liver and kidneys. When the exposure is limited, your body can easily handle this alone without any major help. However, in today's day and age, the exposure is quite overwhelming, and it is prudent to consider helping your body out.

Given excess toxin exposure, one of the most crucial anti-cancer strategies you need to consider is rational science-based detoxification. We're not talking fad weeklong juicing or "water and lemon only diets" which can do more harm than good from the shock to your system. We're also not talking about hooking yourself up to a colon irrigator and flushing stool out of your system once in a while as if that is going to do anything but potentially risk harm. *No!* What we are proposing here is a **DAILY** routine of dietary intake, herbal and supplement use which helps your body's detox mechanisms function at their peak capacity. One has to be careful here because done the wrong way a "detox" program can actually be a "toxin" program and you can damage your organs. Detox is another exception to the diet over whole food rule to some extent. Let's dive into the extensive but important details.

First of all, what exactly is "detox" or "detoxification" when used in the context of cleansing or purifying your body?

Detoxification is defined as the elimination or decrease of accumulated toxins in your body. A toxin can be defined as anything which has a negative effect on your cells, the building blocks of all the organs and tissues of your body. As you've discovered, these toxins can be accumulated from exposure to the environment or produced by your body. The question is how long does it take to "accumulate" these toxins? The answer is, *very quickly!* It only takes seconds to minutes.

Common Detox Practices

An occasional or even a rather frequent periodic "detoxification" has become very popular, but misunderstood, means of trying to proactively "stay healthy" and "boost energy." Some gurus recommend detox on a "seasonal" basis or some equally arbitrary non-scientific recommendation. This may initially involve a liver detox "kit," a colon cleanse, an elimination diet or many other options. However, did you know that this periodic regimen is robbing you of optimal health and longevity? It is important....no, actually it's crucial...for you to know what each of these offers and what you need to do to maintain that boost you got from one these short-term periodic programs. It's easier than you think to get into an anti-cancer constant energy and health-boosting frame of mind by jumping into a three habits daily detox lifestyle. No more ups and downs!

So what's the secret? Well, your body's normal detox processes occur at the cellular, molecular and even epigenetic level. Huh? Don't worry, while it's important for you to understand why this is important, it is not necessary for you to become a molecular biologist or doctor or anything like that. However, we do live in a modern world and the scientific level of understanding about how the human body works is now at a very deep level. By reading this, you are setting yourself apart from the crowd. The sad statistic is that at least 75% of all adults are "health illiterate," which means they do not know how their body works. This leads to personal health decisions that range from bad to terrible. At least as far as your decisions regarding health improvement through detox go, you will be part of the health literate group after reading this. You will be able to make better detox choices in general and for anti-cancer specifically.

Isn't Intermittent Detox Enough?

Let's move on with some fallacies about intermittent detoxification. You will learn why periodic colon cleanse or liver detox is NOT lasting detox and will not carry you through healthy daily life for very long. Much of your body moves along on a biological time-clock measured by seconds to minutes, not days to months. An occasional detox "tune-up" won't cut it. This is especially true if you live the high paced partly junk food and entertainment "good life" between your detox tune-ups.

In fact, by the time you finish reading a few pages of this book, your body will have internally produced enough toxic biochemicals to kill several small animals. If you add a bit of exposure to household toxins that you are currently consuming, breathing or sitting near to, perhaps those animals can be a bit bigger: maybe even your size. Think of what this might be doing to you on a daily basis. You will begin to appreciate how a daily onslaught of external and internal toxins can accelerate the development of fatigue, susceptibility to infections and degenerative diseases like cardiovascular problems, Alzheimer's and cancer.

It has been estimated that ultimately up to 95% of disease is toxin related, cutting heavily into that 120-year lifespan we should be enjoying. This is highly believable when you consider that you are warding off a daily onslaught of external toxins as well as fighting internal toxic compounds that your body makes all day long, every minute and every second. The good news is that you can significantly control your exposure to external toxins and highly modify how your internal toxins are produced and processed.

Detox And Ancient History

Let's briefly review the history of detox. Historical, cultural vignettes for simple periodic detoxification abound. In fact, the premise of body cleansing is based on the Ancient Greek and Egyptian concept of autointoxication. This held that food, as well as the essential "four humours," can putrefy in the body and produce harmful toxins. These could be absorbed and linger. Early 20th-century knowledge, which was still centered on the humoural theory of health, supported this. Entire colons were surgically removed to "cure" autointoxication.

The Hippocratic theory of humoural medicine held that these four humors in the body were black bile, yellow bile, phlegm, and blood. When these humours were in balance, you were considered healthy. This theory survived for centuries, but in the 20th Century we learned so much more about the human body. Now we think in terms of cells, molecules and genes. Thus we have drilled down much much deeper into each of the humours and well beyond.

Today it is a big mistake to think of your body as a container which fills up with toxins that can be easily purged on a weekly, monthly or quarterly basis, instantly restoring lasting energy and youthful health. You are not a car which needs periodic tune-ups and oil changes. You are an extraordinarily complex human being, whose body requires constant attention. Give yourself what you deserve!

It's Not About "One Thing"

Before we get into the principles of ongoing effective detoxification, I urge you to think globally about health and concerns regarding toxins. In my opinion, it is a huge mistake to listen to some of the "experts" out there who focus on one environmental problem like Mercury poisoning (i.e. dental fillings or tuna in cans), as if eliminating that one thing will restore health or prevent and cure cancer. Instead of looking at the big picture, one can see how an overweight diabetic individual with a BigMac and Super Sized fries in hand might be scared into calling their dentist to have all their old Mercury amalgam fillings pulled and by so doing expect to become healthy and cancer-proof all of a sudden. Taken in perspective, while avoidance of heavy metal exposure is something to keep in mind, there are far more pressing detox issues at hand in the vast majority of people. That burger and fries habit, undoubtedly full of a gazillion preservatives, is far more likely to kill you than a few Mercury fillings. It's most definitely not just "one thing" to stay detoxed, healthy, vibrant, and as cancer-proof as possible.

How Does Your Body Detox Itself?

The major organs involved in active detoxification are the liver, kidneys, skin and lungs. The intestine is also the first line of defense in many ways, so it should be considered part of this essential group, but NOT in the way most people think in this day and age of "colon cleanses." It is far more complex than periodic colonic irrigation from below or swallowing of psyllium or other herbals to try to flush all "built up" toxins.

This book can't be a complete text in anatomy, physiology or biochemistry. However, some basics are important to review to understand how things work and how fast they work, to understand the need for daily detox. Let's quickly run through some of the most important ways our body's main detox systems try to keep us out of trouble.

Liver Detox Processes

Bile is produced by the liver cells (hepatocytes) to help digestion of fats or lipids in the small intestine. In the absence of bile, fats are not digested, creating a condition called steatorrhea in which the stool is grayish white and greasy. More importantly, this leads to deficiencies in fat-soluble vitamins (A, E, D, and K) and essential fatty acids. So, bile is not vile in the sense that is has very important functions.

Approximately one liter (1/4 gallon) of bile is produced per day. Liver cells add alkaline fluid with salts to the bile, almost all of which are reabsorbed in the small intestine to come back to the liver via the bloodstream to get reused. This cycles up to 2 – 3 times per meal, which give you an idea of how rapidly things happen in intestinal digestion and liver function at a biochemical level.

From an internal detoxification perspective, excess cholesterol is dissolved in the bile fluid and carried out into the intestine. When someone has high cholesterol, due to the way the biliary gallbladder storage is regulated using a valve at the small intestine, it can backup, accumulate, solidify and form gallstones.

Bile also helps in detoxifying natural processes by binding and excreting bilirubin, which is a byproduct of the red blood cell hemoglobin breakdown and regeneration process. Otherwise, elevated bilirubin levels are toxic to the brain, and we see people slip into hepatic coma and jaundice at the extreme.

Short of something like Gilbert Syndrome, which is a rare high bilirubin condition more often found in men, high bilirubin and toxicity in adults results only with major system breakdown or disease. On the other hand, Gilbert syndrome can go undiagnosed. Fasting, often used in periodic detox routines, can convert a mild Gilbert syndrome to severe.

Just so you do not come away thinking bilirubin is all bad, at low levels unconjugated bilirubin is a powerful antioxidant. So, here is another example of the body naturally keeping a delicate balance. It is possible to make things worse when doing things marketed as being "healthy."

Furthermore, because the bile is *alkaline*, it also helps keeps the intestinal contents acid-base balanced when excess stomach acid enters the duodenum or the first section of small intestine. Finally, biliary fluid salts are antibiotic in function and help kill some of the bacteria that may enter your system from food.

Elimination Of Bile

The liver has millions of bile ducts interweaving with tiny blood vessels which filter venous blood mainly from intestinal absorption. These ducts all join into the common hepatic duct which joins the cystic duct from the gallbladder, forming the common bile duct. Just before it connects with the duodenum, it also joins with the pancreatic duct which carries digestive enzymes. There is a tiny sphincter valve just at the entrance to the bowel called the sphincter of Oddi. When closed, the bile backs up into the gallbladder where it is stored and concentrated between meals. Later, when food enters the duodenum from the stomach, the duodenum secretes a hormone called cholecystokinin (CCK) which causes the gallbladder to release bile for digestion. When the sphincter is open, bile flows freely from the common bile duct into the duodenum.

So in short, liver cells process everything that gets into the blood stream as well as producing bile which takes fat soluble toxins and transports them into the small intestine. Once there, dietary fiber binds to toxins and carries them out through defecation. If the fiber content in the diet is inadequate, the toxins can be incompletely bound and reabsorbed into the bloodstream.

Toxin Biotransformation

The liver's first job is to take everything that comes through it via the blood stream and process it, neutralizing toxins (Phase I) and then making them easier to eliminate by converting from a fat soluble to a water-soluble state. This is called conjugation (Phase II).

Phase I Enzymes

The cytochrome P450 enzyme system involves over a hundred enzymes. Each of these enzymes is specific for one or more general type of toxins, drugs or herbals. Whoah! Before we go further, what is an enzyme? Enzymes are proteins that immensely accelerate the speed of chemical reactions. In this case, the chemical detoxification processing reaction is accelerated by these enzymes. The types of enzymes present in a cell help define what kind of metabolic process occurs in that cell. The P450 enzymes essentially dictate that the liver cells are aggressive detoxification machines.

The bad news is that individuals may be lacking in certain specific P450 enzymes and therefore can be more sensitive to specific toxins, drugs or herbals. For example, we can all see that some people are much more intolerant to alcohol than others. Fortunately, enzymes are neither created nor consumed in the detoxification process, which leaves the liver able to defend against continued toxin assaults. Also, enzymes can be "induced," which means that the total amount of enzymes available can be increased by certain chemicals, foods or herbals. This can be helpful in general detox, but it may interfere with cancer chemotherapy if the drug is metabolized too rapidly. An example of this is grapefruit, which induces detoxifying enzymes. Again, this is great, except when you are undergoing chemotherapy. Not all chemo drugs are affected but check with your oncologist or pharmacist. Essentially the body reacts to the presence of certain chemicals by saying, "hey we need more enzymes to get rid of these toxins."

An unfortunate byproduct of Phase I neutralization is the formation of free radicals, which damage cells and create an inflammatory reaction. When Phase I activity is inefficient or operating at extreme levels by trying to perform daily detox of too many toxins, enzymes in the Phase II conjugation process can be overwhelmed. In that case, free radical damage to body tissues is increased.

Phase II Enzymes

There are six main "conjugation reactions" which make up Phase II activity towards rendering the Phase I neutralized toxins water soluble. To be complete, their names are acetylation, amino acid conjugation, glucuronidation, glutathione conjugation, methylation, and sulfation. Each of these involves different enzymatically accelerated chemical processes, the details of which are very complex. The main thing to remember is that a "conjugation reaction" attaches various substances to the toxin which makes it water soluble and easier for the body to eliminate via the urine or in bile via feces.

Lung Detox

Your lungs perform two related but separate functions. One is taking in oxygen or respiration. The other is ventilation or release of potentially toxic carbon dioxide as part of your acid-base balancing system. The lungs can also clear the blood of any toxins which can take on a gas form, which is what the alcohol "Breathalyzer" test is based on. Both respiration and ventilation strongly influence other physiologic processes, like your heart function.

When properly functioning and not damaged by severe pollution, inhalation of toxic fumes, or smoking, the surface of the lungs can effectively ward off bacteria and viruses. On the micro-anatomic level, tiny filaments called cilia line the surfaces of the lung airways, and Goblet cells produce mucus. This mucus traps and the beating cilia sweeps or transports foreign substances back to the upper airways or pharynx where they can be expelled by coughing. On the micro-physiologic and biochemical level, the surface is highly active with macrophages and other immune system components to combat the invasion of inhaled toxins.

Shallow, subconscious and relatively rapid "chest" breathing is a typical pattern for many people. This is not efficient and reduces oxygen and carbon dioxide exchange, compared with abdominal or "diaphragmatic" breathing. This, in turn, influences the quality of tissue oxygenation, acid-base balance, heart rate variability, lymphatic flow and other effects. These changes are within a range your body seemingly handles well. However, on a micro level small chronic abnormalities may impact your health in the long run.

Skin Detox

Your skin has a dual job. It is the largest organ in your body and helps with both respiration (your skin basically breathes) and toxin elimination. Through evaporation that goes on every minute, accelerated through sweating, it can eliminate many toxins in your body. Your skin also has to protect itself against the toxic effects of radiation, including damaging rays from the sun. For this, it has a sophisticated protection and repair system. You can see this in action when you cut, scrape or burn yourself. As you get older, the skin starts to lose this ability to repair, particularly at the DNA level, and you start to get cumulative toxicity and visual changes like wrinkles and cancer.

Kidney Detox

The kidneys are very complex in microanatomy, physiology, and biochemistry. Here are the basics about how they work to clean your blood. Every time your heart beats, about 20% of the blood is pumped through the renal artery directly to the kidneys. The blood then enters the nephrons, which are microscopic filtering structures. There are about a million of those in each kidney. Each nephron reabsorbs useful components in the correct amount to keep balance in the body (e.g. salt), keeps the volume of fluid in the body as constant as possible, and filters out toxins and metabolic waste.

Once cleansed, the blood exits the kidney via the renal vein and goes back to the heart for circulation to the rest of the body. The waste products from the nephron system then exit the kidney into the urine, which is secreted by the nephrons in just the right amount to maintain fluid balance. In other words, if you are dehydrated you make less urine, and if you drink tons of water, you will pee like a racehorse to avoid overloading your body with fluid.

The kidneys also help maintain the body's acid-base balance, help maintain blood pressure and calcium balance, and secrete a hormone (erythropoietin) which keeps the production of red blood cells going.

Specifically regarding acid-base balance, the average American diet leads to a daily net acid load averaging 50–100 mEq/d. While it is scientifically debatable if developing a low grade "acidosis" in the body leads to chronic disease, the body still has to neutralize excess acid via the kidneys and the lungs through complex biochemical reactions. The lungs just blow off excess CO_2, but the kidneys may need to use up your body's natural antacid stores of magnesium, potassium, and calcium to neutralize the acid for excretion into urine. That, in turn, may affect your bone health and vitamin D activation.

The kidneys clear toxins in the urine which are initially water soluble or rendered water soluble by liver detoxification Phase II. Generally, drinking six to eight 8oz glasses of fluid per day allows the dilution of toxins and accelerates their departure from your body. The more you drink the faster you filter your blood and make or pass more urine. However, be careful. It is possible to overdo it. Your urine should be light yellow not entirely clear.

These toxins are both the external kind and the internal products of normal metabolism and nitrogen production. Key measures are your blood creatinine (muscle energy creation system byproduct) and blood urea nitrogen (BUN), which is a byproduct of the protein digestion process. When these are elevated, either there is an overload or an inefficient process in metabolism or kidney disease which reduces clearance. If it is kidney disease, then clearance of external toxins and their metabolites is also reduced. The kidneys must, therefore, be in peak working order or all the liver detoxing in the world will not help you very much.

Unfortunately, chronic kidney disease (CKD) affects over 20 million adults, which is up by more than 25% over the past decade. The cause is high blood pressure and diabetes in the overwhelming majority of cases, which is caused by "internal toxicity." Those tiny little nephrons we just discussed are extremely delicate and this it is almost impossible to detect significant damage until it is too late. So, even though Type II or adult onset diabetes may be reversible, the toxicity damage it induces like CKD is often not. It is, therefore, crucial to prevent this cumulative damage by keeping your internal toxin production (i.e. high sugars, inflammatory products) as low as possible. This is only possible through a daily program, which is what rational detox is all about.

Intestinal Detox

Our bowel, both small and large intestine, on average is about 25-28 feet long (20-23 ft for small and about 4-5 ft for large bowel or colon). It can be much shorter in women. When you swallow, food comes down the esophagus, drops into the stomach, then passes through the small intestine, then enters the colon (ascending, then transverse then descending) and exits via the rectum and anus. The small intestine (duodenum, jejunum, and ileum) is about 1.5 inches in diameter, and the colon is about 3 inches in diameter.

As already discussed, the common bile and pancreatic ducts enter the first part of the small intestine (duodenum), allowing bile from the liver & gallbladder and pancreatic juices to enter and help digestion. Bile of course is also carrying bound toxins from the liver. Digestion and nutrient absorption are largely completed in the small intestine, leaving the colon to resorb water mainly. So, if there is enough fiber to finish the detox process, very little of the toxins that come in are reabsorbed in the small intestine. They move on to the colon and out of your body.

If you artificially packed the bowel full of average foodstuff you might succeed in quite temporarily cramming in up to forty pounds, with the colon being able to hold about fifteen pounds max. However, the key is that, without severe disease, this is not possible through normal eating. Your intestine constantly moves on its own with strong, coordinated muscle contractions called peristaltic waves. It constantly pushes food all the way through for an average of about 1.5 bowel movements per day.

The average amount of time food spends in your intestine can vary widely. It is mainly a colon problem as far as food getting "stuck" inside you is concerned. Roughly, it takes about two to three hours after you eat for half of stomach contents to empty into the small intestine, and the process is usually complete by about four hours. Following this, half of the small intestine contents are emptied into the colon by about three hours. However, stool can stay in your colon for forty or fifty hours or even more, which might become a problem if this is your usual pattern.

Some of us have one or two bowel movements per day, but many people are relatively constipated and empty their colon once every few days. We know that foods degrade and a lot of metabolic byproducts are toxic, not to mention the chemical preservatives you take in every day. Since digested food transit time is mainly slowed in the colon and since we know that cancer of the small intestine is extremely rare a theory developed. Keeping your colon moving and emptying it at least daily is a very good thing and protects against cancer and other diseases like diverticulosis and inflammatory conditions. This "transit time" theory has not been universally accepted and the scientific evidence is rather weak, but it is plausible. Other related issues may be the reason for disease. People have different mixtures of intestinal bacteria types, different dietary consumption of toxins (natural and synthetic), different genetic resistance to disease, etc. However, while it is not proven, even mainstream doctors strongly suggest regular bowel habits as a good health goal.

Most of the above are related to mechanical passage and emptying of stool. The intestine also has an extremely complex and delicate balance of microscopic and biochemical processes which affect how food and associated toxins are broken down and absorbed. Some of this is handled through thousands of cellular biochemical processes in the lining of our intestine, the mucosa. Also, under normal circumstances, the bacteria in our intestines actually communicate with us on a cellular level to help maintain health in numerous ways including a major role in detox. This is a hot area of research.

Your small intestine contains very low levels of micro-organisms or bacteria compared to the colon. Normally in the colon, there is a delicate balance of a massive amount of "good" bacteria which prevents colonization or infection by disease-causing or pathogenic bacteria. There are many thousands of species, but the majority is made up of about fifty types or species. Did you know that the bacterial micro-organisms in your colon account for more than 90% of all the cells in your body? These bacteria are your friend and are there to help maintain the immune system part of your gut. They help prevent toxins from being absorbed, metabolize toxins, guide absorption of nutrients and much more. The particular species of bacteria varies by individual, varies by the area you live in and is largely determined during the first year of life. At birth, the intestine is free of bacteria. Then bacteria from the environment, including food, start to establish themselves in the colon. Once established it is not always possible to reliably change this balance very much over your lifetime under normal circumstances. However, cancer, chemotherapy and radiation are not "normal circumstances."

Here's a little more about the degree to which your intestinal immune system is important to your health. The intestinal internal surface area is very large, which means that it has a large area to expose to the outside world. Tons of toxins, viruses, external bacteria, fungi and parasites come streaming by every day. It turns out that this is where 80% of the lymphatic immune activity occurs in your entire body, through what is called the Gut Associated Lymphoid Tissue (GALT). Most people do not know that this is where the line is drawn regarding your first defense against the outside world. This is where much of your detox and disease fighting action is.

So, a critical takeaway lesson is simply this. It is not like your food goes through a rigid plastic pipe that empties into some septic reservoir holding tank and gets stuck there for months. You might find this in your home's plumbing, not your body. It is infinitely more complex than that and represents even more natural cleansing power on the microscopic level. If you interfere too much on this biochemical level, you can easily do yourself harm by throwing your body out of balance.

Looking at all of the processes we just covered, especially if you include more details about the immune system which are also critical, your body is already a highly tuned high performing symphony orchestra. It can be hard to outsmart and "do better" than mother nature designed things to be. However, you can still help your body in some fundamental ways. The key is to make this part of a daily constant gentle routine and also not to accidentally interfere with ongoing detoxification. This is where some people completely miss the boat, fall short of best results and risk harm by temporarily and periodically throwing their body seriously out of its very delicate routine and balance.

Intermittent Liver Detox Problems

The liver faces toxins every single second of every hour of every day. This means chronic exposure and therefore second by second work is required to adequately detoxify your body. A brief week to ten-day detoxification routine is simply not going to last and will not reverse the ongoing chronic damage. The good news is that the liver is a remarkably resilient organ and can regenerate very well. So, a longer term strategy can help you achieve maximum detox-ability of liver cells! We will get to how this is possible shortly.

Intermittent Colon Cleansing Problems

The next point is also worth repeating because you can badly hurt yourself with colon cleansing in oh so many ways. People seem to be fascinated because clean-ing a "dirty place" seems to make all sorts of sense. However, don't forget the healthy microbiome concept that we keep referring to. Bacteria, viruses, and even some parasites can be beneficial to your health. A balanced microbiome is central to your health and can be disrupted. Also, a major and dangerous misconception is that you accumulate garbage and gunk in your intestines that can be lost in there somewhere for years or decades. Folklore holds that people hold forty to fifty pounds or more of stool in their systems which includes food they may have consumed months or years ago. This is simply not true. The intestine is quite ef-ficient at propelling bile and stool forward, and the walls are metabolically active, both absorbing and producing mucus to help move things along.

The bowel is not like a rigid plastic sewer pipe that you need to take a bristle brush or high powered water irrigation to clean off the sidewalls of so-called "plaques." It just does not happen. How do I know? Aside from the science of anatomy, physiology, and biochemistry which completely debunks this, I have surgically operated on thousands of intestines over the last thirty years. As long as the patient has been having normal bowel movements and not constipated, the walls are often visibly squeaky clean. There is stool in there, but it is not attached with hooks or velcro or duct tape to the bowel walls. It is moving along. Going to the microscopic level, disrupting the bacteria attached to the bowel wall is disrupting your microbiome's health. Colonic irrigation and aggressive colon cleanses disrupt both bacteria within the stool and the bacteria on the intestinal sidewall. This sidewall bacterial microbiome is what you do not want to mess with because your health depends on it. I am going to repeat this until you get sick of reading it. *This is a very bad idea!*

Detox gurus often suggest periodic bowel cleansing to remove parasites. In the

United States parasite infections are rather unusual, estimated in the 5% range in the general population, and is mainly a problem if you live under conditions known as "waste to face." In other words, if you practice terrible hygiene or drink stool infected water or in some cases get a little too friendly with animals, you can get infected with parasites. Some parasites, like tapeworms, can go unnoticed with the only symptom being weight loss. However, with most other types you would feel pretty sick and not simply have some temporary symptoms of intestinal upset.

Parasitic infections do not lead to weight gain. If anything, they may result in weight loss! So colon flush detox will simply not work to drop a few pounds towards the goal of getting healthy. A rare and severe overgrowing infection by certain parasitic worms *can* cause an intestinal obstruction. However, in this case, you might not only be constipated, but you would also be very sick with nausea and vomiting.

To get rid of parasites would require a whole lot more than just a colonic flush. Some alternative herbal remedies may work, but often extremely slowly. Effective treatment usually requires some pretty big time anti-parasitic medicines unless you want to spend a long time being uncomfortable. Also, although this may sound unpleasant, keep your microbiome in mind and what it is made up of. Yes, it can contain some parasitic worms (helminths) or at least eggs thereof. It has recently been shown that the presence of helminths in the colon acts as an immune modulator, may actually reduce leaky gut and lead to less allergic and inflammatory-based diseases such as asthma. Since this can reduce inflammation, it may reduce the risk of cancer as well. This is something to consider when you are artificially messing with and altering the balance in your body. As usual, if you try to outsmart Mother Nature, you may be hurting yourself in a big way.

If you decided to indulge in the almost useless concept of colonic irrigation, you should know that colon perforations and serious infections have occurred, especially in the presence of diverticulosis (a common finding in older adults). This can lead to death. Also, this therapy, as with any artificial means to stimulate bowel elimination, can result in dependence on that treatment to normally defecate. Further, irrigating out normal bowel bacteria, which help elimination and detox, can result in repopulation of the colon with abnormal bacteria and infections which would require antibiotics to treat. You've heard of people getting nail bacterial and fungal infections after a manicure and pedicure in less than reputable establishments right? Well, getting an infection "where the sun don't shine" is significantly worse. Even good institutions can have a break in sterile technique and fail to kill bacteria from the last customer. Why risk this when there is no known scientific benefit and only marketing driven hype?

Herbal bowel cleansing preparations may be safer than irrigation, but this also alters the microbiome composition. Herbals can also lead to alteration in metabolism of common prescription drugs. If you are taking any medications, check with your doctor before proceeding. This might be a big problem if you are taking critical life-sustaining medications such as blood thinners or cardiac medications. Short of that, you still can't get away from the fact that the microbiome that you should be nurturing can instead be damaged by mindless colonic cleansing. This can alter your immune response and potentially put you at greater risk for just about everything related to intestinal microbiome dysbiosis.

Having said all of the above, remember the theory regarding "transit time." While stool is not trapped in the bowel for years, it can sit in the colon longer than it should for optimal health. Promoting regular bowel movements, as naturally as possible and ideally on a daily basis, is a major health goal.

Chelation Therapy

Chelation therapy works, when you need it for true poisoning with iron, mercury, arsenic, lead, copper and other heavy metals and toxins. The idea is to bind the toxic heavy metal and convert it into a chemical form that can be readily excreted by your body. This needs to be administered under very careful medical care. There have been fatalities reported directly related to chelation agents like EDTA. Furthermore, it is synthesized from formaldehyde and cyanide, both potent toxins. Having said that, there are botanical chelation agents but they are far less effective. There is nothing gentle and natural in this story. Practically speaking, 99.9999999% of the time you do not need chelation.

As far as fighting cancer, feeling good, being disease free and improving your longevity, you will get 80-90% of the way to where you want to be using way less dangerous and exotic therapies. Unless you have been diagnosed with clinical toxicity from heavy metal poisoning, you can consider exploring this option (carefully) when you are already 95-99% of the way to superhuman detox level, or you are offered to be part of a legitimate anti-cancer clinical trial. If you undergo a toxin panel assessment and higher than normal levels are found the best answer is to avoid those toxin sources rather than undergo expensive and possibly dangerous treatment.

Let's single out copper for a second because there is too much attention paid to this heavy metal in alternative cancer therapy. It is true that serum and tumor copper levels are elevated in multiple malignancies. So, chelation treatments with d-penicillamine have been proposed, but not proven, to decrease cancer progression. However, hold on a second, a new anti-cancer drug actually contains copper as the active cancer-fighting molecule. What's going on? Copper is a trace element essential to human and plant health and is critical to natural antioxidant activity. However, too much or too little leads to disease. Before pulling out the dangerous chelation cannons to eliminate copper from your body as if it were a villain, maybe a gentler approach might help. First, get your blood levels checked for copper and its carrier protein, ceruloplasmin. If they are normal, this is most definitely not your problem and focusing on the bigger picture will get you a lot further. If copper or ceruloplasmin is elevated a little, then how about reducing your intake first? Does your house have copper pipes or fixtures that might be leaching copper into your water? I bet it does. If not, look at other potential sources, but you may be forced to consider removing health promoting legumes and mushrooms from your diet. That may not be a good tradeoff. Get the picture? Don't fall for alternative hype regarding chelation and respect the balance Mother Nature has set up. Rather than blow it up, reinforce it the best you can.

SUPERCHARGING YOUR DETOX-ABILITY

This is where the rubber meets the road using identification and avoidance, prolonged dietary mods and boosting detox-ability. I would simply define detox-ability as your body's ability to detoxify. You can amplify your detox-ability a *lot*!

Liver Detox Potentiation

Supplementation can theoretically help enhance some liver detoxification processes, and provide antioxidant protection from free radicals. We know that these can contribute to the biochemical processes discussed. The question is how much supplementation in each individual is really needed. As in other areas discussed in this book, it is highly individualized, and accurate scientific data simply does not exist. It is plausible to consider supplementation based on the nature of the biochemical reactions, but the details are simply not worked out with respect to risk vs. benefit. In moderation, this is highly unlikely to cause harm and the theoretical, or proven upside is huge. The following information is at least partly repetitive from what you find in other parts of this book. I am including it here for continuity's sake and because these supplements are central to an ongoing detoxification. As also mentioned before, whenever you can get these nutrients from diet… you should.

Fish Oils And Omega Fatty Acids

The detox effects related to fish oil are based on limiting inflammation, which can lead to increased internal metabolic toxin production and chronic disease. Even though Omega-3 fatty acids are anti-inflammatory and Omega-6 fatty acids are pro-inflammatory, they are both considered "good" and essential for you in the right balance. Fish oils from wild cold water fish are the best-balanced source since wild fish eat more algae which are a rich source of the Omega-3 variant. Recommended total fish oil dose ranges from 1 gram/day to 2-4 grams/day. However, be careful. Excess intake can lead to intestinal disturbances, bleeding, and in very high doses even Omega-3 fatty acids become oxidants. In that case, antioxidants are recommended including vitamins C, E, and selenium, which are sometimes found packaged together in a capsule for this reason. The best strategy is not to overdo it.

If fish oil supplements are your choice over fresh fish, keep in mind that the dosing is NOT all the same despite similar looking labels. A 1g capsule of fish oil typically contains about 120 mg of docosahexaenoic acid (DHA) and 180 mg of eicosapentaenoic acid (EPA), but the total amount of Omega-3 can vary from 100 to 300mg per gram depending upon the type of fish oil.

The best marine sources of Omega fatty acids are lower on the food chain. Along those lines, New Zealand Green Lipped Mussels or Krill, which is a tiny shrimp-like organism, are some of the best. The higher you go up in the food chain, the more likely it may be contaminated with Mercury and other toxins. Of course, supplements are often monitored for toxins, but if you are looking at dietary intake, this is something to consider. Also, unless you have several million dollars worth of testing equipment in your kitchen, you will never know if the toxin levels are as reported on the supplement bottle or not.

Finally, you can also supplement your Omega-3 needs from flaxseed, which contains about 700mg per gram of oil in the form of alpha-linolenic acid. Other plant sources include green leafy vegetables, algae, soybeans and hemp seeds. These are not considered to be as good for heart health as marine sources, but they are still a good option overall. We covered more on this in Chapter 13 if you would like to cross reference.

Alpha Lipoic Acid (ALA)

Alpha-lipoic acid is an antioxidant that is made and found in practically every cell in the body, where it also helps turn glucose into energy. This should not be confused with another ALA, which is alpha-linolenic acid, an Omega-3 fatty acid. Unlike other antioxidants, which work only in water (e.g. Vitamin C) or fatty tissues (e.g. Vitamin E), alpha-lipoic acid is both fat – and water-soluble and can work throughout the body. It assists synthesis of glutathione, which is a potent antioxidant and helps the liver with detoxification.

In general, a healthy body makes enough ALA, but supplementation might help fight damaging free radicals and the dose range generally reported is between 100 and 600 mg per day. Animal models have shown ALA to have a protective role against heavy metal or chemical toxicity. Keep in mind that it's a very potent antioxidant, so consider avoiding it during chemo. This is mainly a post-treatment survivorship detox suggestion.

Vitamin C

Ascorbic acid is a storied vitamin. Unfortunately, there are many exaggerations along with the scientifically proven or plausible effects. As far as enhancing detoxability, vitamin C is an antioxidant and free radical scavenger, which means that it neutralizes them. Like ALA it helps increase glutathione synthesis, which you remember is important as part of Phase II liver detox.

As far as dosage, this is where part of the hype and exaggeration comes in. Grams and grams of vitamin C may lead to more side effects and toxicity than benefit. At approximately 500mg per day, 63% is absorbed. Absorption of powder is most efficient. Your tissues will achieve all that they need at about 200mg/day for a relatively short period, which is individual. Beyond this oral consumption, the excess is simply passed into the urine. Remember, we are talking detox here, not cancer therapy. Higher-dose intravenous vitamin C is being investigated, once again, as an anti-cancer therapy. That's a different story.

Vitamin D

Regarding detox, vitamin D has recently been discovered to help dial down fat. In that way, it can reduce the amount of toxins bioaccumulating in your body. Vitamin D can also directly affect upper respiratory infections, rheumatoid arthritis, multiple sclerosis, type 2 diabetes, and has an anti-cancer effect. Vitamin D is synthesized by the skin when exposed to sunlight but is activated in the kidney assuming enough magnesium is present. A solid day in the sun, assuming you did not block it all, can produce 10,000 to 25,000 International Units (IU) of vitamin D. Having said that, please avoid sunburn as this can lead to melanoma which is deadly. Also, keep in mind that many people who live in the "sun belt" are still deficient.

Assuming your sun exposure is not consistently at a high level on an every-day basis, supplementation is best. The Institute of Medicine has recently raised the daily minimum requirement recommendation to the range of 600-800IU daily, depending on age and sex. However, other expert organizations feel that is too low based on best evidence. A range of 2000IU to 10,000IU per day leads to the following effects: 1) promotes fat metabolism by reducing parathyroid hormone output and increasing fat breakdown by the liver, 2) activates receptors on fat cells, suppressing fat cell growth, 3) increases sensitivity to leptin, which tells your brain that you are not hungry, and 4) reduces fat accumulation in muscles. If you are not sure that you have "enough" circulating vitamin D, you can have it measured. Levels of 30-50ng/ml are considered sufficient to optimal, but it can be reported in different units. So beware of that when comparing results. For optimal anti-cancer effect, a higher level in the normal range might be better but unproven. The best strategy is to get your blood tested and not exceed the normal range. Liver toxicity can occur.

Vitamin E

Otherwise known as alpha-tocopherol, vitamin E is a fat-soluble vitamin and is a potent antioxidant, which is critical to daily detox activity and may support liver cell health. The average dose is 400IU per day and it best absorbed with meals. Excess dosage can thin your blood and make you prone to bruising and bleeding. This is why the upper limit recommended dose is between 1000 and 1500 IU. While this might be one of the least toxic of the fat soluble vitamins, other side effects like intestinal disturbances, weakness, fatigue and double vision have been reported. As with other strong antioxidants, use during chemo may be counter-productive. Also, there is no data that says more is better.

Magnesium

Magnesium is an earth metal element essential to the human diet. Over 300 enzymes require magnesium to function properly, including those in the liver. It is also critical for the formation of cyclic adenosine monophosphate (cAMP) which helps move ions across cell membranes. Rich sources include spices, nuts, cereals, coffee, cocoa, tea, and vegetables and green leafy vegetables such as spinach. Aging, excessive chronic alcohol intake and stress increase requirements. Magnesium citrate is available as the most bio-available oral supplement, but the dose varies. Higher doses (3-5 grams) can cause diarrhea and resulting dehydration. Ideally, replacement should be done based on lab values showing you are deficient. Although it is not a toxin, very aggressive dosing can cause you to stop breathing because at high concentrations it paralyzes muscle. It's a better strategy to maintain levels based on adequate intake of the foods mentioned above. Due to kidney regulation, it is almost impossible to overdose on dietary amounts, but it is certainly possible with aggressive supplementation.

Selenium

Selenium is an essential trace element. It represents a great example of how a toxic chemical is essential to life, and it is all a matter of degree. In tiny quantities, it is essential for cellular function and specifically for glutathione peroxidase enzyme activity in Phase II detox. In larger quantities, it is toxic and increases cellular oxidation. Good dietary sources include garlic, broccoli, onions and Brazil nuts. The daily dose range is 100 to 200 micro-grams, which can be accomplished by consuming one or two Brazil nuts. At only 910 micrograms acute toxicity symptoms like nausea and vomiting can occur, and a few grams (still a pretty small amount) is deadly.

Although controversial in many cancers, it appears to have a significant preventative effect against prostate cancer. There is one negative study which supposedly proved that selenium promotes prostate cancer, and that was the Selenium and Vitamin E Cancer Prevention Trial (SELECT). This study has since been criticized for its methodology and largely debunked. As such it's a great reminder that a single study, positive or negative, should never be used for treatment recommendations.

Glutathione

Glutathione is a vital antioxidant tri-peptide (i.e. essentially a tiny protein) and helps protect cells against free radicals and peroxides. In fact, the ratio of reduced glutathione to oxidized glutathione within cells is often used as a measure of cellular toxicity status. It is synthesized within the body. Thus it is not an "essential nutrient" like some other antioxidants which must be consumed as a nutrient (i.e. essential). Glutathione is crucial for liver detox function.

The best source of supplemental glutathione is through consuming fruits and vegetables. Taking synthetic supplement formulations is not recommended as they are not very bioavailable. Intestinal and liver enzymes deactivate them readily.

Taurine

Also known as 2-aminoethanesulfonic acid, taurine is an amino acid which is synthesized in the pancreas and then conjugated to become a component of bile. From a detox perspective, it stimulates bile flow. It is also an antioxidant and scavenges free radicals. It tends to be present in lower concentrations in vegans. So, even though it is not essential in the diet, if one were looking to optimize their detox plan it can be supplemented. Average dose reported in studies is 2 grams per day, taken in three divided doses.

SAMe

S-adenosyl methionine is a chemical compound synthesized and used throughout the body, but mostly in the liver. It is a "methyl group donor" in the chemical process of detox by methylation (e.g. one of Phase II reaction types in the liver). It is also helpful in bile flow stimulation and can help regenerate glutathione when levels fall. Nutrients required for its synthesis are choline, folic acid, and vitamin B12. Concentrations decrease with age.

Supplementation dose range for liver disease is 400-1600 mg per day, best absorbed on an empty stomach. However, caution should be used if you have bipolar disorder or Parkinson's disease. Also, there are possible other severe side effects if vitamin B6, vitamin B12, and folic acid levels are inadequate. These include increased risk of heart attacks, strokes, liver damage, and possibly Alzheimer's disease.

SAMe supplementation can also produce anxiety, insomnia, various intestinal side effects and dry mouth. This can occur with as little as 50mg per day supplementation. Based on this, perhaps the better strategy for many people is to maintain cofactor B vitamin supplementation and depend on your own body's synthesis of SAMe. Otherwise, it is best to consider this supplementation under medical supervision.

Milk Thistle

Otherwise known as Sylibum marianum, milk thistle is a flowering plant native to the Mediterranean region. It has been used for over 2000 years to help various liver problems. With modern science, we know that the active component is silymarin, which contains four flavonolignans. These are powerful antioxidants and enhance liver regeneration. The dose range is 140-210 mg per day of Milk Thistle, assuming it contains 70-80% silymarin.

Schisandra

Otherwise known as Schisandra chinensis, the fruit of schisandra contains the active flavonolignans which have the anti-inflammatory and anti-oxidant effects. Schisandra also improves liver detox by improving Phase II enzyme activity. The dose range is 500-1500mg per day of boiled schisandra tea.

Dandelion

Taraxum officinale may improve digestion and stimulates bile flow, while also exhibiting antioxidant and anti-inflammatory activity. Its leaves also contain various vitamins and minerals, especially vitamins A, C and K, calcium and potassium, among others. The entire plant has beneficial effects, and the dose ranges are as follows: leaf 4-10mg tea three times per day, root 2-8mg tea three times per day. As with any form of herbal or prescription substance, there may be adverse side effects. For example, at low doses, it may help prevent cancer, but at higher doses, it can promote cancer. Any bile flow stimulants should be consumed with caution in people who have gallbladder or bile duct conditions.

Artichoke

Cynara cardunculus has also been shown to contain compounds that are bile flow stimulants. These include chlorogenic acid, scolymoside, caffeoylquinic acid and cynarine. The dose range of leaf extract preparations is about 600mg three times per day.

Yellow Dock

Known as Rumex crispus, the active components are in the root and rhizome (i.e. the underground portion of the plant stem). Active components include oxalates, tannins, and anthraquinone glycosides. It is widely recommended as a digestive aid and works by increasing digestive enzymes and stomach acid. The dose range is 2-4 grams three times per day as a tea. However, severe allergic reactions can severely damage the kidneys and liver. Anyone with kidney stone problems or on prescription diuretics should avoid this preparation. If you still want to use this, use it only under medical supervision.

Water Fasting

To avoid confusion, please keep in mind that "intermittent fasting" which is very short and down to a twelve-hour eating window, or caloric restriction are not the same as fasting for days or a week or more. Intermittent fasting and caloric restriction have some anti-cancer benefits compared to prolonged fasting, which does not. Overall, as you will see, there is more risk than benefit. So, especially as a survivor, this is not a great strategy. Fasting, in an already depleted nutritional state that comes with cancer, can lead to very serious complications and weaken you further. Prolonged fasting also reduces the liver's ability to detoxify because nutritional depletion lowers production of enzymes. So, do not fast for detoxification and "cleansing" purposes. You will lose far more than you will gain.

Fasting is often recommended as part of an intermittent detox regimen and is defined as a period with water intake only. Keep in mind that if juices are involved, this is a modified fast and may lead to very different results. Also, bear in mind that toxins are more absorbable on an empty stomach, so keep additional chemical exposure to a minimum.

While there is a scientific theoretical basis for brief fasting, it comes with some drawbacks. First of all, when you fast your body rapidly runs out of glucose from your muscle glycogen stores. Other than possibly feeling run down until your body converts to burning your fat stores, your brain screams out and you are likely to experience headaches. When you convert to fat burning for energy you become ketogenic, and the brain has to learn how to run on ketones and not glucose, its preferred fuel. This can take a few days before your brain gets used to it, and this results in headache *pain!* Who needs it? It can be avoided if you approach detox as a daily habit rather than a periodic and unnecessary shocking stress on your body.

So what is the theoretical basis for fasting during periodic detox? Toxins bioaccumulate in your fat cells. Upon starting a detox regimen, these toxins can be released into the bloodstream at a more rapid rate as you burn the fat they are hiding in. So a temporary additional increase in symptoms (i.e. beyond those caused by ketones) can occur because more toxins may be circulating in your body. These symptoms can include fatigue or malaise and just feeling ill. First recognized in the treatment of syphilis, it is known as the Jarisch-Herxheimer reaction and may also occur during parasitic and fungal infections. As the infecting organisms die, their internal and external parts (exo and endotoxins) cause a severe inflammatory reaction with fevers and muscle pain, much like you would experience with the flu. This type of reaction has not been proven with removal of accumulated chemical xenobiotic toxins in your fat cells but remains a theoretical consideration. The reason I mention this is that damage that occurs at the cellular level may be quite severe but not recognized by your body enough to produce acute symptoms. So, even though you may not feel it, bad things can be happening at the cellular level.

So, as in everything else, moderation in approaching detoxification is reasonable. Since we are talking about a long-term detoxification process here for maximum safe effect, there is no reason to risk bad effects by jumping in too fast and too aggressively. First of all, the total toxin amount that you might theoretically purge from fat cells by periodic detox is relatively small unless you intend to mobilize all of your fat in 3-4 days. Of course, this is impossible. Also, instead of periodically risking side effects and increased damage to your cells (which then need repair) why not reduce the amount of fat you carry by longer term strategies of diet and exercise? Although this violates the popular fitness concept of " no pain, no gain," the reality is that in almost all systems continued maintenance is better than periodic emergency shock therapy. As an example, this is true in a simple system like maintaining chlorine levels in your swimming pool. Shocking a pool with high concentrations of chlorine destroys the walls of the pool over time and makes it unusable for periods of time. It is much better to keep the chlorine level in balance. If it's true in this simple example, it is certainly true for an infinitely more complex system like your body.

If you are truly in incredible shape and are looking for that last competitive "edge" to become a super-healthy survivor long past treatment, then looking at radical approaches is possibly for you. However, remember that you risk harm while thinking you are doing good. Keep the Pareto Principle (80/20 Rule) in mind. Stick to the basics. You will get 80% of your results the daily detox way and not suffer for it or do yourself inadvertent damage.

Kidney Detox Potentiation

Fluid Types

The kidneys do not detoxify most substances per se. However, they are a main conduit for toxin release via urine. To that end, dilution is the primary goal. The most commonly seen recommendation is to drink eight glasses of 8oz of water daily. With hot weather, exercise and any sweat-inducing activity this should be increased in direct proportion to fluid losses. However, keep in mind that this recommendation was designed for the average weight man in his 40's with no medical problems. The bigger you are, the more you need and the reverse is also true to some extent if you have a smaller build.

Protectants And Natural Diuretics

Water by itself may or may not be enough for acute or chronic detox needs. It depends on individual physiological age, possible existing conditions or diseases, type and degree of toxins and more. It would require huge studies that are likely impossible to imagine in order to capture all of the information needed. Therefore, any recommendations are totally theoretical and may lead to more harm than good in any given individual.

To keep the kidneys functioning optimally for as long as possible, the best strategy is to prevent and try to reverse effects related to diabetes and high blood pressure due to cardiovascular disease. Beyond that, keeping the urine flowing is key and additional antioxidants in moderate amounts are not likely to hurt.

Along the lines of additional protection, milk thistle containing about 75% silymarin at a dose range of 140-210mg per day has been shown to protect against certain types of kidney damage. This may or may not apply to all damaging toxins, but is a great start. Remember, milk thistle also protects the liver. So this is a "twofer."

Skin Detox Potentiation

Exercise

Exercise increases blood flow to your fatty tissues and by doing so may promote mobilization of toxins from fat cells. Also, exercise intensity which produces sweating allows you to expel numerous toxins from your body. It is likely that the list is greater, but a number of heavy metals, chemical toxins, and various drugs have been proven to be eliminated from your body through sweat. Sweating also loses water and various electrolytes like sodium, potassium, and chloride. So they need to be replaced. However, maintaining internal electrolyte balance is compensated by hormonal regulation through the kidneys, whereas the toxins are eliminated forever.

Saunas

Both the traditional Finnish sauna and infrared sauna have been shown to extend the detox effect of exercise through the same mechanism of sweat production. The Finnish sauna is a bit more controversial because of uncertain physiologic effects in people who have cardiovascular disease. The data is mixed, but the Finnish sauna has been used to actually treat congestive heart failure under close supervision. However, a less intense way to produce the same results is via the infrared sauna. It does not escalate to the Finnish sauna high temperature, thereby easing the concerns for people with some degree of heart disease. A number of routines involving exercise, sauna, and cool-down have been described. It can be a shock to the system, so be careful. Make sure you speak with a doctor about whether or not your body can handle this shock. You may need to work up to it.

Other than feeling good, repeated sauna sessions of 15 minutes/day over time is safe and effectively reduces oxidative stress based on reduced levels of 8-epi-prostaglandin-F2alpha. Therefore, this is a scientifically proven method to improve detox-ability through your skin, in addition to simply sweating out toxins.

However, caution is still necessary if saunas are routine. Dehydration needs to be avoided, and electrolytes (sodium, potassium, and chloride), and trace elements such as copper, zinc, nickel, chromium and manganese need to be replaced as well. Those with cardiovascular disease should be cautious and under doctor's supervision.

Massage

We know that specialized massage can mobilize lymph fluid quite effectively. Theoretically, this means that toxins moving through the lymphatic system might be accelerated by such massage. Of course, most of your lymphatic system is deeper than your skin. There are many more potential beneficial effects of massage including stimulation of acupressure points. Lymphatic toxin removal by massage remains unproven but might theoretically help if it were frequently used.

Lung Detox Potentiation

Breathing exercises can improve deep efficient diaphragmatic breathing and thus improve the ability of the lungs to clear toxins in addition to numerous other physiologic benefits. Breathing is an unconscious autonomic nervous system activity (i.e. you do not have to think about breathing, it just happens). However, the quality of breathing can be voluntarily influenced. This is the reason many cultures have regarded the breath as the core force of life. It is central to the whole concept of mind-body connection.

Through training to achieve diaphragmatic or abdominal breathing, you can achieve the following:

1. Decrease blood pressure and improve cardiac output with each heartbeat

2. Improve lung function, including detox-ability

3. Improve lymphatic and blood flow

4. Improve stress response and sleep patterns

5. Help flush out toxins

Here are a few daily breathing exercise tips:

1. Take one full deep breath every ten seconds

2. Place a hand on your abdomen and chest and when inhaling make sure that your belly rises higher than your chest

3. Take a slow deep full breath through your nose and hold for a count of six

4. Exhale slowly for a count of eight, then make sure you force any remaining air out by contracting your muscles

5. Repeat the cycle four or five times

6. Repeat the exercise several times per day

While you are in the middle of your breathing exercises, you can minimize your inhalation of indoor toxin vapors by making sure you have some plants in the house. Believe it or not, many common building materials used in most homes including carpeting, curtains, plywood and adhesives contain formaldehyde and other toxins. N.A.S.A. published a study some twenty years ago, confirmed by others, that the best plants for improving air quality and removing pollutants are golden pothos, philodendrons, and spider plants. The N.A.S.A. researchers suggested that for the plants to be most effective as "air cleaners" there should be one potted plant per 100 square feet of home or office space. If you are allergic to various airborne particles including plants and pollen, you might also consider a high-efficiency particulate air (HEPA) filter. Of course, if you live near a clean air outside area with lots of vegetation, consider doing your lung exercises there.

Intestinal Detox Potentiation

Stomach

First, when we refer to stomach here, we mean the acid-filled organ that helps digest food and not your "belly" and its associated fat, or love handles. The biggest detox issues facing the stomach are too little or too much acid and infection.

Stomach acid production is regulated by a part of our nervous system and several hormones. In the presence of several diseases, including age-related atrophic gastritis (present in 25% of the elderly), the amount of hydrochloric acid production in the stomach tends to decrease. Also, H.pylori infection can lead to reduced acid production. However, very old studies which suggested that we all start producing less stomach acid with age have been disproven by newer studies, better measurement tools and a better understanding of physiology.

Stress can lead to excess acid production. Therefore, stress reduction techniques are integral to any detox program. Also, there are several phases of digestion during which the degree of acidity in the stomach goes up and down by several pH points (a measure of acidity). The types of food you eat may buffer or neutralize some of this acid, and some may increase it, causing indigestion. This can vary greatly from person to person, and does not depend upon whether or not they "taste" acidic or not. So, best to keep a log and consider something like an elimination diet strategy to see if any given food group leads to excess acid production in you. Also keep in mind that we are only talking about the stomach here, not your total body acid/base balance which is way more complex and depends more on your metabolism, your kidneys, and your lungs.

The main infection problem is with a bacterium called Helicobacter pylori or simply H.pylori. Unfortunately, 80% of infections with H.pylori produce no symptoms, but the inflammation and gastritis it causes can lead to ulcers and even stomach cancer. If you have symptoms of indigestion, you might want to be tested for its presence. If found, the mainstream treatment is proton pump inhibitor antacids and antibiotics. Both are prescription drugs.

Prevention of H.pylori using natural means can be effective and the most likely to work are broccoli sprouts, fermented cabbage (kimchi) and green tea. Although much less effective than triple therapy with antacids and antibiotics, broccoli has also been reported to eradicate H. Pylori. Also, Vitamin C (500mg/day), Vitamin E (200IU/day), probiotics and N-acetylcysteine (600mg once daily), have been reported to help eliminate H. pylori when used with antibiotics.

Small Intestine

Other than coming down with duodenal ulcers (the first segment of small intestine), most people do not suffer much illness related to the small intestine. It contains far fewer bacteria than the colon and is the main site for nutrient absorption, varying somewhat by the intestinal segment (duodenum, jejunum, and ileum).

Although "leaky gut syndrome" has not been fully proven scientifically, there is more and more evidence for its effect in IgG antibody mediated food intolerance and is part of the basis for the "elimination diet" (i.e. elimination of certain nutrients from your diet for specific periods of time to see which nutrient is causing problems). It is plausible that changes in bacteria levels and types, certain drugs like non-steroidal anti-inflammatory agents, some intestinal inflammatory conditions and the like can cause disruption of the delicate intestinal barrier to the blood stream. When that happens, things "leak in" and cause problems, whether they be toxins or allergens in your food. Essentially it can adversely affect the intestinal microbiome, the GALT portion of your immune system and your entire body.

Omega-3 rich anti-inflammatory diets are your mainstay of detox protection in this area.

Colon

By now you should realize that the concept of periodic flushing of your colon by irrigation or enzyme-rich *artificial* psyllium-containing detox concoctions to scrape, irrigate or enzymatically chisel off non-existent plaques in your colon is simply not going to help you very much. At the worst, as mentioned above, it can also be dangerous and interfere with your intestinal microbiome's health. However, tuning up your body to have regular formed but soft daily bowel movements is a desirable daily detox goal.

In most cases, the commercial bowel detox preparations out there will not hurt you, but they are expensive and you will not be able to use them every day. Also, you would not want to because some of the components may disrupt normal colon physiology.

The daily detox goal is to maintain 1-3 bowel movements every day. You can do this by taking in 30 grams of fiber per day from any source you prefer. Simple, cheap and very effective. If you are an average person, you are likely consuming around 10 grams per day. So, what is approximately 30 grams of fiber in plain English? Well, you can look up options in multiple diet and cookbooks, but a simple recipe for achieving 30 grams per day is to eat 5 to 8 servings of fruits and vegetables per day, with a single serving being approximately 1/2 cup.

Probiotics are critical to your colon's health, and that has also been discussed in Chapter 13. Make sure you are taking not only probiotics but prebiotics as well to keep your microbiome well nourished and functional.

Summary Daily Detoxification Plan

In summary, effective detoxification is based on daily maintenance that will contribute to steady high energy levels and improved health. It is highly plausible that limiting your external toxin exposure, reducing your internal toxin production and improving your body's detox-ability will also add years if not decades of healthy vibrant life.

On a *daily* basis your new three step detox solution habits are:

1. Avoid external toxins

    - Shop for non-toxin laden organic foods and personal care items

    - Think before you buy & use household cleaning and maintenance items

    - Monitor your environment and avoid those things that seem "unnatural," as much as possible

2. Reduce internal toxin production

    - Low glycemic index, anti-inflammatory, anti-oxidant rich diet

    - Exercise daily 20-30 minutes cardio minimum

3. Improve your detox-ability through

    *   Daily bowel movements
    *   Diaphragmatic deep breathing exercises daily
    *   Hydration
    *   Selected supplements and herbals
    *   Probiotics & Prebiotics

Your body will appreciate you for your continued daily attention rather than periodic shock therapy like a pool might get with a chlorine shock pack. A daily detox routine is what is most likely to get you to a long life.

CHAPTER 16
EXERCISE

When people think of exercise and why it is a good idea they usually think weight loss and avoiding obesity. Some might be thinking it's a good idea for heart health and possibly avoiding some chronic disease. This is a good start and good points, but as you will discover in this chapter, it is so much more than that regarding direct anti-cancer effects. The most conclusive epidemiologic evidence is for postmenopausal breast cancer and colon cancer. Endometrial cancer is next on the list, but many others are not far behind regarding evidence. Keep in mind that even if the scientific evidence is limited for the claim that exercise can reduce cancer risk by 10-50%, what's the downside risk? This is the cheapest anti-cancer medicine you can find at any point in your journey, from primary prevention to prevention of recurrence.

First, let's cover the weight loss part. Why should you care about slimming down? Obesity itself has been linked to a number of cancers, including prostate, colorectal, breast, ovarian and endometrial cancer. This is likely related to effects on metabolism, diabetes, and reducing a pro-inflammatory disease-producing state in your body. Obesity is defined as having a BMI (body mass index) of thirty or higher. Bringing down your weight-to-height ratio brings down your BMI, which diminishes your risk of acquiring cancer. You cannot alter your height, so the only option left is your weight. Keep in mind that the BMI is only a very rough guide. For example, if you are muscular you can have a high BMI and be in superb shape. There are other ways to determine if you are in a healthy weight range or pushing obesity and related medical issues like metabolic syndrome, diabetes, and cancer.

Fast Tip: Measure your circumference at the belly button, not at your waist. It should be less than half of your height. If it is more, you have work to do.

While BMI (Body Mass Index) or height/weight ratio can give you an idea about healthy weight, measuring your circumference at the belly button is a better indicator. However, there is a lot more to it than this. For example, all other things being equal, obese adult males seem to be more at risk for colon cancer than overweight adult females. Likewise, particular body types appear to influence risk to a higher degree than others. Research indicates that additional fat in the waist (an apple shape) increases colon cancer risk more than extra fat in the thighs or hips (a pear shape).

If I could tell you exactly how to slim down quickly and easily, I would. However, regrettably, I am not aware of any long-lasting, quick fix for slimming down. There is no red pill or blue pill that will get you there, yet. Anti-fat pills are coming, but they may defeat the beneficial effects of exercise in the process. So, for the immediate future, don't look to pills or lap-band surgery or anything artificial. The best benefits will be achieved the old fashioned way: a healthy diet and exercise. The ideal mix depends on your individual situation and your tastes. However, both diet and exercise are staples in any serious anti-cancer strategy.

Precise mechanisms as to how exercise affects cancer are not entirely understood, but it is likely that these effects are multiple and it is most definitely not just related to fat weight loss. In fact, it has been said that calorie burn is really just a side effect of exercise compared to the complicated and broad effects on hormones and signal transduction that affect cells, both normal and cancerous.

Physical activity affects all phases of cancer development, meaning initiation, promotion, and progression. The following are the most likely mechanisms of benefit: (1) decrease of adiposity or obesity (2) effect on sex steroid hormones such as estrogen and androgens, as well as glucose and insulin levels (3) reduction of growth factor levels (4) oxidative stress reduction (5) deactivation of carcinogens and detoxification (6) decrease of systemic inflammation (7) immune function improvement and (8) direct effect on DNA repair and epigenetics. Many of these are highly interrelated, and you can dive far deeper into the molecular and genetic mechanisms, anti-cancer cytokine cascade activation and much more. Let's just say that exercise is not just epidemiologically linked to reduced cancer incidence. There are a ton of plausible and proven biological mechanisms to explain why this is so.

Most of the research and data related to the effect of exercise on cancer is primary prevention. In other words, it prevents cancer in the first place or is at least associated with other healthy behaviors that help reduce the risk of cancer. Does it work to prevent recurrence as well? Yes. We know that at least in breast, colon and prostate cancer, the survival is improved, although the reason why is not clear. It may be related to lower insulin levels, lower IGF-1, reduced oxidative DNA damage or a multitude of other possible mechanisms. It's cheap. It's easy. It's healthy. It might make the difference, and the effect is not minor. In one study, which focused on breast cancer, the risk of recurrence was reduced by 30%. Just do it!

Aim for thirty minutes a day, every day, of *at least* moderate exertion exercise. Studies suggest that 45 minutes every day may reduce the risk even more. If you are able, especially if you are not in the middle of treatment where this can be a difficult accomplishment, aim for *vigorous* sweat producing exercise. In one study that showed exercise improves colon cancer survivorship, the difference between mild exercise activity (3 MET hours per week), which did not help survival, and a vigorous program (27 MET hours per week) that did improve survival was substantial. A MET means Metabolic Equivalent of Task. One (MET) is defined as the amount of oxygen consumed while sitting at rest. Some examples are 23 METs for running at a 4 minute per mile pace, 7 METs for jogging and 3.5 METs for briskly walking. If you do a 3 MET activity for 40 minutes, you have done 3 x 40 = 120 MET-minutes (or 2 MET-hours) of exercise. So, aim for more than light exercise activity.

Exercise and Physical Activities	MET
Light or Semi-Sedentary	**< 3**
Sleep	0.9
Couch potato lounging	1.0
Working at a desk on computer	1.5
Slow walking or strolling	2.3
Walking at moderate pace (2.5 mph)	2.9
Moderate Activity	**3 to 6**
Leisurely bicycling	3.0
Brisk walking (3.0 mph)	3.5
Light home exercise	3.5

Exercise and Physical Activities	MET
Speed walking (4 mph)	4.0
Moderate bicycling, some coasting	4.0
Stationary moderate bicycling	5.5
Active sexual intercourse	5.8
High Intensity Activity	**> 6**
Jogging moderate	7.0
Vigorous exercise with multiple routines	8.0
Jogging aggressive	8.0
Jumping rope	10.0

Emerging research suggests "burst training" or "interval training," meaning rapid bursts of resistance and aerobic training, is better than slogging it out for hours on a treadmill or track. So, those 10-20 minute per day rapid workouts you see on TV infomercials these days actually have a very real scientific basis. You may or may not lose weight with them, but they are good for activating anti-cancer molecular pathways. The problem is that they can be a bit intense sometimes, so check with your doctor to see what you can incorporate. If possible, work in routines that definitely break a sweat. Ideally, work with a fitness and physical medicine professional. However, please remember that anything is better than nothing. If it's less MET intensive exercise or activity, just do more of it per week. Do not sit around.

Components of a good exercise program include resistance training, aerobic exercise, and stretching. It should be tempered by your medical or physical restrictions. For example, are your heart and lungs ready for vigorous aerobic exercise? Do you have physical disabilities which would mean you may have to focus on upper or lower body primarily? Did you have surgery, such as an axillary node dissection for breast cancer, which would modify what you can or should do with your arms? Is your abdominal incision healed enough or do you need to avoid core exercises for now in order to prevent a hernia? These questions and more are the reason you should strategize your individual exercise program rather than jumping into something that may not work or may hurt you.

Aerobic training can be ramped up. In other words, depending upon your limitations and baseline cardiovascular health, you can start lighter and amp it up. Instead of a 30-minute brisk walk, perhaps three separate ten-minute episodes might work better for you. Even gardening and house cleaning provide a work-out of sorts.

When starting resistance training, light weights or resistance bands are enough. Also, even with light weights or bands, you should start with a warm-up or you may tear a muscle or tendon. For strength training and some muscle building, you may not have to increase the weight load at all. It depends on your goal and baseline shape.

Stretching routines are the most neglected aspect of a good exercise program. This keeps your muscles and joints limber. It also helps with balance. In fact, stretching is part of a good warm-up routine before any resistance training starts.

A relatively small number of patients I have taken care of over the years came down with cancer despite being outright athletes. Does this mean exercise does not work against cancer? No, but it does mean that in some situations genetic influence overshadows lifestyle choices. This is not the case in the vast majority of folks. Some of my patients proclaim they have "always been healthy" and yet have cancer. In most cases, there are clear areas for improvement in lifestyle choices and exercise patterns. Generally OK health habits may just not be enough.

When you start in, make sure you: 1) enjoy the program you have decided to follow, 2) mix it up with aerobic, resistance and stretching, 3) dress comfortably, 4) remain hydrated, 5) possibly make it social in a group, 6) do not overdo it. Overdoing it can lead to frustration and giving up. Enhance your exercise incorporating music and meditation (along with Yoga and Tai Chi). There are many ways to go. Just do it!

Chapter 17

Alternative Cures or Discredited, Disproven and Dangerous Therapies?

There is a *huge* difference between the following concepts:

1. Unproven but scientifically plausible treatments

2. Unproven and scientifically *not* plausible treatments

3. Disproven or discredited treatments that have been tested and simply do not work or are dangerous and have no scientific plausibility

The difference between the first and second concept is especially crucial to understand. Something may not be proven in human clinical trials but has basic science, epidemiologic or animal data to suggest it is worth considering as long as it is reasonably safe. These are usually treatments or strategies that are about to be explored in clinical trials or are likely to be studied in the future. Alternatively, they may be low-risk propositions like eating a generally healthy diet to prevent disease. Finally, they may be things that make scientific sense but will never go to trials. For example, there will never be a clinical trial looking at whether or not it makes sense to put on a parachute before jumping out of an airplane.

As an example of what I mean, consider energy medicine. In particular, I am talking about radionics and the Rife bioelectric field generator. Until recently, this was scientifically considered a big stretch. Today, a very related treatment type called electric Tumor Treating Fields (TTF) is FDA approved for a particular kind of brain cancer. It is far more sophisticated but the same idea. You are about to learn about this treatment, and it is in clinical trials against other types of cancer. This is following a legitimate process to evaluate a concept that was considered complete quackery not long ago.

For the second category of unproven and not plausible treatments an example of what is never likely to be tested is full-dose cyanide as chemotherapy. It is an irreversible poison with no antidote. So, it is not a plausible and safe treatment strategy. Over the eons, it has only been used for committing suicide or murder.

What is plausible? It depends on the trail of science. However, by definition, it has not been proven through clinical trials. At the end of the day, it depends on the totality of science as we know it today, including everything from physics and biology through genetics and beyond. As I have said before, we do not know everything. However, we do know a whole lot about how the body works. When something does not make scientific sense within today's level of scientific understanding, it is probably useless. Could there be a finding 200 years from now that negates all or most of our scientific knowledge as we know it today? Sure. How likely is that to happen in the near future? I will let *you* answer that one. All I can say is, your life depends on either choosing between something that fits scientific plausibility vs. nonsensical and sometimes ridiculous conspiracy theory supported drivel.

The last category should speak for itself. Many supposedly "alternative" treatments are proven not to work and/or are dangerous. As mentioned several times in this book, pharmaceutical houses actively look for natural substances that can be used against cancer. These are often refined and are most definitely patentable once they are proven effective. Like many examples in this book demonstrate, they have been. So, if no one in industry is interested in it, it is likely baseless and not likely to help anyone. More on some blockbuster anti-cancer drugs derived from natural substances in a moment.

Natural Cure Miracles?

What is the true story behind patients who say they were "naturally cured"? They seem to be paraded out there as "proof" that natural therapy often, or even always, works. One glib short answer is miracles or near-miracles do occur, and "better lucky than good." However, it is like trying to win the lottery because no reputable published compendiums of rigorously documented "natural cures" exist. Having said that, there have been a few publications documenting spontaneous remissions from cancer and quite a few case reports of variable quality. However, even if you accept every single one as a truly natural or miraculous faith-based cure, a few thousand spontaneous remissions in the face of tens of millions of cancer cases diagnosed in the same time frame are a tiny drop in the bucket. No one doubts that they exist, but the odds of being one of them are indeed at a miracle level.

Let's put one thing to rest, and that is to say that potential natural cures are repressed in some way. To say that natural cancer therapy practitioners are denied publication is a bald faced lie unless they are indeed trying to publish junk or drivel and are refused for that reason after review. Anyone who has something to say, even if controversial, can publish.

These days, because there are thousands of peer-reviewed journals out there, anything even remotely decent can be published. In the worst case scenario, one can pay to be published in an "open access" journal, and it is not an exorbitant fee. It follows that some have failed to publish their results because their documentation is very poor. However, this is reasonable. Would you want to read something and bet your life on it if it were not based on facts or at least some plausibility? It is not that hard to provide the basic facts. Where is the pathology report and has a competent pathologist read it? Where are the labs and scans before and after treatment? What was the exact treatment? That's it for the basics, which is more than adequate for publication. In fact, you don't even need many patients to get your paper published. So-called "case reports" only require *one* patient to be written about along with some background information, and a "case series" usually includes a handful. Mind you that such case reports and case series are not the best science and they actually prove nothing. But they would certainly raise awareness about possible treatments to study further.

The reality is that even good case-series for "natural cures" generally don't exist, never mind randomized trials which can prove that something worked. The randomized trials that ARE published are almost all negative, meaning patients who were given natural therapy fared worse than those receiving mainstream therapy; sometimes far worse.

As oncologists we all have a handful of patients who seem to survive very poor prognosis cancers, defying the odds. Some of these folks have received mainstream therapy and have had "alternative" treatment as well. Which one worked? Quite possibly both had a role, but it is unfair to say that the mainstream treatment was worthless. It is always reasonable to go with natural support to do your part in cancer-proofing your body and trying to influence cancer stem cell dormancy. However, by itself, "alternative" is not enough 99.99% of the time.

In those relatively few well-documented cases where natural methods alone have apparently cured someone, the scientific explanation for this may be that the stem cells were regulated effectively by nutrition and epigenetics while the wayward cancer cells making up most of the tumor essentially burned themselves out. This is scientifically plausible but is just speculation. In other words, getting at the root cause actually may have worked in the sense that no new cancer cells were being produced to replace the dying active cancer cells. This is a very young area of research. While it is true that cancer cells are considered "immortal" by escaping apoptosis (programmed cells death, like normal cells) they are very inefficient and do actually die. So, if they outgrow their blood supply and die and don't have enough replacement from cancer stem cells, this "miracle" scenario is scientifically plausible but not proven. This is entirely speculative and the science of cancer stem cells is just evolving. The concept of epigenetically regulating cancer stem cells into dormancy is more likely to benefit a lot more people after mainstream therapy has eliminated or reduced the number of actively dividing cancer cells. While this may be promising, don't bet your life on it quite yet as the only therapy.

There are a couple more reasons that individual alternative treatment patient testimonials can be misleading. Too often their biopsy and other diagnostic data are not available. So, while I am sure they are well meaning and ecstatic to be alive, some may never have had cancer. Others may have had low-grade forms that don't progress for many years or are cured by a relatively small surgery.

Moreover, if treatment is given as an "adjuvant" to surgery for relatively early cancer (e.g. like chemo or radiation or hormonal treatment after lumpectomy) it is very possible that any treatment beyond surgery was not really needed. Say what?? You mean patients get "poisoned and burned" when they need not have been? The short answer is yes, but this is not based on negligent practice. In earlier stages of cancer chemotherapy is often recommended because it reduces the risk of recurrence. For example, with early ovarian cancer this might be a reduction of recurrence risk from 30% to less than 10%. That is a scientifically documented very significant difference based on randomized controlled trials. What it means is that is the worst case scenario, 70% of patients would not recur if they ignored this advice for chemo. Whether or not they use natural therapy after that point, they will be part of the survivor group no matter what they do. This is a point that is lost or misunderstood by folks who are offered "adjuvant" chemo or radiation after surgery.

The problem is, we do not yet know how to tell if patients need chemo or not after surgery with certainty. We do know when it reduces risk of recurrence from some percentage to a much lower percentage. This is based on research look-ing at hundreds or thousands of patients who received adjuvant treatment or not. Think of it as an insurance policy that is offered. In most cases we all buy insurance that we never use. In this case the insurance can be toxic, but it is a personal choice if that toxicity is worth the 20% reduction in risk of recurrence (30% risk to 10% risk). But to say that natural therapy "worked" when chemo is avoided in this case is egregiously misleading. We do not hear from those who tried natural or alternative treatment only and then die. So, just playing the odds, in this case at least 70% of the time you would be in a position to provide this misleading success-story testimonial. The same goes for adjuvant therapy in many other cancers, including breast, ovarian, uterine, prostate, colon, lung and so on. The degree to which it works to reduce risk of recurrence varies by stage and cancer type.

Contrary to crank naysayers, in the case of early stage ovarian and breast cancer, chemotherapy clearly saves lives. The ovarian cancer situation was noted above. In many women with breast cancer, it reduces the risk of dying from cancer by one-third (stage dependent). This may not be perfect, but it means tens of thousands of women are alive thanks to chemotherapy. In many other cancers, the results are favorably similar.

However, in some cancers, we know that adjuvant therapy does not work well, notably pancreatic cancer. Each situation is different, and a detailed risk-benefit discussion with your oncologist will help you decide which route to take. Keep in mind that as we move towards targeted genomic based precision medicine, chemotherapy will be relegated to the history books. This is not very far away and extremely exciting clinical trials are underway. So, we are moving rapidly towards far more effective and targeted treatments which will eventually also be far less toxic than the chemotherapy of today.

The bottom line is this. Exceptions and miracles do occur. But when trying to determine if something will work for you, testimonials from a few people don't come close to studies which have hundreds or even thousands of patients enrolled in it. The chances that something will work for you when it has worked for tens of thousands of others is far more likely than if it worked for a few random people here and there. For more information about how things are proven, and how this can help you decide what to do, please review the Appendix.

Kinder Gentler Therapies?

Other than the advent of personalized medicine and biologicals and the research noted above, there is no so-called "kinder gentler" or "non-toxic" cancer therapy available today that replaces mainstream treatment options. I wish there were. Such therapies *will* exist, and possibly relatively soon. I think maybe within 5-10 years we will have a reasonable number of these that will put chemo to bed forever. But they are not here yet, period!

Radical alternative proponents might mention Medieval therapy like black salve, or Blood Root, which supposedly can make tumors magically and painlessly "fall out." The damage this substance does is so great that it is incomprehensible how an ethical practitioner could ever recommend it. It is simply a very powerful caustic agent, like battery acid, that burns anything and everything it comes in contact with. As such it is dangerous. If used internally, the wrong dose or formulation can kill you. Wow! Kinder and gentler? More on this later.

Other examples include all sorts of "alternative" concoctions involving herbs, vitamins, extracts, radical food diets, juicing, energy therapy, and so on. Many are not only unproven but possibly dangerous due to unpredictable interactions between natural substances and medications. Also, many of these are provided in a spa setting where many dollars can be extracted from you. Be careful out there. It could cost you your life by delaying a chance for cure using proven therapies.

Having said that, this book is about guiding you towards those integrative and complementary therapies that can help improve your outcomes with mainstream therapy. This might be through strengthening and cancer-proofing your body or minimizing side effects or both. Even some of the supposedly "alternative" therapies out there may be decent to excellent when used as complementary therapies, alongside or after mainstream treatment. The key is to determine which ones those are. Since there are so many possible combinations out there, it is crucial for you to find an integrative oncologist or an oncologist who works with an integrative team. Each and every situation is very different, but science can be applied to guide you towards the best decisions.

There is an ancient Russian saying that loses something in translation, but you will get the idea. It says: **"Live a hundred years. Study a hundred years. Die an idiot anyway."** This implies that no individual can possibly know everything. My personal take from this is that being too rigid in making professional recommendations can be counterproductive to any given patient sitting in front of me. Before dismissing anything that I am hearing about for the first time I will review the merits, the benefits and the risks of it. Then I will provide my recommendation, taking into account everything about the patient in front of me, meaning details about their physical being, their mental and emotional state, and the status of their cancer. Is this primary treatment, recurrence treatment, palliative treatment or something to prevent recurrence? This makes a big difference.

However, having an open mind to newer better alternatives is not the same as having an appropriately closed mind to something "alternative" that simply does not work and possibly was never plausible in the first place. Hopefully, this book is driving home the point that patient-centered integrative cancer care offers a *lot* of improvements over conventional standards of today. At the same time, it steers you clear of quack remedies that can injure you and cost you quite a bit of money due to unethical charlatans being more than willing to take sucker money.

Look, lots of people come up with a range of brilliant to kooky ideas on many topics in life. Some of these go on to be a legend and even win Nobel prizes while others suffer infamy, or should. When life is in the balance, it is not prudent to fool around with kooky unproven and, even worse, disproven ideas. This means you are allowing someone to be their experimental animal based on an "idea" they have, no matter how brilliant their argument is. If an idea is truly meritorious, it is noticed, tested in the laboratory, then in the animal model, then in humans via a series of clinical trials. Many natural products may have some unpredictable but real anti-cancer actions, especially when used in pharmacologic doses. These are noticed. In fact, Big Pharma is more than interested as well. Mainstream cancer chemotherapy agents have been derived from simple enzymes to trees to sea squirts and many more natural resources. This is no different from the apricot pits (i.e. Laetrile or B17) story, except that over 100 years of hype about these amygdalin-containing pits has failed to generate much interest in this based on lack of scientific promise.

In contradistinction, let's look at the major chemotherapy drug Taxol, which was initially isolated from the Pacific Yew tree in 1962. At that time a National Cancer Institute commission was specifically looking for natural cancer cures and identified a promising extract. It took some time to isolate and prove anti-cancer activity in the laboratory, but this was finally completed in 1977. Then it was taken to appropriate clinical trials escalation, from Phase I to Phase III, which takes years to complete so that the proof of effectiveness is clear. By the late 1980's demand skyrocketed due to excellent results and the FDA approved it in 1992. This story has been repeated with other natural substances that have spawned effective cancer-fighting drugs. Most notably, clinical studies are starting to investigate the anti-cancer effect of curcumin, cannabinoids (CBD) and other natural substances against cancer.

The moral of the above story is that if there was something promising, it would generate interest and if it pans out it can certainly be patented. So, those alternative practitioners who are on the conspiracy bus saying that Big Pharma is not interested in "natural cures," are very mistaken. In fact, Big Pharma is laughing at such conspiracy theorists all the way to the bank. By 2000 annual sales of Taxol peaked at $1.6 billion. Since then, several spin-off related taxane drugs have lifted the total international sales to about $4 billion a year. Many components of natural substances can be isolated and purified, and a new cancer drug can be born at any time. So, when there is low or no interest, this should serve as your "bullshitometer" or a barometer of likely ineffective treatments that charlatans and quacks are more than happy to charge you money for.

One more thing on this topic. When a promising substance, natural or synthetic is found, research ramps up. Studies are initially approved and then run under the guidance of scientific and ethical advisory panels called Institutional Review Boards (IRB). These Boards are not full of cigar smoking Big Pharma executives but are composed of doctors, nurses, ethicists, attorneys, clergy and people just like you from all walks of life in the local community. To prevent the awful clandestine human experiments that occurred during the Holocaust under Nazi direction, these Boards protect the rights of human subjects. If an idea is kooky, potentially dangerous, and has no basis in science, it will not be approved and rightly so. Unfortunately, many charlatans out there still go forward and treat people with therapies that are either unproven or disproven, sometimes citing that they are "doing a study" in their offices and that their results are phenomenal. First of all, if it is not an IRB approved study, it is unethical, and they are breaking the law. Secondly, these poorly conceived "studies" have led to deaths. Third, in most cases, these are not real studies at all. They are merely a collection of poorly documented anecdotes. This level of proof is hardly worth risking your life for. As mentioned in several sections of this book, for more insight into how things are "proven," review the Appendix.

Cancer Cure Marketing Charades

As mentioned in the introductory matter of this book I have one other credential, other than being an MD, which is *critically* important to what I have to say and why you should listen. I have an MBA from UCLA, which has been a leading business school for many decades. A few of the core competencies that we learned while attaining an MBA degree were marketing and entrepreneurship. In fact, UCLA excels in entrepreneurship. Entrepreneurs are owners or managers of a business enterprise who find a need, fill it, and attempt to make profits, pretty much at all costs. In other words, I have the training required to sell ice to an Eskimo. It's sort of like a 007 license or credential in the area of spin and hype to make you buy something, whether you need it or not. So, you can rest assured that I can recognize someone else who is exercising their ninja marketing hype skills to try to influence your mind and pocketbook.

You are probably not a cancer research scientist, not an MD or DO, don't have an MBA and are trying to figure out who is telling the truth. What's worse is that your life depends on it! At some point, you have to admit to yourself that you are outside your element and have to trust someone. You are also extremely vulnerable as a cancer patient or survivor who is trying to completely extinguish cancer in your body. Please consider the possibility that the person who is telling you something which sounds too good to be true is a very slick 007 ninja hype marketing huckster. Some are well meaning but deluded or medically undertrained people, and some are outright crooks. In either case, they have a much better understanding of marketing than medicine, and when used unethically this version of 007 is truly a license to kill. I mention this several times in this book, and it is essential for you to understand.

The world is not flat and science had something to do with proving that. Science does understand how the human body works and anti-cancer therapies have to be at least scientifically plausible, if not proven, to help you in the here and now. If you believe otherwise, please do me a favor and throw this book out and go about your business. Excuse my brutal bluntness, but I need to wake you up if you find yourself drifting into dangerous territory. Barring a true miracle, you will not do well, and I can't help you until and if you turn your brain on. Recognize what might be going on when listening to "non-toxic" options that seem too good to be true. You're being had.

OK, let's look at a few outstanding examples of "alternative therapies" out there that are unproven or disproven. Let's explore if there is any plausibility for some of these. You can find out about others at http://cancercureology.com where I personally review the merits, risks, and benefits of many more. We'll conclude this chapter with therapies that may not be proven for all cancers but may have solid pre-clinical evidence or are proven in some cancer models or are in clinical trials.

Amygdalin/Laetrile

Seeds from fruit have long been advocated for prevention and treatment of cancer with overhyped claims of cures. Most of the attention is focused on apricot seeds that contain amygdalin, a cyanogen precursor to cyanide. As the story goes for this cure "they don't want you to know about," low doses of cyanide are supposed to prevent and cure cancer. The problem is that this has been tested up, down, upside down and sideways and the only reputable clinical data out there shows harm and shortened survivorship in cancer patients. To be fair, there may be renewed interest in research because of the much more advanced sciences we have today in testing compounds on gene expression through epigenetics. Also, if you look closely, the formulations of amygdalin extracts differ. So, with the lack of standardization, it is hard to prove safety and efficacy.

There is a reason cyanide was used for extermination in World War II and killing in spy movies. There is no known antidote!!! Unfortunately, there is no way to predict how much is too much. Amygdalin is found not only in apricot pits but also peaches, plums, apple, almonds, and quince. While eating raw seeds from any of these in small quantities is highly unlikely to kill you, extracts that are higher potency certainly can.

If you are unconvinced because of contrary opinions and supposed proof, at the very least, do not consume anything that has been processed and of unknown potency. Mother Nature may very well have put cyanogens like amygdalin in certain fruits and nuts for a reason, but she did not likely mean for this known natural toxin to be consumed by people in pharmacologic processed doses. There are hundreds of available concoctions, many non-reputable sources and an ever-present danger of irreversible toxicity and death. If further research determines safety and efficacy, this may become a real alternative. For now, it is not and remains a very dangerous proposition. For those interested in digging deeper, references are provided and show that while further research is meager it is still going on internationally.

Insulin Potentiation Therapy

Insulin potentiation therapy (IPTLD) with low dose chemotherapy was initially developed in 1932 by Dr. Donato Perez Garcia, Sr. The idea is based on some scientifically faulty statements. First, the theory notes that cancer cells have more insulin receptors than normal cells making them more sensitive to insulin. This is factually not completely accurate. Some do, some don't.

The idea behind IPTLD is that chemo can be used in much lower doses, thus causing less toxicity and allowing this type of chemo to be "kinder and gentler." The idea is great, but it is just an idea or theory. It may or may not be a good theory to research further, but for now, it is dangerous because the insulin can cause dangerously low blood sugar levels to occur, which can lead to death. We also have no credible science to say if this is effective or not. The amount of chemo administered can easily be so small that it is a waste of time and a threat to your life because the treatment is ineffective.

Even the late Dr. Ayre, the major proponent of this approach in the USA over the past 28 years had a very telling disclaimer placed on his website. His practice is still open, run by his physician son, and the following disclaimer verbatim is still on the website as of November 2016. *"DISCLAIMER: Anecdotal case reports from sixty years of use suggest that Insulin Potentiation Therapy (IPT) might be effective in the treatment of cancer. There is, however, no collection of scientific data validating IPT as a treatment for malignant neoplastic diseases, or cancer.*" Please remember that anecdotal case reports are extremely low on the evidence totem pole, just a bit better than "tall tales." A collection of anecdotes is just stories, nothing more. Again, I refer you to the Appendix in this book for details about how scientific evidence is created.

Having said all of the above as a strong precaution, there are a few scientific, clinical papers which have at least documented proof of concept and some degree of safety in the right hands. The references are provided at the end of this book, and they mainly involve breast and prostate cancer. However, keep in mind that these papers are rather poorly documented and if you find yourself considering this approach at a point in time where nothing else seems to be working, find someone who is very experienced in this method. There are some clinics that allege expertise, but demanding more proof would be critical. This is definitely not a recommended way to proceed, can be extremely dangerous but may be worthy of more research.

Lemon Juice And Baking Soda

Lemon juice can act as a mild diuretic and provides some vitamin C to your diet, which has some benefits in dietary doses as we've already covered. Baking soda is supposed to alkalinize your body, but does it? Its chemical name is sodium bicarbonate, and it is certainly a "base," which means it counterbalances "acid." In a test tube, you can perform all sorts of experiments and can adjust the liquid pH (acid-base balance measurement) rather easily. But in your body, the story is much different.

Keep in mind that the standard American diet (SAD) is indeed very slightly acidic. Over time this may add up and have direct metabolic and epigenetic effects. Although this remains unproven, it is prudent and low risk to consider a diet that tends to the alkaline side overall.

As far as direct anti-cancer effect and how much you can influence the pH around the tumor, the story is very complex. Pouring some baking soda down your throat does not immediately "alkalinize" your body, nor does it affect the generally acidic environment that is present around cancer. Your body has many mechanisms to keep your pH balanced in a relatively narrow safe range and strongly resists anything you might do to change it. This is called homeostasis. Your body knows that getting too acidic or alkalotic can lead to death, so it's a matter of survival. For example, when someone has a heart attack and the heart stops, often a state of deadly acidosis develops. Intravenous bicarbonate has to be administered in pretty large doses to counteract this, and a life and death scenario ensues to make sure the body's pH is artificially balanced. Can you do the same with oral baking soda? Yes, but it would be extremely dangerous, and you would have to ingest enormous amounts. You would be needlessly risking your immediate life to do something that has not been shown to limit cancer growth or progression.

An approximate dose of 12 grams of baking soda per day in a 65kg (143 pound) adult might balance the acid produced by a tumor approximately one millimeter in size. This is a little larger than a pinhead. If you have detectable cancer on a scan (e.g. CT, MRI or ultrasound), it is usually at the very least a thousand times that size, and if you have multiple large cancerous tumors then it as a factor of billions more cancer cells. The above estimate also assumes you can get the bicarbonate directly to the cancer at full strength and this will simply not happen because your body metabolizes and adjusts in order to maintain a safe pH range. If you take a dose of thirty grams per day you are likely to cause severe health issues or death and you still would not come close to getting enough bicarbonate to influence the environment surrounding the cancer in any meaningful way. It is simply impossible.

So, the recommendation is to not go to dangerous extremes and simply try to maintain a slightly alkaline diet. As mentioned before, you can look up the acid producing potential of various foods online.

Hydrogen Peroxide

Alternative practitioners recommend hydrogen peroxide for various infectious conditions, including AIDS, emphysema, and cancer. Patients are advised to take hydrogen peroxide orally or get an injection daily. The supposed anti-cancer effect is based on two concepts: (1) cancer, and other pathogenic organisms are anaerobic and can't survive in oxygen-rich environments (2) hydrogen peroxide is naturally produced and used by the immune system. Both of these concepts are partly true, but the meaning is stretched by a country mile in an attempt to try to justify this therapy.

First of all, not all pathogens are anaerobic, and cancer is not totally anaerobic. Although cancer lives in a predominantly anaerobic environment, it does not simply drop dead when oxygen arrives like a vampire being hit by light. Cancer does prefer glycolysis, which can be aerobic and anaerobic, and lactate fermentation over mitochondrial oxidative phosphorylation to derive energy and fuel for growth. This preference for glycolysis even in the presence of ample oxygen is called the Warburg effect, which the Nobel Prize-winning Dr. Warburg described in 1924. It is still unclear why cancer chooses a far less efficient way to derive energy, but it seems that this approach is anabolic and helps tumor growth. Cancer cells do have energy producing mitochondria, albeit they may be defective. Also, we have learned a thing or two over the past 100 years. Through 21st century science, we know that the Warburg hypothesis was oversimplified. Cancer uses both glycolysis and mitochondrial oxidative phosphorylation to satisfy its energy and growth needs.

Looking at this from a slightly different but related perspective, we know that hyperbaric (high pressure) oxygen therapy in patients with cancer shows a variable effect in different cancers. In some cancers it seems to be somewhat inhibitory. In none does it cause cancer to grow like wildfire. But there are definitely some cancers such as bladder and cervical that are resistant to oxygen at the high oxygenation levels achievable through hyperbaric conditions. In other words, some cancers don't care one way or the other and others are inhibited from growing and spreading. None are killed immediately just because they are exposed to more oxygen.

Even if you held on to the vanishing thought that oxygen is the cancer cell's kryptonite and worst nightmare, there is also the problem of oxygen delivery to cancer cells. The blood vessels which cancer forms through angiogenesis are very fragile, malformed and do not reach all of the cells in a tumor. Also, there is no scientific proof that hydrogen peroxide can increase the level of oxygen in cancer cells. In a test tube, it might. In the human body, it is highly unlikely.

Regarding the immune system and hydrogen peroxide, there are white cells that eat invaders like bacteria and cancer cells. They are called phagocytes. These cells kill what they eat using hydrogen peroxide, which is stored in microscopic vesicles (little bags) within the phagocyte. Tiny quantities are released from these vesicles during this process. There is a world of difference between that microscopic local process and drinking hydrogen peroxide to try to kill cancer cells, even if the peroxide could somehow reach the cancer cells directly. In fact, we know that hydrogen peroxide damages any tissue it encounters through oxidative stress, which is a carcinogenic effect. We also know that when applied externally hydrogen peroxide interferes with macrophage function and delays healing in wounds. So, it basically has an adverse immunomodulatory effect.

Ingesting hydrogen peroxide orally may cause irritation and blistering to the mouth, throat, and intestine. So it can cause abdominal pain, vomiting, and diarrhea. Hydrogen peroxide injected intravenously has been linked to several deaths.

What's the bottom line? Taking hydrogen peroxide does not work. It can be dangerous and can kill. But wait, there's more to this story, and it involves our old friend Vitamin C.

Vitamin C

Before we get to the latest and greatest on Vitamin C, let's get one thing out of the way. If you take a small dose of oral vitamin C as an antioxidant, in multivitamin doses or even if you take a couple of grams, it may be healthy and it might help with wound healing, but it does not kill cancer. Also, you have to worry about kidney stones and an upset stomach with possible diarrhea when you take more of it. All of Linus Pauling's and Ewan Cameron's research showed promise but clinically it was discredited because there was no way to get the amount of ascorbate (vitamin C) to the cancer cells by taking it orally. In fact, no matter how much you ingest orally you don't absorb more than 250mg at a time.

So, what's new? As mentioned, the bioavailability of oral Vitamin C is rather poor. But this can be bypassed by administering it intravenously. While this does not prove that Vitamin C is indeed a significant anti-cancer agent, it opens up the need for further research for the following reasons. At the tissue level, where cancer lives, pharmacologic levels of ascorbate are a precursor or generator of hydrogen peroxide (H_2O_2). So, while getting H_2O_2 to the tissue is not possible directly by taking it, H_2O_2 can be generated locally as needed. Now, it is far more complex than that even if you can get H_2O_2 to the cancer cells. It involves a lot of transcription factors and other biochemical factors to fall into place. Also, keep in mind that at this dose Vitamin C is acting as a selective pro-oxidant, like chemotherapy, not as an antioxidant. So, it can cause damage. However, the theory surrounding this is that it may damage cancer cells much more than normal cells. It's a theory, so this is clinically unproven.

In addition to the H2O2 pathway, high dose ascorbate may influence tumor angiogenesis and have direct effects on the cancer cell cycle. The phase of cell cycle influenced is dependent on dose and the cancer type. What this all points to is the need for more research because there is promise when ascorbate is delivered intravenously.

Because Vitamin C is a pro-oxidant in high doses, the whole concern about antioxidant interference with chemo and radiation therapy disappears. In fact, there is laboratory and animal evidence that it may enhance the effects of certain chemo (e.g. gemcitabine, paclitaxel, doxorubicin and more). Unfortunately, in other studies, it interfered with effectiveness. So clearly this opens up another reason for more research.

As far as safety, there is data from several University based small studies that demonstrated it to be well tolerated and with minimal side effects. Quality of life was reported to be better, and the main issues were vein irritation, kidney stones, nausea, and vomiting. However, the studies cautioned that people who have reduced kidney function, glucose-6-dehydrogenase deficiency, or paroxysmal nocturnal hemoglobinuria are at much greater risk for life-threatening complications.

The bottom line here is that oral high dose Vitamin C will only make you sick to the stomach with no significant anti-cancer benefit. Intravenous treatment seems to be relatively safe and may help mainstream therapies to be more effective. However, in some cases, it interferes. So, it is crucial to keep your oncologist and oncology pharmacist informed if you are inclined to proceed with intravenous Vitamin C. Keep in mind that it may be promising and plausible but is not proven.

Chelation Therapy

We've already touched on chelation therapy as part of the detoxification process in Chapter 15. Unless you are diagnosed with a heavy metal toxicity, there is no proven reason to go through chelation therapy. While there are better and better chelation agents being developed, there is a significant safety concern. As far as "safer" natural plant based phyto-agents for chelation, there is no clinical benefit that has been shown. In principle, a robust anti-cancer diet may keep the metals in your body balanced. So, this may be partly how an anti-cancer diet with phy-tonutrients works. However, that approach is way different from a practitioner trying to convince you that specific metal chelation is safe and effective.

Having stated the safety issue and no clinical proof of anti-cancer effective-ness, research is ongoing to investigate drugs called DpT thiosemicarbazones as iron chelating anti-cancer agents. There is nothing natural about this, so it is beyond the scope of this book, except to include it because there are alternative practitioners who offer chelation therapy. Be very wary of these as the indica-tions, safety, agents used, and practitioner expertise are all too highly variable to make this a good idea. Some approaches may be reasonably safe when using basic phyto-agents, but the effectiveness is entirely unproven. Therefore, because this is usually an expensive proposition, don't fall into debt over this currently unproven and potentially dangerous approach. However, stay tuned in to the research because there is interest in this overall and new findings may soon shape a different future.

Immune Modulation And Immuno-Oncology

As we've touched on in Chapter 5, cancer immunotherapy is coming of age and research in this area is booming. At the time of this book's publication, there are over 1300 clinical trials listed on the ClinicalTrials.gov website related to immunotherapy. In fact, we already have effective immunotherapy against some cancers, like renal cell and melanoma, but it is not quite there for most cancers. Treating people with immunotherapy methods that are not yet proven to work and that can hurt you (including death) is not ethical and is illegal for a good reason. Despite this, there are those who engage in this practice for monetary gain, usually in foreign clinics where patient safety is not well protected.

The most well-known "alternative" immunomodulation therapy out there is based on the work of Josef M. Issels, M.D., (1907-1998). He was a German physician who is regarded by some as a "world-renowned pioneer of integrative oncology." While it certainly true that he was involved in the infancy of immunotherapy for cancer, the work was mainly performed from the 1950's to the 1970's. This was before clinical trials and recordkeeping as we know it today were around. At that time in medical history, doctors performed a lot of observational research and tried things on patients "off the cuff." That means they merely collected random data observing how their patients did and tested stuff randomly on patients that seemed interesting. This might seem like a reasonable idea from a lay person's perspective, and for many years that is how clinical research was conducted. But we now know that a ton of observational data in many fields of medicine was proven completely wrong, often harmful, and even deadly, through clinical trials. Once again, better science reflects reality. While Dr.Issels was noted to be an upstanding individual who truly cared for his patients, he was tried and convicted on a manslaughter charge of "homicide by negligence." Why? Because he had three patients die under his alternative care where, according to the published information, they may have lived if they had accepted surgery. This was appealed and reversed because it was felt that, while he was misguided, he truly did care for his patients. That is great, but folks this had no place back then, and it certainly has no place now. Trying random treatment on unsuspecting and vulnerable cancer patients is not ethical and is in fact criminal in this country.

Another important thing to consider is that at the time Dr.Issels was making observations, many of which were quite new and illuminating, he was operating with a mid 20th Century knowledge base about immunology. That is ancient history. The difference between what he knew and what we know now is gargantuan. It's like comparing the complexity of a drive to the local grocery store vs. a trip to a distant galaxy. So, were his observations legitimate? Many may have been, but are now extremely outdated.

The modern day version of Dr.Issels' clinic exists, but to date research supporting their treatments has not being published in any significant peer-reviewed journals. Rather, some old fashioned immunotherapy (Colley's toxins) combined with unproven therapies like dendritic cell vaccines are being dispensed to patients. This approach is reminiscent of why Dr.Issels got into trouble in 1960. This is not compliant with United States ethics, efficacy or safety standards and thus the treatment is mainly administered in their Mexican clinic. That's a shame because they could be adding to the knowledge base of what works and what does not, other than collecting anecdotal testimonials. As always, please refer to the Appendix to discover why testimonials are not very useful to you as proof.

For some historical background, http://skepdic.com/issels.html covers the chronology of their attempts at supportive information publication. Unfortunately, according to them, there is nothing substantial.

There are similar alternative "immune-oncology" clinics which offer very scientific sounding therapies such as Autologous Dendritic Cell Cancer Vaccine, Prostate Cancer Vaccine, Activated Natural Killer (NK) Cells, Autologous Cytokines, Extracorporeal Photopheresis, Lymphokine-Activated Killer (LAK) Cells, Stem Cell and Lymphokine-Activated Killer Cell Procedure and the like. Despite promises that these therapies are individualized towards your particular case, this is not scientifically possible today. Some of these concepts have some laboratory basic science support but are not proven to be safe or effective in humans. Or, if they are proven for one type of cancer it does not mean it will work for another, especially if they are completely different types (e.g. leukemia vs. breast cancer). If any one of these concepts is provided to patients in carefully monitored clinical trials which offer a significant degree of safety, then it is reasonable to participate. But this is worlds apart from going to a foreign clinic that: 1) may or may not be administering what they say they are administering to you, 2) have no published safety record to show you, 3) have no published data regarding effectiveness to show you, and 4) are extracting large amounts of money from you or signing you up for a reverse mortgage on your house or a loan against your life insurance policy. In the USA this is criminal and for a good reason.

Blood Root / Black Salve

Blood root is otherwise known as Sanguinaria Canadensis, and mixed in with other ingredients creates a paste called black salve. As part of the Fell Technique, blood root was topically applied to the breast to remove tumors during the 1800s. You can unbelievably still get this treatment today. But, would you rather have an awful festering mess that takes months to heal with disfiguring scars? Or would you prefer a clean surgical incision and repair with healing that occurs in days to a few weeks at most? The tumor does not just "fall out" and leave the surrounding tissue non-disrupted. Instead, it acts like battery acid that drills down to the tumor and the entire section of breast falls off after it rots. The more tissue is disrupted the less it heals quickly and nicely without a scar. All I can say is, really??

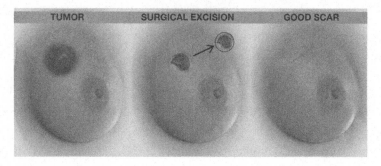

Original artwork

Surgery may be invasive, but with an appropriate incision, the cosmetic effect can be minor. In comparison to the surgical result, the black salve approach is quite inferior don't you think?

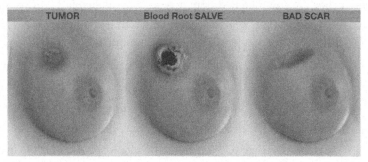

Original artwork

You can Google this and see many more images of people with parts of their face falling off where black salve was applied to treat skin cancer. At the very most, similar escharotics were designed to treat small skin tags with tiny quantities, and not even remotely for cancer. Blood root itself, taken orally in small amounts, causes nausea and vomiting to "clear the intestines." In higher doses, it can kill you. Folks, we don't live in the 1800s anymore. This is an irresponsible treatment that some practitioners, who should be imprisoned, still promote.

Energy Medicine

Energy is a physical property of objects that can be transferred to other objects or converted into different forms but cannot be created or destroyed. Many forms of energy can easily be detected, measured and quantified by various tools. In the human body, brain waves and electrocardiograms are prime examples. Other energy fields are not easily measured or not proven even to exist.

Energy medicine uses various forms of energy to diagnose or treat conditions, whether this energy is generated by devices or by the human body. We will briefly cover both.

No one debates that the human body uses electrical energy in powering your brain, your heart, your muscles and more. At the cellular level, chemical energy creation in the mitochondria is an accepted fact. The MRI uses a powerful magnet to influence the body's natural magnetic properties, mainly the hydrogen nucleus in water and fat, in order to produce anatomically correct images. Ultrasound can be used for diagnosis or treatment. Radiation is a standard mainstream energy therapy. Whether they are produced by the body or applied externally, these are all measurable and scientifically verified or "veritable" electromagnetic, electrical, magnetic, chemical, sound and light energies.

Taking it one step further, no one has measured or even defined human life force or aura with any scientific precision. Yet, many believe in the soul and other energy fields that surround and sustain the human physical body in inexplicable ways. These are "putative" but as yet scientifically undefined energies. They are variably named by various cultures over the eons as Ch'i (or Qi), Ki, Prana, and many more.

There are those energies that are in between veritable and putative. An example of externally generated energy fields that can influence the human body at the cellular and DNA level and even possibly interconnect all of us in a collective consciousness are scalar waves. These were intensively studied by Nikola Tesla.

This book cannot do this topic justice, and I do not mean to either scientifically support or reject this as a form of potential cancer therapy. I am merely suggesting that this is not that far fetched if you look beyond the end of your nose. In other words, no there are no proven internal energy bio-field or life force manipulation medicine cures for cancer. However, there are technologies that are being investigated and healing techniques that are plausible extensions of mainstream energy technology use for diagnosis and treatment. One in particular uses externally applied electrical energy fields and is very promising for numerous cancers. I'll cover that below.

Regarding practitioners who claim to have harnessed life force energy fields in the healing arts of Reiki, Healing Touch, Chakra healing, acupuncture and acupressure and others, it is quite simple. Some are far more likely to be helpful than others because anyone can claim they are a healer in this area. Some have gone through the trouble of studying, apprenticing, mastering and really trying to capture the essence of these arts and some are charlatans who just decided to throw up a sign or a website that says they are an expert in the area. Be careful in selecting. In general, if it sounds too good to be true or is much too expensive you should probably look the other way. In today's world, these healing arts can help cancer patients and survivors regarding stress management, pain reduction, nausea management, and other quality of life and general health areas. To say that they can reliably cure cancer is going very far beyond reality. Perhaps in the future this might change but, short of miraculous events, that is today's reality.

As far as external energy field therapies there are many energy healing "devices" out there that can look quite professional but inside may simply contain a battery and a few basic electronic components that serve no purpose whatsoever. How can you tell the difference between these and the few potentially beneficial ones? Unless you are an electrical engineer with access to millions of dollars of testing equipment, you can't! So don't waste money on unproven or disproven junk that promises "cures."

An energy medicine therapy that does work is based on something called Electric Tumor Treating Fields. This relies on low-intensity electrical fields that act on electrically charged cellular and nuclear proteins and interfere with cancer cell division. The work of Nikola Tesla, Dr. Royal Rife, and others over the past 100 years laid some of the groundwork for this emerging treatment option. Unfortunately, the application of their devices for clinical care did not follow proper research process and devices like the Rife Machine frequency generator are not approved by the FDA. You can buy them, but they are very expensive and who knows what the various manufacturers actually put inside them. You see, when it comes to energy medicine it is all about the appropriate frequencies and other physics properties that have to be exact or they are useless. It is the same as using the wrong chemotherapy for a particular cancer or the wrong herbal for a given condition.

Optune® is an FDA approved energy treatment for a brain tumor called Glioblastoma Multiforme. They went through the appropriate research process to prove effectiveness for very specific electrical field generation. It is considered to be a major advance in the treatment of that disease and is covered by Aetna among other insurance carriers as of the publication date of this book. It is in early clinical trials for ovarian cancer, lung cancer, pancreatic cancer and others. It requires wearing a device for hours at a time but offers an excellent quality of life with little or no side effects. You can't buy it, but you can go to centers that offer treatment for Glioblastoma or are participating in clinical trials for other cancers.

Hyperthermia or heat delivered either to the whole body or locally, is another form of energy medicine that has scientific merit. This is not a new concept but has been refined for many decades and is mainly available in clinical trials. Generally speaking, it works better when used with chemo or radiation therapy. Heat is generated using various devices from sophisticated ultrasound probes to something as simple as thermal blankets. A current extension of this type of treatment is the use of heated intraperitoneal fluid for malignancies that spread in the abdominal cavity like ovarian and some gastrointestinal cancers. This is called Hyperthermic Intraperitoneal Chemotherapy (HIPEC) and is in clinical trials.

Photodynamic therapy uses light energy to kill cancer cells which are exposed to sensitizing agents that are injected into a vein and travel to cancerous tumors. The toxicity is low, but the ability to get light to tumors is a limitation. This is usually done using fiber-optic endoscopes to reachable areas such as esophageal, lung and cervical cancer. For treatment of cancers of deeper organs, such are ovarian, surgery is required. As a bonus, photodynamic therapy also stimulates an enhanced anti-tumor immune response. This is a treatment that has been languishing and is still a research option.

Static magnetic energy therapy has not been proven useful for pain management when compared to placebo. So, if you are going to try to use them anyway, make sure you don't buy some high dollar magnetized gizmo. It would be a complete waste of money. As far as direct cancer treatment is concerned, magnetic nanoparticle research is at the forefront of an emerging field called "theranostics." This field addresses the use of nanoparticles to deliver diagnostic and treatment particles specifically to cancer cells; in this case highly magnetized nanoparticles.

In summary, there is no doubt that putative human energy fields and veritable externally applied energy have biologic effects and offer an exciting direction for cancer treatment. Perhaps eons of "alternative" or non-Western medical practice applications based on both putative and veritable energies have passed by unexplored. But, the beauty of today is that we can apply sophisticated scientific process to determine which of these is better or more effective than the other. It's a work in progress to be sure, especially in the area of putative energy field therapy that of course is not very amenable to scientific method. In the end, some of this will turn out to be trash and in other cases scientific discoveries will verify ancient therapies as being valid. This is indeed an exciting time.

Anti-Cancer Diets

We have already covered a lot about how proper nutrition, diet, various macro – and micro-nutrients are important in fighting cancer. That is all meant to be used as a primary prevention strategy, a support strategy during treatment and as part of recurrence prevention. None of that information is intended to imply that dietary manipulation can replace mainstream therapy, short of a miracle. Having said that, a few diets are reasonable to consider in an attempt to further reduce the risk of recurrence.

Ketogenic Diet

Almost 100 years ago Otto Warburg discovered that cancer cells primarily use inefficient anaerobic glycolysis (not requiring oxygen) to get their energy, even when sufficient oxygen is available. Glucose to lactate conversion, which normally occurs in hypoxic cells, persists in cancer cells even in the presence of oxygen that would normally inhibit glycolysis (Pasteur effect).

This type of metabolic energy production uses glucose to make adenosine triphosphate (ATP) energy packets. It was a curious observation because it is not very efficient and usually a last resort for cells to produce energy. Healthy cells preferentially use a process called oxidative phosphorylation which requires oxygen and normal mitochondria, our energy producing cellular organelles. It was then discovered that most cancer cells have defects in their mitochondria.

So, it is not clear why cancer cells preferentially defer to anaerobic glycolysis. One theory is that this type of energy production is optimal for growth rather than energy needs and cancers do need that constant trickle of fuel. Another theory is that it is based on truly damaged cancer cell DNA and that this leads to defective mitochondria.

It does not really matter because, in the end, cancer cells have a odd way of making energy to survive and perhaps this might be useful to treat or prevent cancer.

Whichever of these is more accurate; the result appears the same – cancer cells almost exclusively utilize glucose to make ATP without the use of their mitochondria. A detailed discussion of which explanation is better is beyond the scope of my word allotment, and it's not the point I want to make. The point is, cancer cells have a metabolic quirk. Regardless of how much oxygen and fatty acid they have access to, they preferentially use glucose to make ATP, and they do it without their mitochondria and oxygen.

So, can this be exploited to treat or even prevent cancer? Well, we already know that it is a way to help uncover metastases and monitor for treatment effectiveness. The FDG-PET scan exploits cancer's sugar preference. When radioactive sugar is injected it makes its way to areas of increased metabolic activity, usually in the form of cancer or intense inflammation or both. The more radioactive sugar is concentrated there, the hotter or brighter the signal. In the image below, the arrow points to a PET-CT "hot spot" where the radioactive sugar tracer was taken up by an enlarge lymph node replaced by cancer. When shown in full color, it ranges from orange to very bright yellow, depending on how much tracer is taken up. This signifies how active the cancer is.

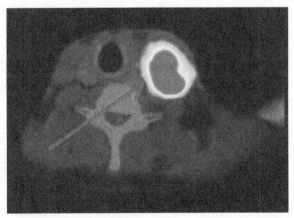

Akira Kouchiyama [CC BY-SA 3.0 (http://creativecommons.org/licenses/by-sa/3.0) or GFDL (http://www.gnu.org/copyleft/fdl.html)], via Wikimedia Commons

On the treatment side, the same idea applies. If cancer prefers sugar that much can we starve it to death if we deprive it from getting any sugar? When we're talking about sugar here, cancer does not care what type it is. There is no such thing as processed "unhealthy" sugar and "healthy" sugar. In fact, cancer's most preferred sugar is fructose, which is the main sugar in fruits and vegetables. The idea is to starve it from all sugar.

The problem with this is that your body needs some sugar to survive. So, even if you eliminated all carbohydrates from your diet, your liver makes glucose from protein. In particular, your brain generally needs sugar to thrive. Therefore, to really drive blood and tissue sugar down to the lowest possible level, you need to eliminate almost all carbs and a large amount of protein. This is, in essence, the ketogenic diet and is quite similar to the Atkin's diet, which has you living mostly if not exclusively on fats. The problem with the Atkin's diet is that fat from bacon and other animal sources poses cardiovascular and other challenges. Remember, Dr. Atkin's died of a cardiovascular event at age 72. While the exact cause of death is still being debated, the point is that most authorities do not recommend a high animal fat diet in general and it is not recommended as an anti-cancer strategy either. Today's ketogenic anti-cancer diet relies on plant fats instead of animal fats but requires a 3:1 to 4:1 ratio of fats to carbs and protein.

The name "ketogenic" is derived from the fact that in the presence of low blood sugar your body still needs fuel. It gets this fuel from forming ketone bodies (acetone, acetoacetic acid, and beta-hydroxybutyric acid) which you can survive on while cancer cells are deprived of the sugar they need and can't use ketone bodies very well for fuel.

Does it work? Its effectiveness against epilepsy is well known, and it seems to be effective against certain brain cancers. Based on that, it is in clinical trials against a number of cancers as of the publication date of this book. The data we have so far suggests that it can help, but it is an imperfect answer. The reason is that cancer does use aerobic glycolysis and oxidative phosphorylation to get part of its energy. So, for any significant benefit, you need to be sure that you are at least depriving cancer of anaerobic glycolysis and are always in a ketotic state. This can be measured with urine dipsticks.

Keep in mind that some researchers think that the reason this diet might work does not have anything to do with Warburg effect. It is possible that the reason the diet may help prevent cancer or recurrence is that it is basically a calorie restrictive diet. There are other metabolic reasons why calorie restriction is anti-cancer, and we have already touched on those.

A big downside is that this is not an easy diet to follow. Initially, almost everyone feels lousy from being fuzzy to outright headaches and fatigue. This can last from days to weeks. Your body adjusts to it, but you should never try this without physician guidance. Especially if you already have metabolic syndrome or diabetes, a rapid shift can lead to hypoglycemia, coma, and death. In the long run, this is a highly acidic diet and for multiple metabolic reasons can lead to sleep disturbances, muscle cramps, diarrhea, constipation, kidney stones, osteoporosis, impaired thyroid function and much more. So, it is doable but certainly has drawbacks.

Is there a way to supercharge the effect of the ketogenic diet? We hinted about this before, and it is related to blocking the conversion of protein to blood sugar, among other strategies in the category of energy disruption.

Several retrospective studies of diabetic patients taking a drug called metformin, which helps lower blood sugar, seem to get less cancer. Also, when they do come down with cancer, they live longer. Metformin has a number of biochemical actions, but a major one is activation of AMP kinase. This is an enzyme that helps reduce the formation of glucose in the liver from protein. In diabetic patients who have cancer, it is possible that their improved prognosis is because they need less insulin. Remember that insulin and IGF-1 help cancers grow. Their improved outcome may also be due to the reduction of glucose. Activation of AMP kinase may have other anti-cancer effects. It may be the energy disruption aspect of this that is the real anti-cancer factor. Research is ongoing, but cancer cell energy disruption appears to be an emerging anti-cancer strategy.

Anti-Cancer Nutraceuticals

The focus of this book is on whole food in the fight against cancer as opposed to isolated and processed nutrients found in supplements. This is because Mother Nature's emphasis is on the synergy between micro – and macro-nutrients found in whole foods. We know that in general when you split out nutrients you can lose effectiveness. Regardless, it may be semantics, but nutraceuticals can be quite different from basic vitamins and supplements.

Is there a role for specific nutraceutical isolates in the fight against cancer? Well, it is true that many of our past and current cancer therapies are based on highly refined isolates from tree bark (taxanes), periwinkle (vinca alkaloids), a Chinese ornamental tree (camptothecins), marine organisms (trabectedin), and many more. But nutraceuticals, a hybrid word bridging nutrients, and pharmaceuticals, are really unrefined and often multi-targeting or pleiotropic substances. Thus the question is difficult to answer. Many nutraceuticals, which often contain multiple products, affect various cellular metabolic processes and affect various epigenetic triggers. We introduced this in Chapter 7 when covering nutrigenomics and nutrigenetics.

If you consider only nutraceuticals that are highly refined, then it is a little different story. For example, the most active anti-cancer component of turmeric is curcumin. Curcumin has relatively low bioavailability, which can be helped with ingestion of black pepper. However, a curcumin analog (difluorinated curcumin) has been synthesized which has better bioavailability and evidence of a better anti-cancer effect. Of course one can say that this is no longer a nutraceutical but a refined pharmaceutical since it is no longer natural. But that is the conundrum. You can certainly take natural substances and tweak them with today's science and potentially make them "better." If you are a purist, you view this with skepticism. If you are progressive and integrative in mindset, you see this as a bridge between reductionist mainstream and natural botanical or herbal medicine.

For both whole food and nutraceutical anti-cancer strategies, a huge commonality lies in the NF-kappa B signaling pathway. Almost all anti-cancer foods and nutraceuticals inhibit this generally pro-cancer pathway. However, the beauty here is that this pathway is activated by many contributing genetic, epigenetic, transcriptional and metabolic processes, all of which can be influenced by various nutrients at different points. This is quite different from highly targeted drug induced blockade of a single point in a pathway like NF-kappa B or any of its related or unrelated signaling pathways. It is a far more global effect on multiple pro-cancer processes and pathways at the same time.

There are a staggering number of pathways and processes that can be affected. Just a few of these are growth factor (EGFR) receptors, Hedgehog signaling,

Ras/Raf signaling, MAPK/ERK and PI3K/Akt/mTOR pathways, Notch family, Wnt/β-catenin signaling, sex hormone receptors, TGF-β signaling, insulin-like growth factor (IGFR) signaling, cAMP signaling, and the STAT3 signaling pathway. As already mentioned, nutrients can modulate cancer stem cells, microRNAs (miRNA), epithelial-mesenchymal transition (EMT) and are central to epigenetic modifications. In theory, this hugely multifocal anti-cancer attack is highly attractive and far superior, but proving its effectiveness and determining which points of blockade are the most important is all but impossible.

We thus circle back to the point that food is superior to man-made attempts to concoct the "right" nutraceutical. Unprocessed synergistic combinations of micro – and macro-nutrients in a whole food anti-cancer diet attack multiple anti-cancer pathways. Who are we to pluck out a few and say that these specific plucked out and processed nutrients in a specific nutraceutical package are "better"? The answer is that we would be arrogant idiots.

The bottom line is that we will continue to find anti-cancer properties in natural substances and refined them into a drug or biological agent. These highly refined pharmaceuticals will save many lives and probably get less and less toxic. However, artificially dreaming up and slamming together a few nutrients that we know have anti-cancer properties, processing them, increasing their dose to pharmaceutical levels and proclaiming success without any research to support this is simply stupid. It is naïve to think you can outsmart Mother Nature.

Cancer Treatment Diets

This book is in a large part devoted to nutrition which can help fight cancer and improve the quality of life in survivorship. There are many anti-cancer diets out there, the most famous of which are Gerson and Budwig. Outside of a miracle, none can replace mainstream cancer therapy. However, these two diets, as well as others that are similar, cover the bases of what you have found in this book. If you need intensive teaching and immersion in reshaping your diet, then programs like this can help you. Some of the included adjunct "alternative" therapies such as colonics, coffee enemas, and magnetics do not have any added value and can be dangerous, as described in other sections in this book. There are no miracles here, and you have to consider what you are getting for what can be an extremely high dollar proposition. Some sell "distance programs," which are also very pricey considering you can get everything included at a much lower cost and not miss out on anything. This book alone is a huge start towards what you need to know to get you at least 80-90% of the way towards improved survivorship. Join us at CancerCureology.com for more.

Section III
Symptom Control & Wellness Cureology

Chapter 18

Introduction to Complementary and Mind-Body Anti-Cancer Support Modalities

During cancer therapy, various treatment or disease-related symptoms may arise. Also, stress is psychologically and physiologically harmful to you and will interfere with your anti-cancer battle and with your overall health. Multiple complementary modalities exist that can help you feel better and reduce stress during treatment and beyond. If anything resonates with you, there is much more written on these topics. This introduction is merely meant to guide you towards help where mainstream medicine may not have a good answer.

Remember, integrative oncology is meant to put *you* at the center, rather than cancer. As the disease is being bombarded with mainstream therapy, it can affect you as well, and the side effects can cause you to feel worse than what you started with. Even if you have chosen a more alternative path at any point in your anti-cancer journey, cancer itself can create a substantial burden of symptoms.

Complementary modalities can help with pain, nausea, physical and mental fatigue, depression, anxiety, insomnia, constipation, diarrhea, neuropathy, hot flashes, sexuality issues, chemo-brain and much more. Everyone is different, but you have to prepare to maintain your health so you can put up the best fight possible. In some cases, Western medicine has good answers, but in many cases it does not.

Here's a little example which shows that even mainstream docs give mind-body advice to their patients. Many people have heart palpitations, myself included. This is very bothersome, but after a thorough evaluation by a doctor, most of the time these are called "benign arrhythmias." Sometimes people are put on drugs to control this. Sometimes a rather invasive "ablation" procedure is recommended.

This means burning a part of the heart's electrical conduction pathways so that these arrhythmias don't occur. Anyway, very often no treatment is needed, but the palpitations are aggravating and scary. What does the doctor usually say? Usually, the advice is "take your mind off of it, and they'll go away." Interesting and true. Sometimes it is hard to do by just not thinking about it while a fish is flopping in your chest, but you can go beyond "not thinking about it" using focused mind-body techniques to keep those arrhythmias or palpitations away.

You are in control of a lot of your body's functions. You just don't consciously realize it. So, mind-body is not just a "feel good" approach but rather a demonstrated clear connection between your mind and a gazillion metabolic and epigenetic processes in your body, some of which help control symptoms and others that may have a direct anti-cancer effect. There are many techniques, and they are well worth exploring in supporting yourself during and after cancer therapy.

Mind-body awareness, connection, and exercise go even further. Due to the science of psychoneuroimmunology, we know that you literally can affect how efficient your cancer-fighting immune system works by practicing mind-body techniques. The healing power of the body is enormous and is vastly untapped.

Stress

Stress is all around us. A diagnosis of cancer certainly does not help. The problem is that stress causes a hormonal uproar in our bodies that is very counterproductive. It suppresses our immune system, allows inflammation to take hold, raises blood sugar which is a pro-cancer condition and leads to many other negative events. So what can be done about that? Quite a bit in fact! Let's go over a few.

Attitude And Gratitude

Very few people would say they feel grateful about getting cancer. However, time and time again I see that patients who do best and live the longest are those with a good attitude. As hard as that may be to cultivate, keeping those things in mind that you *can* be grateful for are crucial to focus on. So, something as simple as keeping a "gratitude journal" has been shown to make stress more manageable. By trying to develop a gratitude attitude, you also get the benefit of boosting your immune system through psychoneuroimmunology and potentially improving your outcome.

Sleeping & Not Couch Potato-ing

If you've been physically working out to reduce your risk of cancer or recurrence, that is simply awesome! But you should recognize that getting those additional hours on the treadmill might not do as much good if you aren't getting enough hours of sleep as well. Research shows that getting at least 7 hours of sleep every night may maximize cancer prevention advantages in physically active adults. There is a lot to mind-body connections in disease prevention and management that we are only beginning to understand. An optimal body is one that physically stresses periodically, but also has the time to replenish and rejuvenate through sleep and specific anti-stress activities.

As part of the "Maryland Study," adult women answered many questions concerning their activity level and typical rest habits. Cancer statistics in the group were then examined over the following nine years. During this period, 604 new cancer cases were described in the group. Who developed more cancer?

In adult women between the ages of eighteen and sixty-five, those who slept seven hours per night in addition to averaging approximately an hour per day of moderate physical exercise were forty-seven percent less likely to have cancer compared to adult women who averaged less sleep and activity level. Why was this the case? Isn't sleep just a lazy activity that doesn't really add anything "physical" to your health? Why not just "relax" in front of the TV for hours on end like a typical couch potato? Is that good too? The answer is no, and there is a good reason for this. You see, even when adults meet exercise guidelines, "couch potato-ing" or sitting and lounging around for prolonged periods can adversely affect your metabolic health. Adequate sleep can help your physiologic and psychological health.

Overall couch potato behavior is an extension of "sitting is the new smoking." Often it is related to sitting or lounging and snacking, which is even worse. Basically, among other biochemical and physiologic events, the loss of muscle stimulation induced through sitting or lounging results in suppression of skeletal muscle lipoprotein lipase (LPL) activity. This is required for triglyceride uptake and HDL-cholesterol (good cholesterol) production. It also reduces glucose uptake. This differs from what happens during sleep because of differences in cortisol, serotonin, and other hormones during the day vs. that during the night.

Also, there is a tendency to snooze in front of the television or on the couch that may keep you up late and interfere with good quality sleep.

In short, an active lifestyle combined with good quality sleep are crucial. Physical activity is important because it reduces your body fat, improves your cardiovascular health and kicks off complex cancer-fighting cytokine pathways. Sleep and a good portion of active relaxation techniques are almost equally important but has to go hand in hand with activity. You see, both enjoyable physical activity and sleep reduce your stress levels. Stress is not just something you "feel." A bad mind-body connection can lead to a biochemical assault on your body's normal biochemistry. Stress leads to physical impairment of cellular activity and oxidative stress, which leads to disease, including cancer. It goes even further. Based on research in psychoneuroimmunology, we already covered that you can actually improve or hurt your immune response by your level of stress and overall psychological health.

You might be thinking; this is all nice in concept but what are you talking about? I'm stressed out!!! I can't rest or sleep very well. I need anti-anxiety and anti-depressant drugs, and even those don't work well. Well, yes, this is a stressful world, and it is magnified if you have been diagnosed with cancer. But there are some natural approaches to getting some solid rejuvenating shuteye. Specifically, you can try valerian root and melatonin. There are many others, but these have good safety records. Also, try to get into a wind-down routine before sleeping, starting up to 3 hours before sleep. Finally, a completely dark and quiet environment helps you sleep better. Even a LED light in your alarm clock is not a good idea. It can interfere with sleep and lower your endogenous melatonin levels, which is not good for fighting cancer. If you can't achieve this completely tranquil environment without help, use earplugs and eye shades.

Massage Therapy

Massage therapy is safe and effective as long as the therapist is trained to work with cancer patients. Regular masseuses are not trained in this regard, so please be careful. There are problem areas that need to be handled appropriately, but the research shows that massage can reduce stress, fatigue, nausea, depression and other related symptoms by over 50%. The effect can last for several days. Not bad for a non-invasive, non-drug therapy. One can even learn how to perform self-massage or have family or caregivers learn focused safe techniques so that you don't need to go into an office for treatment. Common modified approaches are Swedish, Shiatsu, Tuina, and Reflexology.

Music Therapy

Music therapy is documented to work extremely well in reducing stress, anxiety, and depression. Music gets to the root of brain function directly and works without your even knowing it. So, at least consider putting on relaxing tunes that you have found to be supportive and relaxing throughout life. There is much more to it because the idea is to use musical instruments to speak to your body instead of words at a subconscious and conscious level. But just listening to calming music would be a start.

Sound Therapy

Sound therapy is closely related to music therapy. This is an area that is ancient, and yet we are learning so much more about how this works using 21st century science related to sound waves and brain waves. There are crystal singing bowls, Tibetan singing bowls, and many others. Tibetan bowls are more robust and rich and ideally create frequencies which take our brain from beta to an alpha state and sometimes theta.

You have four brain states that are reflected by four different frequencies of brain waves: Beta, Alpha, Theta, and Delta. Beta waves are associated with wide awake and focused alertness. In this state, you are learning, studying for an exam or engaged in other cognition intense activity. Alpha waves reflect relaxation and creativity. You may be deep in Alpha thought but not yet in a meditative state. When you enter a Theta state, you are deeper into relaxation and in various levels of a meditative state. In Delta state you are in the realm of subconscious thought and sleep. When achieved outside of restorative sleep at night you may be in a waking dream, and this becomes a state of deep stress relief, super learning, and self-hypnosis.

Laugh Therapy

The words speak for themselves. How can you be depressed and stressed while laughing? It's almost impossible. This again seems simpleton, but basic science research confirms very real and positive biochemical activity related to the act of laughing. Look up your favorite comedians. Many of their routines can be found on YouTube. If you can't find anything to laugh at, just go to a quiet room and start trying to laugh. Even the process of starting this can quickly snowball into laughter as you laugh at yourself and the concept of standing in the middle of a room mindlessly laughing. If this sounds ridiculous to you, please understand that something as simple as laughter can lead to an increase in natural killer cells among providing many other anti-cancer benefits.

Active Mind-Body Techniques

Active mind-body therapies can also affect many symptoms, reduce stress and help improve breathing. This is simple but extremely effective. Techniques include meditation, yoga, Tai-Chi and Qi-Gong, Reiki, guided imagery, self-hypnosis, mindfulness, mindful movement and biofeedback techniques like HeartMath®. Many of these you can learn from a professional coach and then practice at home.

In the end, stress reduction is a highly individualized thing. For some, getting too far outside their comfort zone doing yoga or something may increase stress. Don't do anything unless it feels right and is putting you in a better state of mind.

Herbal Stress Relief

Herbal remedy promises often far exceed reality. The reality is that herbs are unrefined pharmaceuticals. They may be natural but can have effects similar to prescription drugs, and quite possibly even more side effects because they are not as focused as drugs. The problem is what works and what does not? There are simply too many combinations out there, at too many doses, to prove or disprove effectiveness or safety. Also, various mixtures may not be safe, especially during chemo or radiation therapy or before surgery (e.g. increased risk of bleeding or anesthesia complications). Herbs can interact with prescription drugs and sometimes threaten your life. Anyone who claims this is not true is inexperienced, deluded or is simply lying to you in order to sell something. If you're going to explore herbals or botanicals, it is safer after you have completed your mainstream therapy rather than during. I say this with trepidation because there are certainly some herbs that can help during treatment, but practitioner expertise, dosing, and purity vary widely. There are just too many unknowns, and safety information is incomplete or inaccurate. My advice is usually to generally stay away during active cancer treatment or if you are on a lot of medications for various conditions because the combination can be very adverse. Expert guidance is critical, and there are certainly some proven and generally safe natural symptom relievers out there.

With that rather lengthy admonition, if you are not on a lot of potentially cross-reacting prescription medications, stress relieving herbals may be better than adding to drug polypharmacy. That is certainly also a dangerous situation to steer clear of.

Stress-busting herbals for either aromatherapy or ingestion to discuss with your doctor and pharmacist include lavender, lemon balm, ashwagandha, passionflower, and motherwort. An amino acid, l-theanine, rounds out the short-list.

Chapter 19
Specific Symptom & Syndrome Control

Some cancer and treatment-related symptoms are global, like lack of energy and full-on fatigue. Others are more specific to different types of treatment. So, the amount of time we spend on each will vary, but there are tips for many of the challenges you may have during treatment and in survivorship.

Most of this section is focused on disease and chemotherapy-related symptoms and side effects. Sometimes it is obvious, and sometimes it is not clear if the symptoms are from cancer or the treatment, so the suggestions are focused on the symptoms, no matter what the cause. We will also cover radiation related and surgical recovery tips.

Let's start with general intestinal support to prevent and ameliorate side effects like diarrhea, gastritis and the like. Then we will move to many other symptoms and solutions including nerve toxicity, fatigue, chemobrain and more.

INTESTINAL SYMPTOMS

Nausea

For nausea due to chemotherapy, the most effective remedies are the mainstream medications available such as Zofran®. Beyond that, there is acupuncture or acupressure, from a licensed acupuncturist, which is proven to be effective. Acupressure techniques can be learned and self-applied at home as well. Finally, related to this approach, you can buy acupressure bands that are used for motion sickness and see if those help. The pressure trigger point is called P6 (Nei Guan; 内关). This is located slightly towards the thumb side (with the palm facing up), three to four finger-widths below the wrist between two large tendons. Mild but firm pressure with your other thumb in a circular massage motion should do the trick. It needs to be repeated throughout the nausea episode.

Regarding herbal and botanical solutions, marijuana or THC can be effective. Also, peppermint can help relax the stomach which may reduce nausea. Try sucking on a sugarless peppermint lozenge all day. Ginger can also help. Both peppermint and ginger are readily available in teas. In both cases, make sure it is real peppermint and ginger rather than flavoring. The best solution is to get the natural substance itself. Although nausea is In both cases, make sure it is real peppermint and ginger rather than flavoring. The best solution is to get the natural substance itself.

Gastritis And GERD

Things to consider that may help are raft-forming alginate, black raspberry, berry polyphenol ellagic acid, licorice extract, zinc-carnosine, cranberry, picrorhiza. Make sure your diet is full of broccoli which contains sulforaphane among other beneficial nutrients. Lastly, consider chamomile or slippery elm.

Mouth Sores

Creating a paste from a medication called sucralfate can be helpful along with topical pain reducing ointments. Natural solutions include aloe, curcumin, honey (specifically Manuka honey), glutamine, and deglycyrrhizinated licorice (DGL). These can be topically applied or used as a rinse. In some cases, a superinfection with candida fungus may make matters worse and require specific anti-fungal treatment.

Diarrhea

Cancer itself, chemo, radiation, biologicals or infection can cause diarrhea. It's important to determine which of these is the likely problem, especially regarding infection. A common infection during immune-suppression is with a bacterial type called Clostridium difficile or you may hear C-Diff for short. Although there are natural approaches that *might* eradicate this infection over the long run, it creates a very dangerous situation, and antibiotic therapy is a better choice. Anyone can get a viral gastroenteritis, cancer patient or not. Those can't be treated with any medication and just requires keeping up with fluids until it gets better. However, there are other bacteria and parasites that can cause diarrhea. If diarrhea persists for more than a few days, you need to get your stool analyzed. For prevention, we already covered probiotics, which is the best option. Also, during chemo or biological therapy, it is best to clean your food well (i.e. wash your veggies) and avoid foods like sushi, which carries a risk of getting parasites.

When you have active chemo, biological or radiation related diarrhea, and the prevention measures have failed, the options are limited. If you have not been on probiotics and L-glutamine, you can try to start those. Again, make sure you don't have an infection first. Otherwise, the only effective natural acute therapy for chemo related diarrhea is charcoal, which is usually available in capsules over the counter. Charcoal binds drugs in the intestine and helps them get excreted faster in the stool rather than affecting the intestinal lining.

Keep in mind that no matter why you have diarrhea, you are losing electrolytes as well as fluids. Estimate the fluid volume and replace it. As far as electrolytes, other than buying something like Gatorade®, you can make a natural concoction by adding a half teaspoon of salt into a liter of water, with flavor and other electrolytes by adding some lemon and orange juice. Salt substitute contains potassium, and you can add a little of that too. Flavor with other things, like a bit of honey, to taste. Avoid too much juice because the fructose can worsen diarrhea. Drink this mix over the course of a day, not all at once. If you need it to taste sweeter, use stevia root.

Bananas contain some more potassium and along with applesauce and some toast, may be a good bland diet along with some brown rice. Pectin, a soluble fiber in bananas and apples, will soak up some of the fluid in your intestines and help make formed stools again.

Constipation

Constipation is a symptom, not a disease. However, in the case of chemo related constipation, fixing the symptom is more or less getting at the root cause. Beware that in bowel cancers, or due to metastases in your abdomen from other cancers, constipation may be related to tumors pressing on your intestine. This may or may not be helped with medical or natural remedies. In fact, it may even be a surgical issue. So, if constipation persists or is getting worse, let your oncologist know.

The mainstays of treatment are fiber, hydration, probiotics, avoidance of narcotics, magnesium. Sometimes old school milk and molasses enemas help.

INTESTINAL SUPPORT

Hydration

It is very easy to get dehydrated even without chemotherapy, and this will contribute to constipation. Obviously, the hotter it is in your environment and the more you sweat, the worse it is. If there is nausea and any vomiting, and this is not getting replenished, even worse. So, keep yourself hydrated at all times. Constipation is a minor issue with dehydration compared to more important concerns and bodily functions. How much you should drink varies, and sodas and coffee don't count. These can dehydrate you even more. So, regarding water, it is based on body weight and the conditions you live in (i.e. heat, sweating, exercise, vomiting, diarrhea, urination, etc.), not on a random number. You often see a recommendation for 8-ounce glasses eight times. That may be easy to remember but could be way too little or too much for an individual. The Institute of Medicine recommends what they call an adequate intake (AI). For men, this is roughly 13 cups (3 liters) of total beverages a day, and for women, it's about 9 cups (2.2 liters) of total beverages a day. A mindless recommendation based on body weight is also not ideal. Stay away from those types of generalized recommendations because too much or too little may be crucial when you're getting chemo. For example, if you have some degree of heart failure, you can drink too much and get into trouble. Even for something as simple as water intake, it's all about YOU as an individual.

The Institute of Medicine's AI and the 8x8oz recommendation is not too far off the mark as a baseline, but keep the following in mind. Food is also composed partly of water and can be up to 20% of your fluid intake per day, depending on what you eat. As an example, certain vegetables and fruits are made up 90% of water. If you drink juices or milk, they also contain a high percentage of water. So, you need to take a close look at your diet to determine how much water is in it.

As far as extra losses, we already mentioned covering additional losses like sweating, diarrhea, increased urination and things like that. The adjustment depends.

So, for vomiting or diarrhea, you should be able to gauge what amount extra you need by observing what is coming out. In fact, with larger losses you may need some electrolytes which can be found in drinks like Gatorade® and Powerade® or prescription fluid replacement.

Regarding sweating from exercise or a hot, humid environment, an extra one to two 8oz glasses for sweating an hour or less should be adequate. Scale up from that if you have more significant sweating. If the sweating is related to exercise, drink a little beyond your exercise period.

If you live at a high altitude, you may be breathing more frequently and urinating more often, at least during acclimatization. Also, heated indoor air during the winter may cause your skin to lose more moisture. So, adjust accordingly.

Probiotics

Store bought probiotics, and prebiotic mixes have been covered in the supplementation chapter (Chapter 13). There are also many ways to add probiotics through natural diets. This includes yogurt containing "live cultures" like Lactobacillus acidophilus and Bifidobacterium, kefir, or fermented foods like Kimchi or sour pickles. Other sources include Kombucha, miso, fermented cabbage or sauerkraut (if non-Pasteurized), and tempeh. Theoretically, store bought mixtures, or dietary intake will both work to recolonize your colon with good bacteria and keep your microbiome healthy. However, as with other supplements, beware of what you buy. What's on the label is not necessarily what is in the mixture. Simply focusing on a plant based whole food diet will tilt the microbiome towards a healthy state.

Glutamine

Glutamine can help general intestinal support and was covered in Chapter 13, as well as specific support mentioned in many areas of this book. In the intestinal tract, it helps maintain normal intestinal permeability, mucosal cell regeneration, and structure. So, it can help with reducing "leaky gut." Also, glutamine supports immune function of the gastrointestinal tract. It seems to be much more effective when used intravenously, but oral supplementation is still an option. This is partly because oral supplementation discourages the growth of harmful gut bacteria that promote the secretion of pro-inflammatory cytokines. Therefore glutamine has an anti-inflammatory effect, partly by supporting a healthy microbiome.

Digestive Enzymes

Chew your food thoroughly. This releases the fullest potential for nutrients by activating and releasing your salivary enzymes. This, in turn, helps the stomach digest food and sends a message to the pancreas to secrete other enzymes such as amylase to help with the process down the line.

Bromelain protease in pineapple, mainly in the stem, papain protease in papaya, amylase in mango, multiple enzymes (sucrase, amylase, and protease) in honey and bee pollen (from bee saliva) can all help.

Magnesium

A deficiency of magnesium affects skeletal muscles (e.g. the muscles in your arms) and smooth muscle (e.g. the muscle in your intestinal wall) and makes them weak. With weakness in your intestine, constipation can occur. Magnesium deficiency can occur in anyone and can be due to inadequate intake, extra losses from diarrhea or vomiting, sweating, and due to some types of chemotherapy, especially cis-platinum.

The good news is that you don't have to guess on the amount of magnesium you might need. It is possible to take too much and in the worst case scenario, at a high blood level, stop breathing. If your magnesium is very low, intravenous replenishment is the fastest and best. In a medium low situation, oral supplementation is adequate but due to chemical stability reasons there is no such thing as a pure magnesium supplement. Magnesium must be bound to another substance like chloride, sulfate, hydroxide, and citrate, among others. Magnesium citrate can be taken and if you have constipation it is a good laxative, but it may overstimulate your intestine and cause intense cramping. Magnesium sulfate or hydroxide is found in Milk of Magnesia and is a gentler laxative and antacid, but one can overdose more readily on this due to absorption. Since there is danger here and potential drug interactions, I would strongly recommend that you to talk with your oncologist or pharmacist about the type and dose that is right for you.

For prevention of magnesium deficiency and prevention of the related problems of constipation and weakness, consider going to the best source, food. Foods high in magnesium are also likely to contain calcium, vitamin K2, and vitamin D, which need to be in balance in your body for optimal results. The best foods for magnesium intake are chlorophyll related, like seaweed, spinach, avocado,

Swiss chard, almonds, pumpkin seeds, sunflower seeds, sesame seeds and some beans.

Lastly, if you're trying to supplement magnesium but trying to avoid laxative effect, consider the following variants: magnesium malate, magnesium glycinate, magnesium aspartate, magnesium orotate, magnesium taurate, magnesium-L-threonate.

Fiber

Fiber, from your diet or supplements, are not all the same. We covered fiber for intestinal and overall health in general already. But for constipation, you want the insoluble kind. Try whole-grain bread, cereals, and pasta. Cereal fibers resist digestion and retain water very well. In particular, wheat bran can be an outstanding natural laxative and stool softener. Another good option is ground up psyllium seeds.

There is nothing special about prescription or over the counter stool softener capsules like Colace® or Metamucil®. Some preparations are more natural than others, some are mixed with additional laxatives, but overall it is best to go natural for long term use.

PAIN

Other than anti-inflammatory or narcotic medications, acupuncture is also effective for pain. Although we do not yet know exactly how this works and how nerves, fascial planes, and meridians interact, we know that it is effective and is not based on placebo effect. It is not voodoo. The point is that it works for a wide variety of issues including hot flashes, fatigue, neuropathy, osteoarthritis, sexual dysfunction and some urinary problems. It is well worth a try. Keep in mind that it is as much of an art as it is a science. Not all practitioners will produce the same results. So, look around carefully and select someone who is well trained and has a good reputation.

For minor to moderate pain and depending on your pain threshold, natural therapies can be considered. This includes anti-inflammatories such as omega-3 fish oil and willow bark, which is a natural salicylate. Natural salicylates can also be found in apples, avocados, broccoli, eggplant, peaches, spinach and turmeric spice. However, there is nothing "natural" that is not processed which will handle severe pain. For that, narcotics are almost always necessary. Perhaps the only exception to this is the cannabinoids. But be careful with drug interactions.

NEUROTOXICITY

Neurotoxicity from chemo is hard to treat when it looks like it may be due to multiple factors and is really incompletely understood. So, everyone might be different. Along those lines, nothing has been proven to prevent or adequately treat this. Nothing prescription based and nothing natural. However, as the saying goes "where there's smoke there may be fire." The remedies that have been researched the most include those listed and described below. The best anyone can do is to try these in a sequence, but that also presents a problem because nerves grow very slowly. Trying something for a few weeks or even a month may not produce results, but may have if it was continued for a longer period. In some of these cases, you can try several remedies at a time, but you will not know which one worked if you get relief. The same is true of prevention if you use multiple remedies at once.

The most promising treatments are glutamine, astaxanthin, vitamin E, omega 3 fatty acids, goshajinkigan, CBD oil, acupuncture, alpha lipoic acid, B-complex vitamins and methyl-cobalamin, magnesium and calcium.

In most situations, glutamine is a common first choice. The dose is 10,000mg of powder three times daily.

However, theoretically glutamine may feed cancer and provide it with building blocks, as we previously covered. This is not clinically proven, but some recommend using glutamine during chemotherapy only a day or two before and after chemotherapy.

HAIR LOSS

Cells in your hair follicles divide rapidly, and because chemo mainly attacks rapidly dividing cells like cancer, damage occurs and severe hair thinning or hair loss (alopecia) results in many cases, depending upon which chemo is used. Cold caps (literally ice to the scalp) have not been effective in all cases, but a review of fifty-three studies suggests it is worth trying. Unfortunately, this is a big bugaboo for mainstream and complementary medicine. There are no good reproducible answers for prevention. To accelerate recovery, low-level laser light may be of help. Innovative tools like laser head caps are available but can be expensive.

HAND AND FOOT SYNDROME

No one really knows what causes hand foot syndrome or palmar-plantar erythrodysesthesia (PPE), as it is formally named. It starts with some numbness and tingling on the soles of your feet and/or palms of your hands. Then it can progress to redness, swelling, blistering and peeling, which can become infected and is painful. This can happen early or after many months of treatment.

Not all chemotherapy does this. The agents known to cause this are capecitabine (Xeloda®), fluorouracil (5-FU), liposomal doxorubicin (Doxil®), doxorubicin (Adriamycin®), cytarabine (Ara-c®), hydroxyurea (Hydrea®), sunitinib (Sutent®) and sorafenib (Nexavar®).

The main theory is that tiny blood vessels on your palms and soles rupture which means chemo leaks into the tissues and causes these inflammatory symptoms. Also if your skin is deeply chapped and cracked in the area, this can lead to the same problem. Finally, these drugs may collect in the sweat glands in the palms and soles and then leak onto the surface, releasing chemotherapy-related chemical metabolites.

Prevention includes avoiding tight socks or gloves, excess rubbing, pressure, excess use (e.g. using a screwdriver or garden tools) or heat (e.g. hot water) on your palms or soles. Wear soft comfortable shoes, don't go barefoot, avoid sun exposure in those areas, and apply hypo-allergenic moisturizers to keep the skin well hydrated. Moisturizers containing 10% urea have been shown particularly effective, as has Marpisal®, which is a German natural ointment. Antiperspirant containing aluminum chlorohydrate has been shown to reduce grade 2 to 3 (i.e. more severe) hand-foot syndrome, at least after pegylated liposomal doxorubicin (Doxil). Based on the theory of how this develops, it should work when caused by other types of chemo as well. Lastly, Vitamin E has anecdotally shown some promise as a preventive agent.

If you start noticing the tingling and numbness, let your oncologist know right away. It may be time to change to another chemo agent. If it is further along, do not break blisters as this can lead to infection and if you have a fever, this might mean you need antibiotics. Ignoring this, especially if you have a suppressed white cell count, can land you in the emergency room deathly sick.

Active measures include keeping your skin hydrated with cool water and moisturizers, using pain relievers and ice packs as needed. These should not stay on for more than 15 minutes at a time. Topical steroids may be recommended, but ask your doctor first. Steroids can help for short term but interfere with wound healing in the long run. On the natural options side, topical Henna (Lawsonia inermis) was shown to improve Grade 2-3 symptoms, as has topical DMSO lotion.

Vitamin B6 300mg per day with food has been shown to help some people to prevent this syndrome and possibly accelerate healing. In one small study, Vitamin E therapy (300mg/day) was started if hand-foot syndrome developed. Symptoms improved without the need for chemotherapy dose reduction. After one week of treatment PPE began to disappear.

NAIL & CUTICLE PROBLEMS

Cells in your nail bed divide rapidly, just like hair follicles, so chemotherapy can affect these cells causing lines and indentations, pigmentation changes and brittleness. Overall, the cuticle area may become dry and frayed. Keeping this area hydrated with lotions and avoiding trauma will help minimize worsening and infection. Other than a local problem with pain and swelling, if you get a significant infection in the surrounding tissue (cellulitis) and your white cell count is low, this can lead to a systemic infection and a risk of death. Or, if you have had breast cancer surgery with lymph node dissection in your axilla, this can increase the risk of long-term swelling or lymphedema. So, it's important to keep an eye on something as simple as nail care.

After a number of cycles of chemo, the nail may lift off its bed and fall off. During this time the space in between is increasingly susceptible to infection, so good hygiene is critical. If the nail falls off it will regrow after chemo, just like hair.

For prevention, cut your nails short, don't bite your nails, use moisturizing cuticle cream, don't use acrylic or fake nail wraps which can increase infection risk. If you get a professional manicure or pedicure ask that the instruments be additionally sterilized or bring your own. If your cuticles become dry, use a cuticle remover rather than cutting or pulling or tearing them away. Finally, reports suggest that using "cryotherapy" or cooling the nails on your hands and feet during chemo can minimize blood flow through that area and reduce the risk of nail damage. This is similar to hair preservation attempts by wearing an iced "cold cap" during chemo. Be careful, because excess icing can cause severe burns and worsen the situation. While it is not standard of practice in the United States, there is sufficient global evidence that hair and nail prevention using this method does help some patients.

HOT FLASHES

Premature postmenopausal symptoms of hot flashes, night sweats and mood swings related to cancer treatment is due mainly to a drop in circulating estrogen. Whether or not it is safe to replace estrogen medically or through natural phytoestrogens depends on the type of cancer and presence or absence of estrogen and progesterone receptors. This is a highly complex topic that we covered in Chapter 6.

SEXUALITY

Sexuality issues arise during and after a diagnosis and treatment for cancer. In some cases, there can be a direct effect of cancer or treatment on body image and sexual organs. In other cases, it is an indirect hormonal or psychosexual effect. This is an exceedingly complex issue which requires very personal attention to achieve solutions. This often involves counseling or therapy, not a medication or supplement.

Having said the above, there are some basic support suggestions that may be of help. For men, the most common physical issue is erectile dysfunction (ED) that may be related to surgery or radiation. Mainstream treatment options include medications such as Viagra® or longer acting phosphodiesterase type 5 (PDE-5) enzyme inhibitors. These medications also work by increasing a naturally occurring chemical called nitric oxide. This all leads to an improved erection. Generally speaking, these agents work much better than natural approaches such as Yohimbe bark even without the presence of cancer or cancer treatment related ED. The other mainstream approach in severe ED is surgical cylinder implantation. Unfortunately, natural approaches are not very effective in this area.

For women, common direct physical issues other than body image are vaginal dryness and sexual drive. Cancer, chemo, surgery, and radiation can all affect the vagina if it is a gynecologic cancer. Chemo, radiation, and surgery can also affect the ovaries. Either ovarian removal or damage from the mainstream treatments will eliminate or lower testosterone, which is the main sex drive hormone in both men and women. Vaginal health can be improved or maintained using probiotics, but vaginal lubrication may need to be boosted artificially. Common vaginal lubricants have included coconut oil and aloe based formulations. Water based lubricants are often insufficient, and silicone is as un-natural as possible. They work but are potentially toxic in the long run.

Regarding testosterone supplementation, in most cases this can be done with prescription medications, but sexual desire is more complex than a single hormone. Another problem is that the "right" dose in women is not established, so it is individualized to avoid complications like unwanted hair growth, clitoral enlargement, and a deeper voice. This is a good reason to work with a doctor and not try to self-medicate with bio-identicals. It is prudent to consider the natural approach first. Taking dubious natural testosterone nutraceuticals is not the answer. Try the following, especially if the ovaries are still in place but partly damaged by chemo or radiation: 1) consume ginseng, which may have a hypothalamic adaptogen effect, 2) add quality protein and fats to your diet, mainly from plants and fish, 3) maintain intake of zinc, vitamin C, vitamins B6, magnesium, 4) remain sexually active, 5) limit alcohol intake to red wine and no more than a glass a day. This combination is all favorable to testosterone production, but there is no clinical data for this. The risk is low, but the effect is likely also going to be weak.

FATIGUE

It is impossible to cover everything regarding cancer-related fatigue. However, we're going to cover a lot of ground in this area focusing mainly on situations where no obvious reason for the fatigue exists other than the fact that you are a cancer patient undergoing treatment or a survivor having completed it.

Fatigue can be due to many things, some of which build on each other to overwhelm you. It can be related to cancer itself, the medications and treatment, surgical recovery, or other underlying conditions such as diabetes, cardiovascular disease and much more. You may even have an underlying fibromyalgia or chronic fatigue syndrome that was exacerbated by cancer and treatment. Rather than guess, the very first thing to do if fatigue is getting the best of you is to tell you, oncologist. It is possible that you are anemic from chemo, in which case a transfusion or other ways to boost your red blood cells would help. This requires testing, and the solution is really based on the exact problem.

Cancer-related fatigue can be due to the deprivation of quality sleep, lack of exercise, poor diet, dehydration, and stress. We have already covered a lot of ground about what you can do to improve in these areas. Now we'll dive deeper into some additional factors that can lead to fatigue. It's a process of elimination. But keep in mind that it can certainly be due to multiple factors. Address each of these, starting with stress reduction, better sleep, improved diet and exercise.

Exercise

Exercising might seem like the last thing to do when you're feeling exhausted, but it can help you. It may seem counterintuitive but increasing your physical activity is a great way to boost your overall energy levels. This could mean talking a walk around the block or heading to the gym. Anything is better than nothing.

Recent research shows that short 10-minute walks provide an energy boost that lasts nearly two hours. One study also found that if you continue these walks for three weeks, then you will feel more energized and in a better mood.

Diet

Don't skip meals and keep hydrated. We all know the feeling of sleeping in through the alarm. You rush to get to work or school and are forced to skip breakfast. Or maybe you have too much to get done at work and are forced to skip lunch. Either way, skipping meals isn't the best idea, especially breakfast. At the very least, hydrate when you get up.

Having breakfast in the morning helps restore your body's energy after sleeping all night. If you skip it, then it wouldn't be surprising if you felt completely drained by lunchtime. Research has shown that people who do not skip meals are more energetic and also in a better mood throughout the day.

Power Snacking

Tired of feeling tired in the middle of the day despite eating a healthy breakfast? Try a power snack. Not a useless and dangerous sugar fix but a well-balanced power snack. The best are those that have protein, fiber and a little bit of fat. Examples are peanut butter on a celery stick, whole grain bread or a protein bar. The protein acts to maintain your energy; the fiber gives you a quick boost of energy and the fat makes this boost last.

A great liquid energy booster is Wheatgrass juice or tea. This is a true superfood with multiple benefits, and the many nutrients contained within are absorbed very quickly. An alternative might be green tea with D-ribose as a natural sugar energy filled sweetener. Ribose is manufactured from glucose in the body and is a critical component of adenosine triphosphate (ATP). We've already covered this, but ATP molecules are the energy packets that your body uses for all processes that require energy.

Your body does not recognize d-ribose as a fuel, so there is no caloric value per se. As far as dose, data is limited, but among the few studies that exist dosing did not exceed five grams three times a day. I would not recommend exceeding this. Plus, be aware that d-ribose is being added to some energy drinks, so beware of taking in too much overall from multiple sources.

Finally, there has been some recent attention as to L-tyrosine taken several times per day for improvement of cognition and overall energy. L-tyrosine is an amino acid and is a building block of protein. One of its functions is to make chemical messengers help conditions involving the brain such as improving mental alertness. There are some plausible laboratory and animal study data to support this, but human studies are not consistent.

An interesting smaller study in college students showed that a mixture of nutrients they called CRAM maintained reaction time, and subjective feelings of focus and alertness to both visual and auditory stimuli in healthy college students following exhaustive exercise. In addition to L-tyrosine, the mixture contained α-glycerophosphocholine, choline bitartrate, phosphatidylserine, vitamins B3, B6, and B12, folic acid, anhydrous caffeine, acetyl-L-carnitine, and naringin. It is impossible to tell which of these, if any, are the most responsible for positive effects but all have been suggested as energy boosters in their own right. This is not great scientific proof. But if you are reaching for creative solutions to your mid-day energy drain, these are ingredients that have been tested to some degree vs. pulling others out of the hat so to speak.

As far as the caffeine per se, from an energy perspective, it can lead to a fatigue roller coaster. However, it does have some anti-cancer properties, so moderation is the advice. Ideally, consider green tea where you get anti-cancer EGCG along with a moderate amount of caffeine.

Traditional Chinese Medicine (TCM)

There are a ton of potions, teas, herbs, powders, and other mixtures out there purporting that they contain energy producing medicinal properties. The problem is, many are an expensive black box. Which do you believe and what do you buy? On the one hand, there are thousands of years of "experience" quoted by practitioners of Traditional Chinese Medicine (TCM) for one herbal preparation or another. On the other hand, there is precious little in the way of good scientific evidence supporting the claims. BUT, hold on! There are a ton of laboratory studies which have drilled down and examined many TCM preparations for their medicinal properties using modern technologies. You see, once bioactive components are documented, which could plausibly have a positive effect on metabolic processes, animal studies are done. Parenthetically, this is the way drugs are investigated as well. Drugs don't go from "idea" to human trials either. So, along these lines, there are now quite a few animal studies which really support the plausible claims of thousands of years of TCM "experience" with many herbal preparations.

There are many examples, and one could write a book larger than War and Peace or Shogun documenting all of these. Please keep in mind (review the Appendix discussion regarding the scientific process at the end of this book) that human studies do not always pan out after promising lab and animal studies. However, if you were to pick and choose possible TCM aids for fatigue prevention, it is best to consider those which have relative proof from the historical data, laboratory data, and animal data. Again, this assumes human studies have not been done yet or have not proven efficacy. If good quality human studies have shown that a particular preparation does not work, or can harm you, maybe you should consider some other preparation.

Here is one example. A Chinese herb, Cistanche deserticola, commonly called Rou Cong Rong, has long been used for fatigue-fighting. It has now been proven to contain pharmaceutically active materials. These are known in Chinese as suosuo dayun (索索大元), which are produced by slicing the stems of the plant. As a sidebar, Cistanche deserticola is on the world's endangered species list so if this study about its fatigue-fighting properties is proven to be right on in humans, we may run out. Would it be over? A total loss of "the answer" to everyone's fatigue? NO! This is where technology can assist because we can re-create natural substances *exactly* in the lab (not sort of, but exactly). Purists would argue that this is still "un-natural" and synthetic. Well, that may be true, but it is better than "un-available." Nuff' said and as I mentioned before, this book is not about conspiracies and semantics. It's about getting the best-known options to you. So, just a thought that technology might not be all that bad in some cases.

One particular research study on Cistanche was performed in rats, but what they measured is pretty objective and hard to fake. Specifically, in addition to checking time to exhaustion from swimming, blood tests that measure muscle fatigue were checked. These are common blood tests that might be similarly used in humans. It appears that at least in rats, Cistanche deserticola is very active and prevents fatigue.

One word of caution when exploring this or other herbals for any purpose. Make sure the one that has been studied is the one you're considering for use. In this case, a specific type of Cistanche was tested. Others may not have the same properties (the Japanese Cistanche salsa for example). Also be careful about the purity of anything you consider buying. Active botanicals may be significantly "cut" or diluted by other herbs included in whatever mix is being sold.

A few additional botanicals to mention that may have a fatigue-fighting effect are Rhodiola and Astragalus. There are of course many others, and we cover those in greater detail at http://CancerCureology.com.

Energy Sapping Conditions

Tried all the energy boosting habits and still feeling exhausted? Well, sometimes there is more to your fatigue than just being tired from bad habits. It might be the result of something worse than not getting enough sleep. Today, millions of people worldwide suffer from developing chronic health conditions that cause them to feel tired. If you have found none of the energy-boosting habits to work, then it might be time to see your physician to see if you are suffering from a common energy-draining illness. These may or may not be related to cancer per se.

While fatigue is a symptom of hundreds of diseases, the most common among them that might be complicating a cancer diagnosis or in survivorship include anemia, hypothyroidism, and diabetes or even *pre*-diabetes. Adrenal insufficiency rounds out this list but is less common. These can all be easily tested for and then treated.

Still Tired? Chronic Fatigue Syndrome?

Have we not hit the nail on the head yet? Do the energy-producing tips not work or do the above medical conditions not apply to you? Do you have some of the symptoms of fibromyalgia, but aren't quite sure if you have it? Do you constantly feel exhausted regardless of what you're doing? If this is the case, then your fatigue may be a red-flag for a much more serious condition known as Chronic Fatigue Syndrome (CFS) or fibromyalgia. While it is not life-threatening, it is characterized by chronic, debilitating and prolonged fatigue, with or without myofascial pain. There is no single known cause, but it is a real syndrome or ailment.

Unfortunately, cancer can be associated with CFS, although it is probably not a cause-effect relationship. In other words, CFS does not cause cancer and cancer does not cause CFS. But there are associated concepts that connect the two. If no known reason, like anemia, is found to be causing your fatigue, CFS is a possibility. Let's cover the main CFS theories and how they overlap with cancer, followed by some treatment hints.

How CFS Begins

The majority of those who suffer from CFS say that it started suddenly. It is also incredibly common if these symptoms appeared right after a flu-like illness or after several months of severe and unfavorable stress. Cancer can certainly be such a stressor.

Earlier research studies revealed that some people developed CFS after some sort of infection, which led them to conclude that CFS might actually be caused by a bacterial or viral infection. However, more recent research has not confirmed that infection and stress are possible causes of CFS. So, that remains a plausible but unproven theory this point. Something to think about is that even if an infection or stress does not directly cause this disease, both of these can weaken your immune system. It follows that supporting your immune system, in general, might be a good strategy. You should already be getting an inkling of strongly related issues between CFS and cancer.

Again, the exact cause, or causes, of CFS is still unknown. However, knowing what causes it will help many people prevent it from happening and will also help us find more effective ways of treating it. Here are the main theories.

Theory 1: Infectious Disease: Viral Or Bacterial

It's pretty common for the symptoms of CFS to suddenly appear after flu-like illnesses. There are also more cases of CFS reported during the winter flu season than during any other time of the year. To many experts, this means that there might be a connection between whatever causes the flu and CFS. Today, we know that the flu is caused by a family of viruses. Maybe CFS is caused by a type of virus? Perhaps, but we don't know for sure.

Research has shown that antiviral (drugs that fight viruses) medications don't help. There is also not enough evidence to support the effectiveness of natural antiviral products either.

Not long ago it was thought that a very specific cause was found. It was a virus known as XMRV. At the time, this was incredibly exciting news. The initial research in 2009 suggested the possibility of a link between CFS and this virus. This excitement was relatively short-lived. Follow-up studies did not find an association between the two. Still, as mentioned before, there might be an indirect effect or immune suppression. Much more research in this area is needed and is ongoing.

While many experts still believe an undiscovered virus is responsible for CFS, there are some who believe that it might be caused by bacteria instead. This is because Lyme disease, a bacterial infection, has many symptoms that are similar to those of CFS.

Bacteria and viruses are completely different types of organisms. Bacteria are much more complex than viruses. Because of this, we use two entirely different types of medication depending on whether its a virus (antiviral) or bacteria (antibacterial or antibiotic).

If bacteria causes CFS, this might explain why antiviral medication did not seem to work. However, so far no concrete research evidence has been found supporting a bacterial cause either.

Theory 2: Psychiatric Or Neurologic Illness

Many times when people see psychiatric and illness in the same sentence, they think it means "crazy." So if a psychiatric illness is the cause of CFS, does that mean you're crazy? Absolutely not! Most people with these types of illnesses are anything but crazy.

But many people who develop CFS already suffer from depression and anxiety, both of which are psychiatric disorders. So, is there a connection between psychiatric disorders and CFS? Maybe, but there are many of you who do not suffer from any psychiatric disorders and still have CFS.

For example, it is common for many to have a harder time concentrating on things after coming down with CFS. So, maybe there is a problem going on in your brain?

In order to answer this question brain imaging studies were done on CFS patients. These tests revealed that even people without previous psychiatric disorders had small regions of the brain that didn't look normal. Many think that this supports the theory that CFS at least partly is a disorder of the brain.

Theory 3: An Immune System Disorder

Your immune system is in charge of defending you from most of the things that can get you sick. It's not surprising some believe that you might have CFS because your immune system isn't working the way it should be. In fact, a lot of people with CFS have abnormal levels of lymphocytes. There might also be changes in your cytokine production, the activity of natural killer cells and the reactivity of T-cells.

While it seems like a believable cause, abnormal levels of these cells are only seen in some CFS patients. So, just like the rest of the theories, scientific evidence supporting this theory is inconclusive.

Theory 4: Nutrient Deficiency

Do you have CFS because you haven't been eating right? Well, that's what some experts have proposed. As a result, many have stuffed themselves full of multi-vitamins and minerals. Before you get too vitamin-happy, you should probably know that people with CFS have diets that are surprisingly similar to completely healthy people.

Research has even shown that nutrient levels are not consistently different or abnormal in people with CFS. So what gives? Well, there are a few exceptions to these findings. You may have some sort of nutrient deficiency, like low magnesium levels. In these cases, vitamin supplementation might help. But this rings true only for a small number of people with CFS.

The moral of the story once again is that you should not overload on vitamins or minerals to supra-physiologic levels. Instead, focus on optimizing and maintaining a healthy diet. If you have holes in your diet then, by all means, fill them in with strategic use of supplements. Only *you* can determine what is missing from your diet.

Theory 5: A Problem With Metabolism

Your metabolism is what's responsible for breaking down food for energy and for using that energy to build and maintain your body. Key word: energy. So, at face value, it makes sense that a breakdown in this area might cause CFS. ATP is the energy currency of your body. You 'buy' activities with it. So, if you don't have enough of it, then you won't be able to do much.

You're feeling tired because your body isn't able to keep up with your energy demands. There are many components to energy metabolism. For example, mitochondrial dysfunction in producing ATP energy packets may be the cause.

Theory 6: Accumulation Of Oxidative Damage From Toxin Exposure

Another theory is that CFS may be the result of oxidative damage accumulating in your muscle tissue. There are two ways your body could be exposed to this type of injury, through external and internal toxins, as we have already discussed.

Let's recap the theories and how this closely ties in to cancer.

Theory 1: Infectious disease: viral or bacterial

Theory 2: Psychiatric or neurologic Illness

Theory 3: An Immune system disorder

Theory 4: Nutrient deficiency

Theory 5: A problem with metabolism

Theory 6: Accumulation of oxidative damage from toxin exposure

Some cancers are caused by or are associated with various types of parasitic, bacterial and viral infections. Other than neurologic malignancies, cancer is certainly not a psychiatric or neurologic illness. However, chemotherapy and radiation affect both the central and peripheral nervous system. Cancer possibly develops partly due to a defect in immune surveillance and immuno-modulation, and we know the risk of cancer is higher in those who are immune suppressed. There are a lot of links to dietary impact on cancer development. Cancer affects metabolic processed in your body in many ways. Lastly, we know that internal and external toxins contribute to carcinogenesis. There may or may not be some cause-effect relationships buried here, but it does not take much to notice the associations. It follows that a lot of what we have discussed in this book as anti-cancer strategies, like detox and optimal nutrition, may help in eliminating CFS as well.

All of the options for treating CFS is beyond the scope of this book, but here are some of the major mainstream and natural ways that you might explore.

Prescription Treatments

When there are multiple causes for something, there can't be a single treatment. So, mainstream medicine has nothing to "cure" CFS per se.

Currently, there is also no mainstream medication that your doctor can prescribe to alleviate *all* of your CFS symptoms. However, depending on your symptoms, your physician may be able to prescribe symptom-specific medication that may help.

But what is symptom-specific medication? It's pretty self-explanatory. Symptom-specific medication is designed to alleviate specific symptoms. For example, if you have difficulty sleeping, then your doctor may prescribe sleeping medication. While these medications are not meant to fix all your symptoms, they're certainly a start!

Remember, these medications are designed to treat specific symptoms and are not meant to cure CFS. While this may not seem to be as desirable as finding the root cause and the most effective treatment, it can help take the edge off while you pursue that goal.

Anti-Depressants

One of the common CFS symptoms is depression. If you fall into this category, then your doctor may prescribe a type of anti-depressant to deal with that particular symptom. Sometimes, these antidepressants may also be effective for other symptoms, such as insomnia. Typically, the success of anti-depressants varies and also depends on the type that is prescribed.

The most commonly prescribed antidepressants are monoamine oxidase inhibitors (MAOIs), selective serotonin-reuptake inhibitors (SSRIs) and tricyclics. The type that you are prescribed will largely depend on your symptoms and what your physician thinks is best for you. It is important that you are also aware of their side effects because they can negatively react with many other types of medication.

Remember, antidepressants are not meant to treat for CFS. Rather, they are prescribed because they have been shown to be an effective treatment for your underlying depression and they may also curb some of your other symptoms. Although these have shown promise in treating some of your underlying CFS symptoms, it is important to note that the evidence is still mixed and their use remains controversial.

Monoamine Oxidase Inhibitors (MAOIs)

Monoamine oxi-what? We agree that some medical jargon can be intimidating, not to mention tongue-twisting. It's not all that complicated.

There is an enzyme called monoamine oxidase in your body, which negatively interacts with some of the neurotransmitters that are essential for our general well-being. So, this type of medicine inhibits its release and help you feel less depressed. While more data is needed, some studies show that this type of anti-depressant might also have the effect of increasing energy levels, even if you have CFS and are not depressed.

If your doctor does prescribe this type of medication to you, then you should also be aware of its possible adverse effects, with the most severe side effect being hypertension or high blood pressure. For these reasons, you should avoid some foods such as products with concentrated yeast, aged cheese, chicken liver, dried meats and fish and red wine. Also, make sure your doctor is aware of any and all prescription AND non-prescription medications or supplements you're taking because these antidepressants can negatively react with many of them.

Selective Serotonin-Reuptake Inhibitors (SSRIs)

Another big medical name, but another easy explanation. SSRIs are the most widely prescribed antidepressants. They work by increasing the amount of sero-tonin, which is a neurotransmitter or brain chemical. This may improve overall mood while also reducing fatigue and sleeplessness. Fibromyalgia patients have lower levels of serotonin and the essential branched chain amino acids valine, leucine and isoleucine which contribute to the production of neurotransmitters.

Typically, SSRI medications are only prescribed to a subset of CFS patients: those who report the most severe cases of depression. If you fall into this group, then expect your doctor to prescribe something like Prozac®, Zoloft® or Paxil®.

If you would like a natural way to increase serotonin levels, exercise! Serotonin has been long known as the "happiness hormone," even though it is not a hor-mone, and is partly responsible for the euphoria of a "runner's high." You can also supplement your diet with leucine, isoleucine, and valine but don't over-do it. These amino acids can contribute to the synthesis of inhibitory or more depres-sive neurotransmitters too. As always, balance is everything.

Tricyclic Antidepressants

Tricyclics are another class of antidepressants that may be helpful for individuals who suffer from CFS. Besides treating depression, there is preliminary research evidence suggesting that they may even help reduce pain and promote better sleep!

For example, Elavil®, a type of tricyclic antidepressant, has been shown to alleviate many CFS symptoms. This includes fatigue and insomnia. Other tricyclics include Sinequan®, Norpramin®, Pamelor®, Anafranil® and Tofranil®.

Typically, CFS patients will have good results with lower doses than other individuals with depression. Although you probably won't need a high dosage, you should be aware of their adverse side effects anyway. These include dry mouth, constipation, and cognitive impairment. In other words, your thinking abilities might be slightly impaired. The key word is "might." As with any drug or natural substance, there are always possible side effects. So it is a bit of trial and error because everyone is different and can respond to anything they take differently.

If you are prescribed any tricyclic antidepressant, then you should take them as directed by your physician as an overdose can be life-threatening. You should also inform your physician of any other medications and supplements you are taking because tricyclics can have negative interactions with many of them.

Mild Pain Relievers

Another common symptom of CFS is widespread muscle pain. If you suffer from this, then mild pain relievers may help. In particular, CFS patients find that nonsteroidal anti-inflammatory drugs (NSAIDs) can reduce the pain and swelling. These drugs include Aspirin®, Ibuprofen®, Motrin®, Advil® and Aleve®, to name a few.

Although they generally work well, long-term use of NSAIDs can cause stomach ulcers and bleeding. They may also increase the blood pressure of individuals already being treated for hypertension. Critically important, if you have bleeding and clotting problems or are scheduled for an upcoming surgery, you should discontinue NSAIDs because they can interfere with blood clotting.

A natural alternative to these anti-inflammatory drugs is Omega-3 supplementation. Omega 3 fatty acids provide a lot of other benefits and are found in fish and flaxseed. This is not a treatment specific for CFS or fibromyalgia and can help with any inflammatory conditions. As with drugs, it is possible to take too much and end up with life threatening side effects including bleeding.

Natural salicylates, which are the main ingredient of Aspirin®, can be found not only in willow bark but also in many fruits and vegetables. Examples include apples, avocados, broccoli, eggplant, peaches, spinach and turmeric spice.

Specific Natural CFS Therapies

When it comes to CFS, there is no shortage of supposedly "effective" treatments. In fact, there are thousands of websites and articles in which people claim that so-and-so or such-and-such is the best way to treat CFS. But as we've stressed before, there is no such thing as a universal CFS treatment because there is no single causative factor!

In fact, you should always be wary of people who claim to have an expensive (and useless) CFS "cure." Sometimes, use of these supposed treatments can yield potentially dangerous results. Don't get snookered into buying expensive and useless stuff.

There are, however, some natural therapies that have shown significant potential for alleviating some or all of your CFS symptoms. We have chosen to review what we believe, based on published science, to be the most promising of them all.

Remember, these selections were made based on the best available scientific evidence supporting their effectiveness. This is much better than buying solutions whose reported effectiveness are based on non-specific, user testimonials. Again, I encourage you to refer to the Appendix for further coverage of this issue. There are different levels of scientific or research "evidence" out there.

As always, you should discuss these options with your physician before trying *anything* to avoid any unforeseen health issues.

NADH

As we discussed earlier, it has been suggested that CFS may be caused by some sort of metabolic dysfunction. Scientists theorize that CFS patients feel overwhelmingly fatigued because they are unable to keep up with the energy demands of the body. You might simply not have enough adenosine triphosphate (ATP) energy packets in your cells to carry out the energy-demanding pathways within your body, especially metabolic processes.

So, why is NADH important, and what is it?

NADH is nicotinamide adenine dinucleotide hydride. OK, that has to be the longest tongue twister name yet. However, it is a crucial intermediate in the regeneration of your body's ATP-based energy supply. Therefore, without NADH, you won't be able to effectively regenerate your ATP. So, could NADH supplementation help improve the debilitating fatigue CFS patients experience? Well, preliminary research suggests this might be the case.

A study involving twenty-six individuals with CFS was conducted over a three-month period. During the first month, the patients were given daily doses of either 10mg of NADH or a placebo for a month. During the second month, patients were not given either supplement. During the final month, the patients were given the opposite of whatever supplement they were given during the first month. It's called a crossover study and is pretty good in terms of getting at the truth with a small number of participants.

So, if one patient were given a placebo for the first month, then they would have been given the NADH supplement for the last month. Similarly, those who were first given NADH would have then be given the placebo during their final month of observation. Of the twenty-six individuals, 31% reported improvements when given NADH supplementation, compared to only 8% of patients given the placebo. Equally important, there were no adverse side effects.

Another study involved thirty-one CFS patients who were either given psychotherapy or NADH supplementation over a two year period. Of the thirty-one patients, the twelve that were given NADH reported a significant improvement in their overall well-being.

While the preliminary evidence is promising, much larger studies are needed before any concrete conclusions are made regarding the effectiveness of NADH supplementation in CFS patients.

D-Ribose

As you've already learned, D-ribose is a sugar that is an important contributor in the process that regenerates your body's energy supply in the form of ATP. Some research studies suggest that CFS patients might benefit from D-ribose supplementation.

A study of forty-one patients with either CFS or fibromyalgia were given a container of D-ribose and instructed to take three doses of D-ribose per day until the container was empty. The preliminary results were very promising! Almost 66% of the patients reported significant improvements in energy, sleep quality, cognitive functioning, pain threshold and overall well-being.

Once again, these are promising results, but it is important to know that a much larger study should be conducted before any concrete conclusions are drawn.

Vitamin D

A few studies have found lower Vitamin D levels in those who suffer from fibromyalgia, especially women. Others have contradicted this, but we also know that Vitamin D is essential for bone health, anti-cancer benefits and has been linked with fibromyalgia as well. While treatment studies are limited, there is a plausible reason and preliminary data to suspect that supplementation may help improve muscle strength and reduce pain.

It is possible to overdose with Vitamin D and create significant problems including hypercalcemia and liver damage. We've covered this is several areas in this book. Overall, it's best to optimize Vitamin D levels based on blood test monitoring, which is the safest approach.

Magnesium

Magnesium is one of the most abundant minerals found in your body and is responsible for making many of your body's metabolic processes possible. So, it should be evident that a magnesium deficiency would mean bad news for your body. In fact, without magnesium, your body would have a tough time getting much of anything going.

It should come as no surprise that magnesium deficiencies have been associated with many conditions, including fatigue, insomnia, anxiety and muscle pain. Notice anything?

If you guessed that these separate conditions also happen to be common symptoms of CFS, then you guessed right! In fact, recent research increasingly suggests that CFS may be linked to magnesium deficiencies. It is not the first time that these deficiencies have been linked to general fatigue.

For example, a few studies conducted in the 1960s reported improvements in fatigue when patients were given oral doses of magnesium. One study in particular involved oral supplementation of magnesium and potassium aspartate given to 3,000 individuals, with 75-91% of them reporting a reduction in fatigue.

While these results were promising for reduction of general fatigue, what about the fatigue that CFS patients suffer from? Well, the honest truth is that research involving magnesium supplementation in CFS patients is still limited. The few studies that have been done, however, have been very promising.

One such case study was done using thirty-two CFS patients who had subtle, yet noticeably lower levels of magnesium in their red blood cells. Of the thirty-two patients, fifteen were given intramuscular injections of magnesium sulfate while the other seventeen were given a placebo. Of the patients who received the magnesium injection, 80% of them reported a drastic improvement in their symptoms. They had more energy, experienced less muscle pain and exhibited much better moods. In fact, over half of them said that they no longer felt the same fatigue at all! On the other hand, only subtle improvements were reported by 17% of those who were given the placebo.

Although promising, it is important to note that more research is needed to determine the effectiveness of magnesium supplementation with certainty. Also, especially in this case, caution is very important. Too much magnesium can cause you to stop breathing.

L-Carnitine

L-Carnitine is a naturally occurring amino acid found in your body. Why is it important? If you guessed that it has something to do with energy, then you'd be right!

To be a little more specific, it is responsible for helping transport fatty acids to your cell's mitochondria. Once the fatty acids get into the mitochondria, they are then broken down to produce ATP, the energy currency of your body.

In a way, L-carnitine is sort of like a party invitation. Without it, there is no way the fatty acids are getting into the party, which is the mitochondria in this case. So, if your body doesn't have enough L-carnitine, then your fatty acids won't be transported into the mitochondria, and you won't be producing as much as ATP as you could be. You will also experience symptoms including muscle pain and weakness, post-exercise malaise, fatigue and lower blood-sugar levels.

Several studies have found CFS patients to have L-carnitine deficiencies. Also, the lower the levels of L-carnitine, the more severe the symptoms. L-carnitine supplementation may help CFS patients. For example, one small study found that 1-gram doses of L-carnitine taken 3-4 times a day improved twelve out of eighteen symptoms in CFS patients. Some of these patients experienced a complete remission of symptoms.

Specifically, in cancer patients with fatigue, a small study found L-carnitine supplementation at doses up to 3000mg/day (in divided doses) was safe and effective in reducing fatigue. Acetyl-L-Carnitine is the not same as L-Carnitine, but your body can metabolize them back and forth. The human study above used L-Carnitine. Animal studies suggest that Acetyl-L-Carnitine is better. So, the likelihood is that both are effective as a supplement. Beware that both can cause upset stomach, fishy odor in the urine and sweat, elevate blood pressure, and cause anxiety. If side effects occur, back off on the dose.

Cordyceps Sinensis

For millennia Traditional Chinese Medicine (TCM) has been using the mushroom Cordyceps for purposes of boosting immune function and reducing fatigue. There are some laboratory and animal studies that support plausible evidence for improving cortisol levels and effects on reducing fatigue. We include it because there is such a long history of use and the developing biochemical evidence that it might work. However, other than low-level case reports and anecdotal evidence, human studies are lacking as they are for these other "popular" TCM remedies for fatigue: Paecilomyces japonica (PJ), Phellinus linteus (PL), Ganoderma lucidum (GL), Grifola frondosa (GF), and Panax ginseng (PG).

While there is no good human evidence at this time, under proper supervision, these are all relatively non-toxic and safe. So, if you run out of other options, these supportive remedies are something to consider.

CHEMO-BRAIN OR CANCER-BRAIN

Chemo-brain is a newly recognized condition and is defined as "cancer treatment-related cognitive impairment." It is now at least recognized by mainstream oncology but not well studied. However, it is not uniformly accepted as being the result of chemotherapy. In fact, it is possible that it is "cancer brain" from biochemicals produced by cancer, or at least partly due to that.

Until recently, chemobrain was simply thought of as a form of depression, but it is now clear that it's related to cancer or its treatment. Similar symptoms have been described after radiation therapy to the brain. Other factors in cancer treatment, including stress, which may be related to cortisol secretion, can also be the culprit. No matter what the cause is, newer diagnostic techniques now include neuroimaging through MRI, PET scans, and EEG to study this syndrome. These objective measurement tools show that the cognitive impact is very real and not just a collection of subjective non-provable complaints.

It's been reported in 14% to 75% of cancer survivors in various studies vs. only about 8% with similar symptoms who have never had cancer or been exposed to chemotherapy or radiation. Also, this may be a moving target. As we move more into "personalized oncology," chemobrain causes may be different between types of chemotherapy and biologicals.

The problem is that while we seek to sort out what this syndrome is really caused by, there is no good mainstream medicine solution to help survivors deal with the effects. There are no proven natural therapies either, but some strategies that have helped other cognitive decline (e.g. dementia and Alzheimer's) have been suggested. The difference is that dementia and Alzheimer's are chronic degenerative conditions and chemo-brain appears not to be, although chemotherapy can accelerate beta-amyloid deposition which is a common finding in Alzheimer's. Also, the symptoms can be quite different. Alzheimer's and dementia patients struggle with short-term memory loss. Chemobrain causes inefficiency in the retrieval of information, or what people might call a "senior moment." They will eventually recall the question in mind, even if its short-term information they were just exposed to (i.e. a list of numbers or names). But overall, given the lack of a mainstream solution, it is reasonable to look at natural support used for general cognitive decline. The benefit of these remedies is unclear, but while the risk is not zero it is very low.

Below is a list of natural support therapies that have been used to help with memory loss and brain support that have at least reasonable evidence for their effectiveness. Overall, the more advanced ANY disease process is, the harder it is to reverse. In some cases, it is too little too late. So, it follows that natural supportive therapies for advanced dementias and Alzheimer's have NOT shown spectacular results in clinical trials. On the other hand, there is good laboratory and animal study evidence for plausibility.

If you don't have significant memory disease or simply want to prevent it, these are options to consider. As always, work with your physician.

Alpha-Tocopherol

Alpha-Tocopherol (Vitamin E) has also been shown to slow memory loss in older patients and is currently undergoing additional clinical trials. The caution here is that you can overdose on fat soluble vitamins, one of which is Vitamin E. One of the undesirable side effects can be hemorrhage, which may be life-threatening if it occurs within an organ such as the brain or at least extremely frightening if it is a severe nosebleed for example. However, this is usually only in doses over 4000IU per day.

B Vitamins

A 2010 study found that vitamins B12, B6, and folic acid could reduce levels of homocysteine, an amino acid linked to brain cell damage. The same study found that a regular supplement of B vitamins slowed brain atrophy for elderly people with mild cognitive impairment.

Coenzyme Q10

Coenzyme Q10 (ubiquinone) is an antioxidant naturally produced in the body that may support brain function. It is essential for multiple cellular processes, and its production decreases with age. The synthetic version of coenzyme Q10,

Ubiquinol, is absorbed more effectively as a supplement than its natural counterpart Ubiquinone. Parenthetically, absorption is better when taken with food. Used in conjunction with other treatments, Ubiquinol and Ubiquinone may slow cognitive decline.

Ginkgo Biloba

Ginkgo biloba is a plant extract and has been used for centuries in Chinese medicine. It's now being used in Europe for a variety of brain disorders. In 1994, a standardized dry extract of Ginkgo biloba leaves (SeGb), was approved by German health authorities for the treatment of primary degenerative dementia and vascular dementia. Several studies showed that 120-240mg of Ginko extract daily was effective in slowing dementia. The effect was hypothesized to be related to the reduction of inflammation and oxidative stress, membrane protection and a direct positive effect on neurotransmitters. So, Ginkgo is an option based on such studies. However, while it has very few undesirable side effects, it can increase the risk of bleeding. So, this is one extract you do not want to take during chemotherapy or around the time of surgery.

Panax Ginseng

Panax Ginseng (Asian or Red Korean) has a reputation for memory enhancement and has been confirmed as a potential treatment for Alzheimer's by a 2008 study. While using ginseng, the test groups, measured with both the mini-mental state examination (MMSE) and the Alzheimer's disease assessment scale (ADAS), showed increases in their overall cognitive abilities. These abilities declined back to normal levels when the treatment was discontinued. This evidence suggests that ginseng is an effective treatment for improving cognitive performance of Alzheimer's patients. Whether or not it translates to chemo brain is unknown but plausible. A precaution to consider is that the alertness may come at a price that also causes some degree of agitation. Also, the effects are somewhat dose dependent. So, work up to it and don't over-do it. There is some concern that due to a quasi-hormonal effect it may not be prudent to use ginseng beyond six months.

Green Tea

As discussed previously, green tea is known for its properties as an antioxidant, but in vitro studies (in laboratory test tube type studies rather than human or animal studies) show that it may also function to inhibit the activity of cholinesterases, thereby increasing the presence of the neurotransmitter acetylcholine (similar to existing prescription Alzheimer's treatments). The same in vitro study showed that green tea could also suppress the secretion of beta-amyloid protein.

Huperzine A

Huperzine A (Lycopodium serratum) is a moss extract that has been used in Chinese medicine. It's purported to be beneficial to those with moderate to severe Alzheimer's. A 2005 study determined that Huperzine A possesses the ability to reduce oxidative stress, as well as protect brain cells from beta-amyloid protein.

Vinpocetine

Derived from leaves of the periwinkle plant, vinpocetine increases cerebral blood flow and supports the brain's nerve cell metabolism. It was originally developed in Hungary under the drug name Cavinton. However, in the US it is available as a dietary supplement. It does not exist in nature per se and requires a lot of laboratory biochemical modifications to produce. On the downside, the European Commission E warned that it could cause immune suppression and other significant side effects, such as bleeding.

Omega-3 Fatty Acids

The chief omega-3 in the brain is docosahexaenoic acid (DHA), found in the membranes of nerve cells. Research shows that omega-3 can reduce the risk of heart disease, stroke, and dementia.

Theories about why omega-3 might reduce dementia risk include their benefit for the heart, anti-inflammatory effects, and shielding of nerve cell membranes. Researchers have also found that omega-3 fats excite growth of the nerve branches that connect one cell to another. This rich branching creates a dense "neuron forest," which allows the brain to process, store and retrieve information better.

Phosphatidylserine

Phosphatidylserine is a component of the protective membranes which surround nerve cells. It's available as a supplement and is made from cabbage or soy.

The beneficial effect disappears in Alzheimer's after a few months of use. It may be of greatest benefit in a less progressive disease like chemo-brain. There is research to support this concept in general (not chemo-brain), and the risk is low unless you are also taking anticholinergic medications. As always, check with your doctor or pharmacist about what you are taking and the safety of combining this with your medications. Reported doses for memory enhancement in various studies ranges from 100mg to 600mg/day.

Brain Exercising And Entrainment

Beyond botanicals and supplements, there is something to the concept of "use it or lose it." Treating chemo-brain with increased brain stimulating exercise is a no risk proposition. This may be something as simple as engaging in more activities that require one to think. Even playing more games and crossword puzzles may help. Advanced techniques like brain exercises, brain training, and entrainment are strategies you may want to explore.

Stress And Mind-Body Support

Since cancer treatment-related cognitive decline may be stress related and not chemo-brain per se, de-stressing techniques are essential to implement. These are good for your state of body and mind in any case. Obviously, we have covered a lot of them in other chapters.

SURGICAL DAMAGE AND HEALING

For help with preparation for surgery see the chapter on supplements (Chapter 13) which has a section on things to consider and things to avoid. Beyond topicals and herbals for perioperative conditions, keep in mind that acupuncture can be very helpful for pain. In addition, hypnosis can be effective and virtual reality goggle therapy is being studied as of this printing.

RADIATION DAMAGE AND HEALING

Radiation therapy can certainly damage normal tissues even though cancer is being targeted. This is especially true of healthy cells that divide and reproduce rapidly, like the mucosa in your mouth or intestinal tract. The degree to which normal tissue is damaged is highly variable and depends on the body part, the depth, your body size, and many other factors. This is why the planning phase is ultra-important and uses computer simulation with the help of radiation physicists in addition to the radiation oncology doctors. As we covered in Chapter 9, today's radiation is far less damaging than it was even ten years ago. It's not perfect, but there are things you can do to help avoid complications and to help heal after radiation.

Keep in mind that radiation, just like chemotherapy, is a pro-oxidant treatment. This means that antioxidants can help but may also interfere with the effectiveness of the radiation in killing cancer cells. In general, you will be asked to refrain from using any higher dose antioxidants because studies are conflicting. Some raise concerns. On the other hand, there is no evidence of harm from consuming an antioxidant diet during radiation therapy.

Amifostine (WR-2721), dexrazoxane, and mesna are all used as synthetic protectors against both chemotherapy and radiation damage, are all synthetic antioxidants and have been tested to see if they interfere with treatment. Amifostine is the most commonly used and has proven useful in limiting toxicity during treatment of head and neck, thyroid, lung, breast and uterine cancers, without an apparent reduction in anti-cancer radiation effect. Unfortunately, some people get nausea from this medication. Ask your radiation oncologist if these medications are right for you.

As far as specific natural supplemental antioxidants are concerned, they may work to help, or they may interfere with your treatment. No one knows for sure because safety and efficacy studies are largely missing. So if you choose to use these during radiation, you may be helping or hurting yourself. Having said that, let's review what we do know.

Astragalus is a very potent antioxidant and has been recommended during radiation therapy. A meta-analysis of 29 studies in lung cancer arrived at a favorable conclusion. It was found that Astragalus-containing Chinese herbals may improve effectiveness while reducing toxicity during radiation treatment of this disease. This is not spectacular evidence for effectiveness or safety, and it can't necessarily be extrapolated to other cancers, but is listed for your consideration.

Any antioxidant may be radioprotective, but the following have been named specifically with varying levels of laboratory, animal, and limited human evidence. The bioflavonoids quercetin and genistein/soy, resveratrol in lower doses, curcumin, omega-3 fatty acids, melatonin and glutamine in high doses (15 grams per day). For other reasons related to improved blood flow in the radiation field, gingko biloba and niacin have been recommended.

For certain areas when skin toxicity is the primary concern, notably the breast, head and neck, and vulva, topical applications of certain lotions may help prevent or minimize skin damage. These include calendula lotion, boswellia, coconut oil and aloe vera gel.

When radiation produces non-healing radiation-induced skin ulcers or damage to the bone called osteoradionecrosis, or similar healing issues, other options come into play. The one that is most tested is a combination of vitamin E 1000U and pentoxifylline 800mg per day for weeks to months. Both of these thin the blood, and the presumption is that better blood flow is the reason for wound healing benefit, but the exact mechanism by which this works to heal is unclear. Both are required for there to be an effect, and this combination has been used for prevention as well. Unfortunately, serious side effects can occur including bleeding, irregular heartbeats, chest pain, dizziness, nausea and more. With regard to skin ulceration, a wound expert should be involved because before attempting to enhance healing the wound sometimes needs to be cleaned or debrided. This may be done mechanically with surgery or using enzymatic ointments.

Topical treatments for enhancing healing include silver sulfadiazine, steroids, dexpanthenol (a form of pantothenic acid) emollient cream, medical honey, aloe gel, calendula lotion, coconut lotion in various combinations. None of these are outstanding but are all options to try in addition to oral therapy. Before applying any of these to an already injured area, it is best to test a topical on a small patch of healthy skin for allergic potential. Lastly, hyperbaric oxygen treatment is certainly an option to consider. An independent Cochrane review was favorable for head and neck and pelvic radiation injury, meaning that it can help but not in all cases.

Specifically regarding digestive system radiation protection and treatment, berberine, slippery elm bark and glutamine have both been used to help reduce colon symptoms during pelvic radiation. Both have been used for various irritable and inflammatory bowel conditions. Lactose intolerance becomes more pronounced during radiation, so staying away from most dairy products, or use of lactose-free versions, during radiation is prudent.

Damage to the salivary gland from radiation to the head and neck regions is common. This leads to dry mouth (xerostomia) and can increase mouth ulcers. Various saliva replacements and stimulants are available, including chewing gum, vitamin C, and malic acid, which is found in fruits such as pears and apples. The latter two can lead to demineralization of your teeth so be careful and rinse after eating or chewing vitamin C and malic acid containing fruits. On the mainstream side, a drug called pilocarpine can be effective for xerostomia. For mouth sores per se, the treatments are the same as those used during chemotherapy-related sores. Creating a paste from a medication called sucralfate can be helpful along with topical pain reducing ointments. Natural solutions include aloe, curcumin, honey (specifically Manuka honey), glutamine, and deglycyrrhizinated licorice (DGL). In some cases, a superinfection with candida fungus may make matters worse and require specific anti-fungal treatment.

Obviously, the radiation location and type combine with many other factors to make each situation unique. This is not an exhaustive list of remedies but rather an attempt to make it clear that there is help available when radiation complications occur. These can also be used to minimize complications, both acute and late.

CHAPTER 20
ANTI-CANCER RECIPE STARTER KIT

The following recipes are courtesy of Chef Joyce Vasilev, a Le Cordon Bleu trained chef and my wife. We work together as an integrative physician and chef towards making all this information palatable and as much of a pleasant culinary experience as possible. I don't have to tell you that chemo and sometimes radiation can change your taste buds radically. But this is usually temporary. So, if something does not appeal during treatment, try it again after chemo and radiation are over. Experiment and enjoy.

There are some controversial areas in dietary intake that may depend on personalized nutrigenetics in the end. In other words, what works for some might be a problem or even disaster for another. We can't predict it all yet. However, keep the major controversies of dietary nutrients in mind. You may just love something (e.g. cheese) and not want to give it up unless there was incontrovertible evidence about harm. Perhaps you want to play the precautionary principle to the hilt and exercise caution at every turn. It's really up to you. Here are some options to consider in modifying any diet.

If one were to cut out all dairy products, organic or not, from any animal, here are some suggestions to replace them:

Replace dairy milk with coconut, almond, soy or rice milk.

Hard cheeses can be replaced with tofu or bean curd, soft cheese with hummus. Yogurt from dairy can be replaced with soya or coconut yogurt.

Crème fraiche, fromage frais and dairy cream can be replaced with coconut or soya cream. Butter and margarine which contain dairy can be replaced with soya spreads, hummus, peanut or other nut and seed butter.

Dairy based ice cream can also be replaced with coconut or soya based ice cream. Milk chocolate can be replaced with dark chocolate.

Other potential modification advice includes replacing refined and processed oils with extra-virgin olive oil; refined and man-made sugars with stevia root; refined white bread, pasta and rice with unrefined wholegrain products.

Consumption of animal meat (other than fish), poultry and eggs should generally be limited. Ideally, red meat should be severely limited or eliminated. Largely replace these with fish, unrefined carbohydrates, legumes, nuts, vegetables, and fruit. Standard table salt can be replaced by multiple herbs. Instead of coffee consider white or green tea.

Remove all potential toxins from cooking, including plastic cookware, preservatives, artificial colors and food flavorings.

Without further ado, here are the sampler recipes to try:

MUSHROOM BARLEY SOUP

Ingredients:

1. ½ c. pearl barley

2. juice of a ½ fresh lemon

3. 2 tablespoons extra virgin olive oil

4. 1 small onion diced

5. 1 cup finely diced fresh carrots

6. 1 cup of finely diced celery

7. ½ pound of fresh shitake mushrooms thinly sliced

8. 2 cloves garlic

9. ¼ teaspoon dried oregano

10. ¼ teaspoon dried thyme

11. ¼ teaspoon ground caraway

12. 9 cups of vegetable or low sodium beef broth

13. ¼ cup of loosely packed chopped fresh Italian parsley

14. salt and pepper to taste

Directions:

1. Soak barley in a bowl of water, and lemon juice overnight

2. Drain and rinse barley

3. Heat the extra virgin olive oil in a soup pot over medium heat, add onion, S&P tt and sauté until translucent, about 4 minutes. Add the carrots and celery, sauté 3 more minutes. Add the mushrooms, garlic, oregano, thyme, caraway, and barley, sauté for 3 – 4 minutes or until the mushrooms release their juices. Pour in 1 cup of the broth to deglaze the pan and continue cooking until the liquid has reduced by ¾. Add the remaining 8 cups of broth and bring to a boil, then lower heat to simmer for 25 minutes. Stir in the parsley and taste for seasoning.

PREP TIME: 20 minutes (if barley soaked overnight)

COOK TIME: 45 minutes

CHEF JOYCE'S TIP: If you have leftover soup, you'll see the barley will soak up the broth due to expansion, so keep an extra cup or two aside to heat up the leftovers.

CREAM OF BROCCOLI AND POTATO SOUP

Sautéing the broccoli in the extra virgin olive oil, then adding the broth, then blending, releases all the sweetness and cancer-fighting properties.

Ingredients:

1. 2 tablespoons of extra virgin olive oil

2. 1 cup finely diced onion

3. 2 cloves chopped garlic

4. 2 cups peeled and finely diced Yukon gold potatoes

5. ½ teaspoon salt

6. 3/4 pound cut-up broccoli florets (bite size)

7. 4 ½ cups vegetable broth

8. 1 dash of nutmeg

9. Shredded Organic cheddar cheese, for garnish (optional)

Directions:

1. Heat extra virgin olive oil in a large sauté pan over medium heat; add onion and sauté lightly until golden, about 3 minutes. Stir in the garlic and then the potatoes along with the salt and sauté until potatoes are just tender, about 5 minutes.

2. Pour in ½ cup of the broth to deglaze, and turn down the heat to medium-low, and cook until the liquid is reduced by half. Add the broccoli and cook until the broccoli is bright green and just tender, about 3 to 4 minutes.

3. Pour 2 cups of the remaining broth into a blender, add half of the broccoli mixture and blend until smooth. Pour mixture into the soup pot, and repeat the process with remaining broth and vegetables. Add nutmeg.

4. Gently reheat the soup over low heat, and check for seasoning. You may want to add a little extra salt, some fresh ground pepper and a dash of lemon juice.

5. Serve garnished with a sprinkle of the cheese.

PREP TIME: 20 minutes

COOK TIME: 20 minutes

CHEF JOYCE'S TIP: For more "YUM" factor, use roasted garlic instead of sautéed garlic.

COLD AND COOLING AVOCADO
AND CUCUMBER SOUP

For those into cold soups, the clean and fresh feel of this soup will delight those with swallowing difficulties and or mouth sores, with its velvety texture.

Ingredients:

1. 2 cups water

2. 2 pounds English cucumbers, peeled and cut into small chunks

3. 2 ripe avocados, pitted and peeled

4. 3 tablespoons fresh lime juice

5. ¼ teaspoon agave nectar

6. Sea salt

7. Dash of Cayenne

8. 1 tablespoon of fresh mint chopped

9. 1 tablespoon of fresh cilantro chopped

Directions:

1. Pour 1 cup of water into the blender, add cucumbers, avocados, lime juice, agave nectar, ¼ teaspoon of salt, and cayenne. Blend until very smooth, then gradually adding more water until the desired consistency is reached. Taste and adjust the amount of sea salt.

2. Chill for at least 2 hours, then add the mint and cilantro before serving.

PREP TIME: 15 minutes

COOK TIME: 2 hours in the refrigerator

CHEF JOYCE'S TIPS: Only use the English cucumbers, they make a huge difference in this soup. They're less watery and will add more substance to the soup.

LEMONY LENTIL SOUP WITH SPINACH

Lentils provide excellent sources of two types of B Vitamins, iron, potassium and folate, just to name a few. This soup is a fabulous and filling main course full of protein and fiber.

Ingredients:

1. 1 1/2 cups red lentils, rinsed
2. 1 cup chopped tomatoes with their juice
3. 3 tablespoons extra virgin olive oil
4. 1/4 teaspoon turmeric
5. 6 whole garlic cloves, peeled
6. 4 slices fresh ginger (each about the size of a quarter)
7. 1 sprig fresh rosemary
8. 2 bay leaves
9. 1 10 – ounce bag washed baby spinach
10. 2 tablespoons freshly squeezed lemon juice
11. Coarse sea salt or kosher salt to taste
12. Freshly ground black pepper

Directions:

1. Combine 6 cups of water with the lentils in a 3 – to 4-quart saucepan over high heat. Skim off the foam as the lentils begin to boil. Add tomatoes, oil, turmeric, and garlic. Reduce the heat to a simmer. Wrap ginger, rosemary, and bay leaf in a piece of cheesecloth, tie it closed with kitchen string and add to the pan. Simmer until the lentils are tender and the garlic is soft; discard the cheesecloth.

2. Add the spinach and simmer until wilted. Stir in the lemon juice. Crush the garlic against the side of the pot with the back of a spoon and stir so that it melts into the soup. Season with salt and pepper to taste, and serve.

PREP TIME: 20 minutes

COOK TIME: 30 minutes

CHEF JOYCE'S TIPS: Serve this soup with wedges of whole wheat pita for dipping and making sure to mop up all the yummy goodness.

WHOLE WHEAT ENGLISH MUFFIN WITH SALMON

Smoked salmon and eggs on a toasted whole-wheat English muffin is the perfect power breakfast. For more protein and a still substantial meal, use egg whites and pair that with a piece of fruit or a glass of 100% juice.

Ingredients:

1. 1/2 teaspoon extra-virgin olive oil

2. 1 tablespoon finely chopped red onion

3. 2 large eggs, beaten

4. Pinch of salt

5. 1/2 teaspoon capers, rinsed and chopped (optional)

6. 1 ounce smoked salmon

7. 1 slice tomato

8. 1 whole-wheat English muffin, split and toasted

Preparation:

1. Heat olive oil in a small nonstick skillet over medium heat. Add onion and cook, stirring, until it begins to soften, about 1 minute. Add eggs, salt and capers (if using) and cook, constantly stirring, until whites are set, about 30 seconds.

2. To make the sandwich, layer the eggs, smoked salmon and tomato on English muffin.

PREP TIME: 10 minutes

COOK TIME: 10 minutes

CHEF JOYCE'S TIPS: For a bit of freshness and crunch, you can add or substitute sliced cucumber for the tomato.

CREAMY OATMEAL WITH BLUEBERRIES AND PECANS

In this satisfying, on-the-go oatmeal recipe, protein-rich Greek yogurt, crunchy pecans, and sweet berries make this the perfect healthy breakfast.

Ingredients:

1. 1 cup water

2. Pinch of salt

3. 1/2 cup steel cut oats

4. 1/2 cup fresh blueberries

5. 2 tablespoons nonfat plain Greek yogurt

6. 1 tablespoon toasted chopped pecans

Preparation:

1. Bring water and salt to a boil in a small saucepan. Stir in oats, reduce heat to medium and cook, occasionally stirring, until most of the liquid is absorbed, about 5 minutes. Remove from heat, cover and let stand 2 to 3 minutes. Top with blueberries, yogurt, and pecans. Use stevia root for more sweetness.

PREP TIME: 10 minutes

COOK TIME: 10 minutes

SCRAMBLED EGG BURRITO

Ingredients:

1. 4 8-inch whole-wheat flour tortillas

2. 4 large eggs

3. 1/8 teaspoon salt

4. Freshly ground pepper to taste

5. 1 teaspoon extra-virgin olive oil

6. 1 4-ounce can chopped green chiles

7. 1/2 cup grated Cheddar or pepper Jack cheese

8. 1/4 cup reduced-fat sour cream

9. 1 cup prepared salsa

Preparation:

1. To prepare burritos: Preheat oven to 350°F. Wrap tortillas in foil and heat in the oven for 5 to 10 minutes.

2. Meanwhile, blend eggs, 1/8 teaspoon salt, and pepper in a medium bowl with a fork until well combined. Heat 1 teaspoon oil in a medium non-stick skillet over medium-low heat. Add green chiles and cook, stirring, for 1 minute. Add the eggs and cook, stirring slowly with a wooden spoon or heatproof rubber spatula, until soft, fluffy curds form, 1 1/2 to 2 1/2 minutes.

3. To serve, divide eggs evenly among the tortillas. Sprinkle each with about 2 tablespoons cheese and roll up. Serve with sour cream and the salsa.

PREP TIME: 10 minutes

COOK TIME: 20 minutes

CHEF JOYCE'S TIPS: For a smoky and spicier burrito use a can of chipotle chile peppers in adobo sauce.

ORANGE BERRY SMOOTHIE

This meal-in-a-glass smoothie is bursting with berries and orange juice, healthful sources of carbohydrate and powerful antioxidants. Getting plenty of antioxidant-rich foods makes sense since free radicals are produced any time the body's cells process oxygen.

Ingredients:

1. 1 1/4 cups fresh berries

2. 3/4 cup low-fat plain yogurt

3. 1/2 cup fresh blended oranges (retain pulp)

4. 2 tablespoons nonfat dry milk

5. 1 tablespoon toasted wheat germ

6. 1 tablespoon honey

7. 1/2 teaspoon vanilla extract

Preparation:

1. Place berries, yogurt, blended orange juice, dry milk, wheat germ, honey and vanilla in a blender and blend until smooth.

PREP TIME: 5 minutes

CHEF JOYCE'S TIPS: Add a ripe banana for a thicker added richness. Can also add ice to minimize the thickness.

BUCKWHEAT PANCAKES

Ingredients:

1. 2 1/2 cups buckwheat flour

2. 1 cup buttermilk powder, (see Note)

3. 5 tablespoons dried egg whites, such as Just Whites (see Note)

4. 1/4 cup sugar

5. 1 1/2 tablespoons baking powder

6. 2 teaspoons baking soda

7. 1 teaspoon salt

8. 1 cup flaxseed meal, (see Note)

9. 1 cup nonfat dry milk

10. 1/2 cup oat bran

11. 1 1/2 cups nonfat milk

12. 1/4 cup vegetable oil

13. 1 teaspoon vanilla extract

Preparation:

1. Mix well or whisk the flour, buttermilk powder, dried egg whites, sugar, baking powder, baking soda and salt in a large bowl. Stir in flaxseed meal, dry milk, and bran. (Makes 6 cups dry mix.)

2. Combine milk, oil, and vanilla in a glass measuring cup.

3. Place 2 cups pancake mix in a large bowl. (Refrigerate the remaining pancake mix in an airtight container for up to 1 month or freeze for up to 3 months.)

4. Make a well in the center of the pancake mix. Whisk in the milk mixture until just blended; be cautious not to over mix. (The batter will seem quite thin but will thicken up as it stands.) Let stand for 5 minutes.

5. Coat a nonstick pan or griddle with cooking spray and place over medium heat.

6. Whisk the batter. Using 1/4 cup batter for each pancake, cook pancakes until the edges are dry and bubbles begin to form, about 2 minutes. Turn over and cook until golden brown, about 2 minutes longer.

PREP TIME: 20 minutes

COOK TIME: 10 minutes

CHEF JOYCE'S TIPS:

Additional notes: Buttermilk powder, such as Saco Buttermilk Blend, is a useful substitute for fresh buttermilk. Look in the baking section or with the powdered milk in most markets.

Dried egg whites are convenient in recipes calling for egg whites because there is no waste. Look for brands like Just Whites in the baking or natural-foods section of most supermarkets.

You can find flaxseed meal in the natural-foods section of large supermarkets. You can also start with whole flaxseeds: Grind 2/3 cup whole flaxseeds to yield 1 cup.

BUTTERNUT SQUASH SOUP WITH GINGER

Butternut squash is delicious pureed with apple and ginger. This soup is a perfect way to get the inflammation-fighting properties of ginger and turmeric.

Ingredients:

1. 2 tablespoons extra virgin olive oil
2. 1 large onion
3. 2 cloves of garlic, minced
4. 1 teaspoon turmeric
5. 1 butternut squash peeled, seeded, and cubed
6. 4 cups vegetable broth
7. 2 large apples, peeled, cored, and chopped
8. 1 tablespoon grated fresh ginger
9. ½ teaspoon salt

Directions:

1. Heat oil in a large saucepan over medium heat. Add the onion and cook stirring, until translucent and lightly browned, about 4 minutes. Stir in the garlic and turmeric and cook for another minute. Add the squash and vegetable broth and bring to a boil.

2. Reduce the heat to low, cover and simmer until the squash is tender, about 20 minutes. Add the apples, ginger, and the salt and cook until the squash and apples are very tender, another 10 to 20 minutes. Remove from heat and cool for 15 minutes.

3. Working in batches, place the cooled soup mixture in a blender and process until smooth.

PREP TIME: 20 minutes

COOK TIME: 45 minutes

CHEF JOYCE'S TIPS: For a fancy finish, swirl a dollop of plain yogurt on top before serving.

CHOPPED SALAD

Chopped Salad is a classic – it's just plain good and good for you. Here is the basic set up, whatever your craving to make it more of a meal, go for it. Just keep it fresh, organic, or wild caught.

Ingredients:

1. 3 cups roasted or poached chicken or salmon, cut into ½ inch dice

2. 2 firm ripe avocados, cut into ½ inch dice

3. 3 medium ripe sweet tomatoes, seeded and cut into ½ inch dice

4. 2 medium hard cooked eggs, sliced

5. 1 bunch watercress, stems trimmed

6. 1 heart of romaine lettuce, cut into ½ inch squares

7. 1 cup of fresh chives, cut at an angle crosswise into ¼ inch length

Vinaigrette:

1. 1 clove of garlic pressed

2. 1 tablespoon Dijon mustard

3. 2 tablespoons red – wine vinegar

4. 1 tablespoon lemon juice

5. ½ cup extra virgin olive oil

6. salt and pepper to taste

To make the vinaigrette, combine the garlic, mustard, vinegar, lemon juice, and a pinch of salt in a small bowl. Let it sit for 5 to 10 minutes. Whisk in the ½ of olive oil, taste with a leaf of the romaine and add more salt or vinegar if necessary. Set aside.

Directions:

1. Place the chicken or salmon, avocado, tomato, and eggs in a large bowl. Season with the salt and pepper. Add the watercress, romaine, and chives and toss gently to combine.

2. Pour lightly and gently the vinaigrette over the salad and with a delicate hand, transfer the salad to a platter or individual serving plates.

PREP TIME: 25 minutes

COOK TIME: 35 minutes

CHEF JOYCE'S TIPS: To poach chicken or salmon (skinless and boneless), bring meat to room temp for 20 minutes. Bring the slightly salted water to a boil, add chicken or salmon and reduce the heat to maintain a gentle simmer, 10 – 12 minutes. Remove and let cool to room temperature. Then dice.

SPINACH SALAD WITH CHICKPEAS

This fresh and delicious salad is packed with antioxidants, fiber, and cancer – fighting ingredients.

Ingredients:

1. 2 medium red onions, thinly sliced

2. 1 15 ounce can of chickpeas, drained, rinsed, and patted dry

3. ¼ cup of fresh lemon juice

4. 2 tablespoons of flaxseed oil

5. 2 tablespoons extra virgin olive oil

6. 1 garlic clove minced

7. ½ teaspoon salt

8. ¼ cup of crumbled feta cheese (optional)

9. 1 5 ounce package of baby spinach

10. 2 red apples, cored and sliced

11. 2 tablespoons ground flaxseed

Directions:

1. In a measuring cup, whisk together the lemon juice, flaxseed oil, olive oil, and salt. Stir in the cheese (optional)

2. Place the spinach in a large bowl and toss with the onions, chickpeas, apples, and flaxseed. Drizzle on the vinaigrette.

PREP TIME: 10 minutes

CHEF JOYCE'S TIPS: To add a toastier flavor to this salad, roast the onions and the chickpeas in the oven for 10 minutes at 400 degrees.

BROCCOLI SALAD

Broccoli is the all-star cancer fighter, packed with potent anti-cancer compounds that flush out carcinogens.

Ingredients:

1. ¼ cup balsamic vinegar

2. 2 tablespoons Dijon mustard

3. 2 tablespoons honey

4. ¼ teaspoon salt

5. ¼ teaspoon black pepper

6. 2 tablespoons flaxseed oil

7. 3 tablespoons extra virgin olive oil

8. 2 heads of broccoli

9. 1 small red onion, thinly sliced

10. ½ cup slivered almonds

11. ½ cup dried cranberries

12. 4 ounces of crumbled goat cheese (optional)

Directions:

1. In a large bowl, whisk together the vinegar, mustard, honey, salt., and pepper. Whisk in the flaxseed and olive oils until blended. Set aside.

2. Remove the florets from the broccoli and trim the ends with a vegetable peeler, then add to the vinaigrette.

3. Add the onions, almonds, and dried cranberries to the bowl and toss well. Top with cheese (optional).

PREP TIME: 20 minutes

CHEF JOYCE'S TIPS: If the raw broccoli is too tough for you, steam it for 4 minutes, then rinse in cold water and drain well before adding to the salad.

TUNA AND WHITE BEAN SALAD

Delicious salads dressings don't have to always contain fats. Vitamin-rich tomato juice is the base for this amazing salad.

Ingredients:

1. 1/3 cup tomato juice

2. 3 tablespoons lemon juice

3. 3 tablespoons Extra virgin olive oil

4. 1 tablespoon fresh basil

5. ¼ teaspoon salt

6. 1 6 ounce can of albacore tuna, drained (better is fresh if you can find)

7. 1 15 ounce can of white beans, drained and rinsed

8. 1 medium cucumber, peeled seeded and chopped

9. ¼ cup of pitted Kalamata olives, chopped

10. 6 cups of fresh mixed salad greens

Directions:

1. In a large measuring cup, whisk together the tomato juice, lemon juice, oil, basil, and salt.

2. In a medium bowl, toss the tuna, beans, cucumber, olives and 1 tablespoon of the vinaigrette.

3. In a large salad bowl, add the salad greens and top with tuna mixture, and drizzle the rest of the vinaigrette.

PREP TIME: 15 minutes

CHEF JOYCE'S TIPS: Sneak beans into some of your favorite dishes, just drain and rinse well. Add them to soups, salads, stews, and casseroles.

We hope that these recipes are to your liking. There are many more in development for presentation and tasting on http://CancerCureology.com if you join us.

CONCLUSION
PROACTIVE ANTI-CANCER ANTI-RECURRENCE STRATEGIES AND MINDSET BEAT HOPE ALONE

Your future is largely what you make of it, even in the face of cancer. There is a lot in this book, and it might be confusing, but here is a synopsis to help you develop a personal roadmap to success in survivorship. Remember, there is more than one path to success. However, once you have initially beaten cancer, what next?

First of all, you do not want to have defeated one cancer, only to be diagnosed with a second or third or more. I have personally taken care of individuals who have suffered through 7 different cancers in their lifetime. Screening for colorectal, breast, prostate, and cervical cancers may reduce illness and death by early detection of cancers and pre-cancers. These are largely preventable. Unfortunately, some other cancers, notably ovarian cancer, have no good screening tools to date. There are specific recommendations for screening which you should be following. You should also be screened for other diseases which can be inflammatory and pro-cancer in origin, such as diabetes. Don't win one battle to develop and lose another.

Beyond screening, which is better for your psychology? Hoping that things work out or proactively seeking safe and effective avenues to achieve as long a quality-filled life as possible? I am not knocking "faith," but if you are a believer, there is nothing wrong with doing your pro-active part as well. Remember, how you think and emote follows a path through the mind-body connection or psycho-neuroimmunology to either strengthening or weakening your body. This is a fact. There are specific action steps that you have learned about in this book and can be taking which range from general health support to immune support to direct anti-cancer strategies. Everyone is an individual, but there are some commonalities. Devise your best-personalized plan in collaboration with your oncologist and integrative support providers.

After beating cancer, you want to anti-cancerize and otherwise disease-proof your body. When you complete your treatment, your oncologist is likely to say something like, "we'll watch your closely, do scans and tests when needed and hope it doesn't come back." This is called "watchful waiting." To fall into this psychological and biological mind-set trap is certainly not the most proactive thing you can do. This book is a primer about what you can safely take into your own hands. There is also a ton of developing research which suggests a more proactive approach will improve your quality of life and possibly increase longevity.

You want to be in a state of body and mind that celebrates life in your survivorship, don't you? It's a continued journey, whether you are trying to gain back energy from throes of fatigue, regain better memory in defeating chemo-brain, addressing lingering effects like numbness in your hands or feet, and discovering a better life after weathering a potentially life-threatening disease. It is really akin to a rebirth. I hope the information in this book will help as a guide.

Diet and lifestyle modifications, such as exercise, are cornerstones and can go a long way to help strengthen your body and help prevent recurrence. These are no brainer activities when your life hangs in the balance. It's often a gift for a second chance. Take it!

Many cancer-causing agents have now been discovered by researchers, and we are exposed to these almost daily. Most forms of cancer can be prevented by making a few primary lifestyle alterations, such as exercising and eating healthy, averting too much sun exposure, avoiding environmental toxins and refraining from no-brainer deadly tobacco and junk food use.

Cancer is a disease that touches more and more of us. I have been touched by it in my immediate family twice, and I have taken care of thousands of patients with cancer as an oncologist. There are many success stories out there, and I can attest to the fact that the ones who seem to do the best have the best proactive attitudes and approaches to life.

While standard mainstream therapy is a cornerstone to your best chance for a cure, it is equally important to support your body and make it as cancer-proof as you can. With the anti-cancer strategies covered in this book, I hope you will find success in your journey. This book is just the beginning of something greater and is the basis for the **Cancer Cureology Anti-cancer Five Step System**, which is a dynamic, integrative guide and surrounding community towards thriving in survivorship. Join us at http://CancerCureology.com

Appendix
What is SCIENTIFIC "Proof"?

How do you know if what you read in this book can really help you? Another way to say this is, how do we know something is true or totally false? Putting it even more bluntly, does this book contain things that are likely to help you or is it full of garbage? Although some of us retain more healthy skepticism than others, in general, we are all programmed to believe what we read and see in various media, including TV, radio, newspapers, books, websites, etc. It's sad that we are so suggestible but rest assured that this is perfectly normal! Still, when you clear your head, it's important to know how to drill down through the BS and get to the good stuff. The truth! Science is objective and usually a good proxy for the truth when scientific evidence is available. In some form, it usually is.

As far as resources to look at in order of objective importance it would be medical peer-reviewed health journals followed by abstracts (i.e. preliminary results reports) of research presented at medical or other healthcare meetings. There are thousands of international journals listed in Index Medicus® and MEDLINE® on PubMed®, including mainstream and alternative. So there are plenty of opportunities for researchers to have their work published. Those that say they were "banned" because their material was too controversial are bald faced lazy liars.

It is true that any given journal can reject a submitted research paper for many reasons. Perhaps it does not fit the readership, or there are quality issues. For example, you generally can't get cancer research papers published in a journal which covers psychiatric issues. The authors have a chance for rebuttal or submission to at least hundreds of other related journals. These days, if you can't get your work published in traditional journals, there are also "open source" avenues, some of which require A small payment to covers costs to get published. The point is, if you have something even remotely decent to publish, it will get published. But this speaks to only part of the problem. There is actually a lot of junk published every day. So, just because the research was published does not mean it was good research. There is a way to discriminate between the good, bad and ugly as you will find out.

Books are not a great resource unless they are referenced with scientific studies. That is why we added a lot of specific references in this report, and you can rest assured that if you studied those references there are thousands more in their reference section. Without such references a book is merely a collection of opinions and, as you will see as you read on, this is considered to be the lowest level of evidence possible. Literally, anyone can write a book or a magazine article or blog post or even be interviewed on fairly prominent radio and TV shows. Unless grounded in good scientific evidence, it is just an opinion and should be taken with a grain of salt. There is no question that this book contains opinions as well, and that is noted as much as possible.

In the end, the practice of medicine is largely based on professional opinions of physicians who have digested all the information available to them, looked at your specific situation and offered an opinion as to the best course of action. This is especially true if you follow the mantra of holistic medicine and consideration of the whole person. Nonetheless, the more there is a scientific basis for opinions the better, when compared to making things up as you go along.

Please keep in mind that this is a primer on "grading" the quality of scientific evidence and not a textbook on how scientific processes are optimized. We're also going to leave aside conspiracy theories about "Big Pharma" and the FDA in this review and focus on facts about the process.

You can rest assured that there are checks and balances at all levels, from laws to peer review to ethics and institutional review boards which are required to have non-medical citizens as members. This step is intended for review before a study is even started. Then experienced research physicians in independent practices and universities (often international) are recruited and assigned the role of "principle investigator." Or the study may be designed and initiated by a principle investigator and their team at a university or other research center, independent of sponsorship. So, very often the research is disconnected from direct funding by any drug companies.

During the study, even more checks and balances are in place including a third party contract research organization (CRO) which is responsible for monitoring the safety of patients and details of study conduct. Finally, after the study is completed, a peer review process is initiated to ensure that the study met criteria to get published.

This is an extremely brief overview but raises the point that it is hard to imagine the whole international research structure to be somehow fake. Tens of thousands of well-meaning physicians, researchers, statisticians, universities, and citizens just like you are not all "being paid off" to approve, perform and publish bogus or "fudged" research or something crazy like that. Even if this were remotely possible in some isolated instance, all of these levels of scrutiny provide ample opportunity for "whistleblowers" to come forward and state that there was wrongdoing. Clearly, even the best processes fail sometimes, but that is why you need multiple scientific references if possible before deciding what is fact and what is fiction. Finally, there is no question that some studies that are planned, executed and published are far better than others. Some journals are far better than others regarding publication quality. That is what this primer is about. It should be able to help you recognize that the evidence behind something may not be so hot, just like the medical community can. Enough said on this.

Einstein once said that "Imagination is more important than knowledge." Clearly, "out-of-the-box" thinking can be advantageous. However, ignoring proven principles from biology, physiology, anatomy, genetics, biochemistry and physics can be counterproductive. These scientific disciplines are the basis for how all stuff works, and your body is no exception. On the other hand, there is surely a LOT yet to be learned, which will continue to require innovative thought. But there have also been *huge* strides over the past 25 years in medical science, and this does not simply mean the development of newer and more drugs. It means understanding how things work in the human body. Based on this growing knowledge one can hang their hat on scientific evidence as a good basic platform from which to make decisions about improving health. However, as already alluded to, the following is a critical point.

Scientific evidence is NOT all created equal!!! Many quality medical journals require authors to include a level of evidence these days, based on the type of study design, and the summary of this (paraphrased to minimize medical jargon) is as follows:

Level I: Evidence obtained from at least one properly designed and powered randomized controlled trial (RCT). Randomization means a "flip of the coin" (heads or tails) as to which treatment group A vs. group B got when comparing results and outcomes between group A and group B. This "flip of the coin" is now done by computer but the idea is the same. If you are participating in a clinical trial, you are randomly assigned to treatment A or treatment B. This completely removes any bias that a research investigator might have, and the results are much cleaner to interpret.

The "power" of the study is a statistical term which addresses whether not enough people are enrolled in the clinical trial to make a meaningful statement about the results from a statistical perspective. This calculation is done in advance to determine how many people are needed to prove or disprove an idea or treatment. Sometimes underpowered studies are done and even published, which make a claim that something works. If underpowered, the study result is likely to be due to random chance alone and not to the treatment used.

The best possible evidence is often summarized in a rigorous review, called a meta-analysis, of at least several RCTs which seem to indicate the same result. In other words, more than one research group has independently shown the same result, especially if Level I, making it far more compelling and believable.

Level I evidence is the only level that can absolutely prove that a specific intervention works. It is the only level of evidence that can prove cause-effect relationships vs. an association between things. Having said that, not everything requires Level I evidence to be accepted.

Level II-1: Evidence obtained from well-designed controlled trials without randomization. Although randomization is the ideal, sometimes it is not feasible. So this is the next best study design. Many factors and patient characteristics are still "controlled" so that group A and group B are similar in nature (e.g. age, sex, other medical issues, etc.). This makes it more likely that the resulting difference between treatment A and B is due to the treatment and not one of these other factors.

Level II-2: Evidence obtained from well-designed cohort or case-control studies, preferably from more than one center or research group. Cohort studies can be either prospective (forward in time) or retrospective (looking back). In each case a group of subjects/patients/people is followed through time, usually comparing exposed and unexposed subjects to some risk factor or treatment intervention. Case-control studies look back in time. First, the research question is identified and explicitly stated (e.g. why did a certain group do better or worse than another group when living in some area or different geographical areas). Then the objective is to identify subjects with and without a disease or condition. A sample population ("cases") is defined as well as a matched sample population without the condition ("controls") but with similar demographics. The background and exposure to various things (e.g. diet or toxin exposure) of each group are then reviewed to find out why the "cases" developed a given condition whereas the "controls" did not. These epidemiologic studies are very important to reveal interesting associations, but they cannot prove cause and effect. Sometimes the associations are very strong and it may be wise to use that evidence if it is the best we have. But weak association studies, which are unfortunately published all the time, are a waste of paper. These are often quoted as factual proof, and that is extremely misleading.

Level II-3: Evidence obtained from multiple time series with or without the intervention. Dramatic results in uncontrolled experiments could also be regarded as this type of evidence. For example a doctor may compare a series of patients, some of whom received a treatment and others did not. Or perhaps they received a different treatment. When compared to some of the above study types this is a far less rigorous study design. This means a lot of other factors may be present between the groups of patients that might explain the difference in outcomes other than the actual treatment. For example, a doctor gives some patients two different diet enhancing supplements and compares how many end up with diabetes without looking at the possibility that one group was more overweight than the other. The diabetes development may have been more related to the weight and patients' metabolism than the supplements that they received.

Level III: Opinions of respected "expert" authorities, based on clinical experience, descriptive studies, or reports of expert committees. This is the weakest type of evidence but is sometimes the best there is. Think of this as being similar to a collection of expert testimonials from verified and credible sources. The key to this is that the "expert" is verified and credible by some objective criteria.

Plenty of people are out there sporting MD, Ph.D., ND, NMD, OMD, DOM, DC or other degrees from schools that are not accredited or respected by anyone. In other words, there are diploma mills out there which are happy to "sell" degrees for money. Others have bona fide MD or other health professional doctorate degrees from accredited universities but keep in mind that medical school or equivalent is "kindergarten for doctors." When you graduate, you only know the very basic ABC's theoretically. You're still on very shaky training wheels! Then you have to spend time practicing under senior mentors in residencies and fellowships, lasting from 3 to 10 years or more, to actually safely and effectively apply what you learned in medical school. Some doctors receive only very basic internship or residency training making them generally competent but not especially expert in any area. Also, not all residency hospitals are of the same quality; in fact, far from it. This all may seem like dirty laundry coming from a doctor but think about it. Are all mechanics the same? Lawyers? Anybody? Of course not. It is no different in healthcare. Depending on what you are looking for in terms of an "expert," be careful. Check credentials carefully before believing what anyone says. Oncologists, depending upon sub-specialty, often have between four and nine years of training after medical school. Those that do not have an MD or DO degree, like ND or NMD graduates, often have between zero to two years of residency or apprenticeship. This is why looking for a FABNO designation is helpful when you are working with a naturopathic doctor. These doctors have done some residency training in oncology after completing naturopathic medical school. As far as cancer care goes, anyone other than board eligible or certified MD or DO oncologists are on training wheels and can certainly be part of a highly effective team but cannot independently offer safe treatment or counseling. Choose wisely. The level of training as well as competence in research, for which there is additional training, correlate with quality of published research.

EVIDENCE GRADES

When scientific evidence for anything is reviewed, a letter grade may be assigned based upon the overall strength of evidence from all published studies. In other words, there might be a mixture of all of the types of studies we just reviewed supporting or refuting a treatment recommendation. The following are technical descriptions regarding the grades, but the important takeaway lesson is that the sum total of scientific evidence is ultimately "grade-able," based on how many good studies there are and how meaningful the conclusions are in terms of actually helping individuals.

Grade A: Consistent Level I studies showing very similar results. There is high certainty that the net benefit is substantial. In other words, a number of high-level studies show that the treatment is highly likely to help a lot.

Grade B: Consistent Level II or III studies or extrapolations from Level I studies. There is high certainty that the net benefit is moderate or there is moderate certainty that the net benefit is moderate to substantial.

Grade C: Level IV studies or extrapolations from Level II and III studies. There is at least moderate certainty that the net benefit is small. At this point, the recommendation for a remedy might be very cautious.

Grade D: Level V studies or troublingly inconsistent or inconclusive studies at any level. There is moderate or high certainty that the service has no net benefit or that the harms outweigh the benefits. This means that the treatment should not be recommended.

In addition to the above, the United States Preventive Services Task Force (USPSTF) recently issued an additional level of evidence.

I Statement: The USPSTF concludes that the current evidence is insufficient to assess the balance of benefits and harms of the service. Evidence is lacking, of poor quality, or conflicting, and the balance of benefits and harms cannot be determined.

In the case of an "I Statement" body of evidence or proof for something, one has to either guess or rely on how plausible something might be, based on preclinical lab and animal studies as well as knowledge about how the human body works.

WHAT IS THE "BEST" EVIDENCE?

There is no consensus about which evidence rating system is ideal or which should be universally applied. Additional systems have been proposed, based on the field of medicine or are journal specific. You may find any of these, or a combination hybrid, in use by any given medical journal.

It bears repeating that the "best" source of high-quality evidence is generally considered to be the randomized controlled clinical trial (RCT), which is Level I. This study design provides very useful information with the least risk that preconceived bias may taint the accuracy of results, but it is not the appropriate answer to all questions. Many interventions or other clinical questions have not, nor ever will be, investigated at that level. Or the clinical question being asked may not be appropriate for evaluation in a randomized controlled fashion. Examples are abundant and include low prevalence conditions (i.e. rare), or overwhelming results from other study types. For example, the Pap smear for cervical cancer screening was never evaluated by RCT. However, enough observational epidemiologic evidence exists such that its role in reducing the incidence of cervical cancer is not questioned. No one doubts that the Pap smear has saved millions of women's lives.

Healthcare is evolving to where we have better evidence levels for everything we do. Unfortunately, we still have a long way to go. RCTs are undeniably the scientific gold standard of "proof" in medicine when looking for a cause-effect relationship between a very specific treatment and the outcome. However, not all potential and promising treatments require a randomized controlled trial (RCT) to consider starting to use them. As mentioned several times in this book, it is unlikely that anyone would require a randomized trial to determine if parachutes reduce the risk of death from skydiving. In fact, in mainstream medicine, only about 30% of what we do is based on Level I RCT evidence. So, if you run across a doctor that is too rigid about "evidence" and "proven," they might need a refresher course about how firm the ground they're standing on really is.

Some treatments are simply plausible and "should work," based on pre-clinical scientific knowledge regarding how the body works. Although this sounds logical, please understand that literally thousands of plausible mainstream and natural treatments of yesterday have been *proven ineffective or dangerous* by well designed and run scientific studies. So, not everything is the way it seems. Scientific plausibility should not be ignored when no better evidence is available, but just beware of its limitations.

So, why don't we have better scientific evidence for natural therapies? I'll leave aside the fact that there's "no money in it," which may be a factor but not totally true. While Big Pharma is a multi-trillion dollar business, Big Nutra which sells vitamins and supplements is a multi-billion dollar business. So, there is money in natural remedies. However, many natural remedy companies would rather blame "conspiracy" rather than investing in science and research. Having said that, consider the following as well. Natural therapies often really involve more than one "intervention" at a time. For example, a herb contains multiple bio-active plant substances contained within it. It's extremely hard to prove cause-effect when unknown synergies are in play between hundreds or thousands of ingredients or nutrients. Another example is treatment combining acupressure plus aromatherapy plus herbals. This is not amenable to an RCT, which usually examines one specific bioactive factor at a time (e.g. a drug) for a cause-effect relationship. Herbal mixes usually carry a number of different bio-active ingredients, which means they can work together in a very complex synergistic way (i.e. they can amplify the overall positive effect) or even work against each other in some cases. The total effect can also vary based on metabolic differences between individuals. Also, keep in mind that some herbal components can actually be toxic. In other words, some parts can be good, and others can be dangerous or at least cause side effects, just like drugs can.

All of the above makes it extremely difficult to look for a clear cause-effect relationship between one problem and one active ingredient. So, while the RCT is the standard, other scientific research study models are also important, and pre-clinical physiologic plausibility should not be written off in the absence of optimal clinical trials. While awaiting proof through clinical trials, a plausible intervention is something to consider as long as there is no clear or theoretical but plausible and likely harm. Safety data is often not readily available. It is also always good to consider the probability and plausibility of the risk you are willing to take vs. the benefit you are likely to get from something. Unfortunately, in the herbal or botanical remedy world, this information is often not readily available.

Here is a critical factor. The less high-quality evidence there is, the more the scientific plausibility must be pristine and based on solid scientific factors and not "pseudo-scientific" jargon and opinion. When there is a risk of harm, there is no room for seat of the pants creative medicine. You might as well ask your plumber, CPA or lawyer to treat you for cancer because that is the level of help you are likely to get.

In the end, there is a continuum between the extremes of proven and disproven that includes possible & plausible, and it is important to know the likelihood of harm within this continuum as well. The questions boil down to how likely is it that a remedy will help me, how much is it likely to help me and what are the chances that it can harm me? You need all three pieces of information if possible and then look for the best balance for your specific situation. This makes for an informed discussion with your oncologist and other treating health care providers. Finally, don't forget to check credentials and what they mean. Doctors are not all built the same.

RESOURCES & REFERENCES

The following resources and references are meant to stimulate further research should you so desire to pursue it. This is NOT meant to be an exhaustive literature search for everything to do with integrative oncology. Nor are these presented as necessarily the "best" out of the tens of thousands of references out there. New studies are published every day. Every effort was made to ensure that these are representative references. Other than multiple Level 1 randomized trial data, which is often lacking, interpretation of "best" is a bit subjective in any given situation.

As exciting new findings come up and new studies support better recommendations, updated references will be applied in upcoming editions of this book. However, a more dynamic resource for updates and additional information can be found on our complementary website at http://CancerCureology.com. There we review the latest and greatest on an ongoing basis if you elect to join us. Unless you are a health professional, many scientific references may be difficult to understand, if not impossible. Our mission is to simplify and explain.

SELECTED BOOKS:

Modern Nutrition in Health and Disease (Modern Nutrition in Health & Disease (Shils)) Eleventh Edition by A. Catharine Ross PhD (Author), Benjamin Caballero MD PhD (Author), Robert J. Cousins PhD (Author), Katherine L. Tucker Ph.D. (Author), Thomas R. Ziegler M.D. (Author)

The Blue Zones: Lessons for Living Longer From the People Who've Lived the Longest Mass Market Paperback – Deluxe Edition, October 19, 2010 by Dan Buettner (Author)

The China Study: The Most Comprehensive Study of Nutrition Ever Conducted And the Startling Implications for Diet...May 11, 2006 by Thomas Campbell and T. Colin Campbell

The Cancer-Fighting Kitchen: Nourishing, Big-Flavor Recipes for Cancer Treatment and Recovery Aug 25, 2009 by Rebecca Katz and Mat Edelson

Anti-cancer: A New Way of Life Dec 31, 2009 by David Servan-Schreiber

Whole: Rethinking the Science of Nutrition May 6, 2014 by T. Colin Campbell and Howard Jacobson

SECTION I: CANCER CAUSATION AND YOUR BODY

Chapter 1: What is Cancer?

Vineis P, Schatzkin A, Potter JD. Models of carcinogenesis: an overview. Carcinogenesis. 2010 Oct;31(10):1703-9.

Burnet, F.M. (1957). "Cancer—A Biological Approach: I. The Processes Of Control. II. The Significance of Somatic Mutation". Brit. Med. Jour. 1 (5022): 779–786. (historical perspective vs today's perspective)

Bizzarri M, Cucina A. Tumor and the microenvironment: a chance to reframe the paradigm of carcinogenesis? Biomed Res Int. 2014;2014:934038.

Bellamy, C.O.; Malcomson, R.D.; Harrison, D.J.; Wyllie, A.H. (1995). "Cell death in health and disease: the biology and regulation of apoptosis." Semin. Cancer Biol. 6 (1): 3–16.

Thompson, C.B. (1995). "Apoptosis in the pathogenesis and treatment of disease." Science 267 (5203): 1456–1462.

Igney, F.H.; Krammer, P.H. (2002). "Death and anti-death: tumour resistance to apoptosis." Nature Reviews Cancer 2 (4): 277–288.

Nistal E, Fernández-Fernández N, Vivas S, Olcoz JL.

Factors Determining Colorectal Cancer: The Role of the Intestinal Microbiota. Front Oncol. 2015 Oct 12;5:220.

Leibovitz BE, Siegel BV: Aspects of free radical reactions in biological systems: Aging. J Gerontol 1980; 35:45-56.

Pinnell SR: Cutaneous photodamage, oxidative stress, and topical antioxidant protection. J Am Acad Dermatol 2003; 48:1-19.

Venarucci D, Venarucci V, Vallese A, et al: Free radicals: Important cause of pathologies refer to ageing. Panminerva Med 1999; 41:335-339.

Yeh CC, Hou MF, Tsai SM, et al: Superoxide anion radical, lipid peroxides and antioxidant status in the blood of patients with breast cancer. Clin Chim Acta 2005; 361:104-111.

Chapter 2: Prevention and Screening

Cancer Screening Guidelines: http://www.netce.com/coursecontent. php?courseid=1005 Accessed Nov 2015

Moyer VA; U.S. Preventive Services Task Force. Vitamin, mineral, and multi-vitamin supplements for the primary prevention of cardiovascular disease and cancer: U.S. Preventive services Task Force recommendation statement. Ann Intern Med. 2014 Apr 15;160(8):558-64.

PDQ Screening and Prevention Editorial Board. Cancer Prevention Overview (PDQ®): Health Professional Version. PDQ Cancer Information Summaries [Internet]. Bethesda (MD): National Cancer Institute (US); 2002-2015 Jan 30.

Shah M, Denlinger CS. Optimal post-treatment surveillance in cancer survivors: is more really better? Oncology (Williston Park). 2015 Apr;29(4):230-40.

Chapter 3: From Inflammation to Cancer

Hoesel B, Schmid JA. The complexity of NF-κB signaling in inflammation and cancer. Mol Cancer. 2013; 12: 86.

Okada F. Inflammation-related carcinogenesis: current findings in epidemiological trends, causes, and mechanisms. Yonago Acta Med. 2014 Jun;57(2):65-72. Epub 2014 Jul 30.

Levy Nogueira M, da Veiga Moreira J, Baronzio GF, Dubois B, Steyaert JM, Schwartz L. Mechanical Stress as the Common Denominator between Chronic Inflammation, Cancer, and Alzheimer's Disease. Front Oncol. 2015 Sep 17;5:197.

Flower RJ, Perretti M: Controlling inflammation: A fat chance?. J Exp Med 2005; 201:671-674.

Baer DJ, Judd JT, Clevidence BA, et al: Dietary fatty acids affect plasma markers of inflammation in healthy men fed controlled diets: A randomized crossover study.Am J Clin Nutr 2004; 79:969-973.

James MJ, Gibson RA, Cleland LG: Dietary polyunsaturated fatty acids and inflammatory mediator production. Am J Clin Nutr 2000; 71:343S-348S.

Herder C, Illig T, Rathmann W, et al: Inflammation and type 2 diabetes: Results from KORA Augsburg. Gesundheitswesen 2005; 67(Suppl 1):S115-S121.

Rakel DP, Rindfleisch AL Inflammation: Nutritional, botanical, and mind-body influences. South Med J 2005; 98:303-310.

Seaman DR: The diet-induced proinflammatory state: A cause of chronic pain and other degenerative diseases?. J Manipulative Physiol Ther 2002; 25:168-179.

Uribarri J, Cai W, Sandu O, et al: Diet-derived advanced glycation end products are major contributors to the body's AGE pool and induce inflammation in healthy subjects. Ann N Y Acad Sci 2005; 1043:461-466.

Schulze MB, Hoffmann K, Manson JE: Dietary pattern, inflammation, and incidence of type 2 diabetes in women. Am J Clin Nutr 2005; 82:675-684.

Mozaffarian D, Pischon T, Hankinson SE, et al: Dietary intake of trans fatty acids and systemic inflammation in women. Am J Clin Nutr 2004; 79:606-612.

Chapter 4: Insulin Resistance Connection

Vigneri PG, Tirrò E, Pennisi MS, Massimino M, Stella S, Romano C, Manzella L. The Insulin/IGF System in Colorectal Cancer Development and Resistance to Therapy. Front Oncol. 2015 Oct 15;5:230.

American Diabetes Association: Evidence-based nutrition principles and recommendations for the treatment and prevention of diabetes and related complications. Diabetes Care 2003; 26:51S-61S.

Anderson JW, et al: Carbohydrate and fiber recommendations for individuals with diabetes: A quantitative assessment and meta-analysis of the evidence. J Am Coll Nutr. 2004 Feb;23(1):5-17. Review.

Augustin L, Gallus S, Franceschi S, et al: Glycemic index and load and risk of upper aero-digestive tract neoplasms. Cancer Causes Control 2003; 14:657-662.

Augustin L, Gallus S, Negri E, La Vecchia C: Glycemic index, glycemic load, and risk of gastric cancer. Ann Oncol 2004; 15:581-584.

Barclay AW, Brand-Miller JC, Wolever TM: Glycemic index, glycemic load, and glycemic response are not the same. Diabetes Care 2005; 28:1839-1840.

Brand-Miller JC, et al: Physiological validation of the concept of glycemic load in lean young adults. J Nutr 2003; 133:2728-2732.

Brand-Miller JC: Glycemic index in relation to coronary disease. Asia Pac J Clin Nutr 2004; 13(Suppl):S3.

Ebbeling CB, et al: Effects of an ad libitum low-glycemic load diet on cardiovascular disease risk factors in obese young adults. Am J Clin Nutr 2005; 81:976-982.

Folsom A, Demissie Z, Harnack L: Glycemic index, glycemic load, and incidence of endometrial cancer: The Iowa Women's Health Study. Nutr Cancer 2003; 46:119-124.

Foster-Powell K, Holt SHA, Brand-Miller JC: International table of glycemic index and glycemic load values: 2002. Am J Clin Nutr 2002; 76:5-56.

Harbis A, et al: Glycemic and insulinemic meal responses modulate postprandial hepatic and intestinal lipoprotein accumulation in obese, insulin-resistant subjects. Am J Clin Nutr 2004; 80:896-902.

Higginbotham S, Zhang ZF, Lee IM, et al: Dietary glycemic load and risk of colorectal cancer in the Women's Health Study. J Natl Cancer Inst 2004; 96:229-233.

Holmes M, Liu S, Hankinson SE, et al: Dietary carbohydrates, fiber, and breast cancer risk. Am J Epidemiol 2004; 159:732-739.

Kelly S, et al: Low glycaemic index diets for coronary heart disease. Cochrane Database Syst Rev (4):CD004467, 2004.

Liu S, et al: Relation between a diet with a high glycemic load and plasma concentrations of high-sensitivity C-reactive protein in middle-aged women. Am J Clin Nutr 2002; 75:492-498.

Ludwig DS: The glycemic index: Physiological mechanisms relating to obesity, diabetes, and cardiovascular disease. JAMA 2002; 287:2414-2423.

Mantzoros CS, Li R, Manson JE, et al: Circulating adiponectin levels are associated with better glycemic control, more favorable lipid profile and reduced inflammation in women with type 2 diabetes. J Clin Endocrinol Metab 2005; 90:4542-4548.

Michaud D, Liu S, Giovannucci E, et al: Dietary sugar, glycemic load, and pancreatic cancer risk in a prospective study. J Natl Cancer Inst 2002; 94:1293-1300.

Michaud DS, et al: Dietary glycemic load, carbohydrate, sugar, and colorectal cancer risk in men and women. Cancer Epidemiol Biomarkers Prev 2005; 14:138-147.

Oh K, et al: Carbohydrate intake, glycemic index, glycemic load, and dietary fiber in relation to risk of stroke in women. Am J Epidemiol 2005; 161:161-169.

Opperman AM, et al: Meta-analysis of the health effects of using the glycemic index in meal-planning. Br J Nutr 2004; 92:367-381.

Pereira MA, et al: Effects of a low-glycemic load diet on resting energy expenditure and heart disease risk factors during weight loss. JAMA 2004; 292:2482-2490.

Qi L, et al: Dietary glycemic index, glycemic load, cereal fiber, and plasma adiponectin concentration in diabetic men. Diabetes Care 2005; 28:1022-1028.

Rizkalla SW, et al: Improved plasma glucose control, whole-body glucose utilization, and lipid profile on a low-glycemic index diet in type 2 diabetic men: A randomized controlled trial. Diabetes Care 2004; 27:1866-1872.

Schulze MB, Liu S, Rimm EB, et al: Glycemic index, glycemic load, and dietary fiber intake and incidence of type 2 diabetes in younger and middle aged women. Am J Clin Nutr 2004; 80:348-356.

Slyper A, et al: Influence of glycemic load on HDL cholesterol in youth. Am J Clin Nutr 2005; 81:376-379.

Spranger J, Kroke A, Mohlig M, et al: Inflammatory cytokines and the risk to develop type 2 diabetes: Results of the prospective population-based European Prospective Investigation into Cancer and Nutrition (EPIC)—Potsdam Study. Diabetes Care 2003; 52:812-817.

Wolever T: The glycemic index: Aspects of some vitamins, minerals, and enzymes in health and disease. World Rev Nutr Diet 1990; 62:120-185.

Silvera SA, Jain M, Howe GR, et al: Dietary carbohydrates and breast cancer risk: A prospective study of the roles of overall glycemic index and glycemic load. Int J Cancer 2005; 114:653-658.

Michaud DS, Fuchs CS, Liu S, et al: Dietary glycemic load, carbohydrate, sugar, and colorectal cancer risk in men and women. Cancer Epidemiol Biomarkers Prev 2005; 14:138-147.

Mohanty P, et al: Glucose challenge stimulates reactive oxygen species (ROS) generation by leucocytes. J Clin Endocrinol Metab 2000; 85:2970-2973.

Chapter 5: Cancer Immunology

Dunn, G.P.; Bruce, A.T.; Ikeda, H.; Old, L.J.; Schreiber, R.D. (2002). "Cancer immunoediting: from immunosurveillance to tumor escape." Nature Immunology 3 (11): 991–998.

Kim, R.; Emi, M.; Tanabe, K. (2007). "Cancer immunoediting from immune surveillance to immune escape." Journal of Immunology 121 (1): 1–14.

Dunn, G.P.; Old, L.J.; Schreiber, R.D. (2004). "The Three Es of Cancer Immunoediting." Annual Review of Immunology 22: 329–360. doi:10.1146/annurev. immunol.22.012703.104803. PMID 15032581.

Odunsi, K.; Old, L. (2007). "Tumor infiltrating lymphocytes: indicators of tumor-related immune responses." Cancer Immunity 7: 3.

Obeid, M.; Tesniere, A.; Ghiringhello, F.; Fimia, G.M.; Apetoh, L.; Perfettini, J.L.; Castedo, M.; Mignot, G. et al. (2007). "Calreticulin exposure dictates the immunogenicity of cancer cell death." Nature Medicine 13 (10): 54–61.

Steinman, R.M.; Mellman, I. (2004). "Immunotherapy bewitched, bothered, and bewildered no more." Science 305 (5681): 197–200.

Lake, R.A.; der Most, R.G. (2006). "A better way for a cancer cell to die." N. Engl. J. Med. 354 (23): 2503–2504.

Zitvogel, L.; Tesniere, A.; Kroemer, G. (2006). "Cancer in spite of immunosurveillance: immunoselection and immunosubversion." Nat. Rev. Immunol 6 (10): 715–727.

Zitvogel, L.; Casares, N.; Péquignot, M.; Chaput, N; Albert, M.L.; Kroemer, G (2004). "The immune response against dying tumor cells." Adv. Immunol. Advances in Immunology 84: 131–179.

Buckwalter MR, Srivastava PK (2013). "Mechanism of dichotomy between CD8+ responses elicited by apoptotic and necrotic cells". Cancer Immun. 13: 2.

Veiga P1, Pons N2, Agrawal A3, et.al. Changes of the human gut microbiome induced by a fermented milk product. Sci Rep. 2014 Sep 11;4:6328.

Chapter 6: Hormones and Cancer

Gharwan H, Bunch KP, Annunziata CM. The role of reproductive hormones in epithelial ovarian carcinogenesis. Endocr Relat Cancer. 2015 Dec;22(6):R339-63.

Diep CH, Daniel AR, Mauro LJ, Knutson TP, Lange CA. Progesterone action in breast, uterine, and ovarian cancers. J Mol Endocrinol. 2015 Apr;54(2):R31-53.

Cojocneanu Petric R, Braicu C, Raduly L, Zanoaga O, Dragos N, Monroig P, Dumitrascu D, Berindan-Neagoe I. Phytochemicals modulate carcinogenic signaling pathways in breast and hormone-related cancers. Onco Targets Ther. 2015 Aug 6;8:2053-66.

Brisken C, Hess K, Jeitziner R. Progesterone and Overlooked Endocrine Pathways in Breast Cancer Pathogenesis. Endocrinology. 2015 Oct;156(10):3442-50.

Wu X, Zhou T, Cao N, Ni J, Wang X. Role of Vitamin D Metabolism and Activity on Carcinogenesis. Oncol Res. 2015;22(3):129-37.

Chapter 7: Epigenetics, Nutrigenomics & Cancer Stem Cells

Tollefsbol TO. Dietary epigenetics in cancer and aging. Cancer Treat Res. 2014;159:257-67.

Verma M. Cancer control and prevention by nutrition and epigenetic approaches. Antioxid Redox Signal. 2012 Jul 15;17(2):355-64.

Li Y1, Wicha MS, Schwartz SJ, Sun D. Implications of cancer stem cell theory for cancer chemoprevention by natural dietary compounds. J Nutr Biochem. 2011 Sep;22(9):799-806.

Kim YS1, Farrar W, Colburn NH, Milner JA. Cancer stem cells: potential target for bioactive food components. J Nutr Biochem. 2012 Jul;23(7):691-8.

Yoshida GJ, Saya H. Therapeutic strategies targeting cancer stem cells.

Cancer Sci. 2015 Sep 12.

Yeh AC, Ramaswamy S. Mechanisms of Cancer Cell Dormancy-Another Hallmark of Cancer? Cancer Res. 2015 Sep 9.

Ayman Zaky Elsamanoudy et al The role of nutrition related genes and nutrigenetics in understanding the pathogenesis of cancer Journal of Microscopy and Ultrastructure Volume 4, Issue 3, September 2016, Pages 115–122

SECTION II: CANCER TREATMENT & SUPPORT CUREOLOGY

Chapter 8: Beyond Basic Diagnostic Testing

Ajani UA, Ford ES, Mokdad AH: Dietary fiber and C-reactive protein: Findings from National Health and Nutrition Examination Survey Data. J Nutr 2004; 134:1181-1185.

Brighenti F, Valtuena S, Pellegrini N, et al: Total antioxidant capacity of the diet is inversely and independently related to plasma concentration of high-sensitivity C-reactive protein in adult Italian subjects. Br J Nutr 2005 May;93(5):619-25.

Ford ES, Mokdad AH, Liu S: Healthy eating index and C-reactive protein concentration: Findings from the National Health and Nutrition Examination Survey III, 1988 – Eur J Clin Nutr 2005; 59:278-283.

Freese R, Vaarala O, Turpeinen AM, et al: No difference in platelet activation or inflammation markers after diets rich or poor in vegetables, berries, and apple in healthy subjects. Eur J Nutr 2004 Jun;43(3):175-82.

Fung TT, McCullough ML, Newby PK, et al: Diet-quality scores and plasma concentrations of markers of inflammation and endothelial dysfunction. Am J Clin Nutr 2005 Jul;82(1):163-73.

Gao X, Bermudez OI, Tucker KL: Plasma C-reactive protein and homocysteine concentrations are related to frequent fruit and vegetable intake in Hispanic and non-Hispanic white elders. J Nutr 2004; 134:913-918.

King DE, Mainous AG, Geesey ME, et al: Dietary magnesium and C-reactive protein levels. J Am Coll Nutr 2005; 24:166-171.

Liu S, Manson JE, Buring JE, et al: Relation between a diet with a high glycemic load and plasma concentrations of high-sensitivity C-reactive protein in middle-aged women. Am J Clin Nutr 2002; 75:492-498.

Lopez-Garcia E, Schulze MB, Fung TT: Major dietary patterns are related to plasma concentrations of markers of inflammation and endothelial dysfunction. Am J Clin Nutr 2004; 80:1029-1035.

Ridker PM, Stampfer MJ, Rifai N: Novel risk factors for systemic atherosclerosis: A comparison of C-reactive protein, fibrinogen, homocysteine, lipoprotein(a) and standard cholesterol screening as predictors of peripheral arterial disease. JAMA 2002; 285:2481-2485.

Czerska M, Mikołajewska K, Zieliński M, Gromadzińska J, Wąsowicz W.

Today's oxidative stress markers. Med Pr. 2015;66(3):393-405.

Chapter 9: Mainstream Treatment Core Concepts

Shah DJ1, Sachs RK, Wilson DJ. Radiation-induced cancer: a modern view. Br J Radiol. 2012 Dec;85(1020):e1166-73.

Berrington de Gonzalez A1, Gilbert E, Curtis R, et al. Second solid cancers after radiation therapy: a systematic review of the epidemiologic studies of the radiation dose-response relationship. Int J Radiat Oncol Biol Phys. 2013 Jun 1;86(2):224-33. doi: 10.1016/j.ijrobp.2012.09.001. Epub 2012 Oct 24.

Yu Sun, Judith Campisi, Celestia Higano, Tomasz M Beer, Peggy Porter, Ilsa Coleman, Lawrence True & Peter S. Nelson; Treatment-induced damage to the tumor microenvironment promotes prostate cancer therapy resistance through WNT16B" NatureMedicine, Published online 05 August 2012

Chapter 10: Nutrition Core

Simopoulos AP. The Mediterranean diets: What is so special about the diet of Greece? The scientific evidence. J Nutr. 2001 Nov;131(11 Suppl):3065S-73S. Review.

Wolk A: Diet, lifestyle and risk of prostate cancer. Acta Oncol 2005; 44:526-528.

Ramon JM, et al: Dietary fat intake and prostate cancer risk: A case-control study in Spain. Cancer Causes Control 2000; 11:679-685.

Diet and Cancer Lampe JW. Dairy products and cancer. J Am Coll Nutr. 2011 Oct;30(5 Suppl 1):464S-70S.

Chrysohoou C, et al: Adherence to the Mediterranean diet attenuates inflammation and coagulation process in healthy adults: The ATTICA Study. J Am Coll Cardiol 2004; 44:152-158.

Chagas CE1, Rogero MM, Martini LA. Evaluating the links between intake of milk/dairy products and cancer. Nutr Rev. 2012 May;70(5):294-300.

Brottveit M1, Lundin KE.[Cancer risk in coeliac disease].[Article in Norwegian] Tidsskr Nor Laegeforen. 2008 Oct 23;128(20):2312-5.

King DE: Dietary fiber, inflammation, and cardiovascular disease. Mol Nutr Food Res 2005; 49:594-600.

Kellen E, Zeegers M, Paulussen A, et al: Fruit consumption reduces the effect of smoking on bladder cancer risk: The Belgian case control study on bladder cancer. Int J Cancer 2006; 118:2572-2578.

Panza F, Solfrizzi V, Colacicco AM, et al: Mediterranean diet and cognitive decline. Public Health Nutr 2004; 7:959-963.

Negri E, La Vecchia C, Franceschi S, et al: Intake of selected micronutrients and the risk of breast cancer. Int J Cancer 1996; 65:140-144.

Nomura AM, Kolonel LN, Hankin JH, et al: Dietary factors in cancer of the lower urinary tract. Int J Cancer 1991; 48:199-205.

Chapter 11: Anti Cancer Super Foods

Agarwal S, Rao AV: Tomato lycopene and low density lipoprotein oxidation: A human dietary intervention study. Lipids 1998; 33:981-984.

Gann PH, Ma J, Giovannucci E, et al: Lower prostate cancer risk in men with elevated plasma lycopene levels: Results of a prospective analysis. Cancer Res 1999; 59:1225-1230.

Zhang S, Hunter DJ, Forman MR, et al: Dietary carotenoids and vitamins A, C, and E and risk of breast cancer. J Natl Cancer Inst 1999; 91:547-556.

Yen WJ, Wang BS, Chang LW, et al: Antioxidant properties of roasted coffee residues. J Agric Food Chem 2005; 53:2658-2663.

Ariga T: The antioxidative function, preventive action on disease and utilization of proanthocyanidins. Biofactors 2004; 21:197-201.

Chapter 12: Alcohol: The Good, Bad and the Ugly

Ferrini K, Ghelfi F, Mannucci R, Titta L. Lifestyle, nutrition and breast cancer: facts and presumptions for consideration. Ecancermedicalscience. 2015 Jul 23;9:557.

Varoni EM, Lodi G, Iriti M. Ethanol versus Phytochemicals in Wine: Oral Cancer Risk in a Light Drinking Perspective. Int J Mol Sci. 2015 Jul 27;16(8):17029-47.

de Menezes RF, Bergmann A, Thuler LC. Alcohol consumption and risk of cancer: a systematic literature review. Asian Pac J Cancer Prev. 2013;14(9):4965-72.

Bagnardi V, Rota M, Botteri E, et al. Light alcohol drinking and cancer: a meta-analysis. Ann Oncol. 2013 Feb;24(2):301-8.

Hosseini A, Ghorbani A. Cancer therapy with phytochemicals: evidence from clinical studies. Avicenna J Phytomed. 2015 Mar-Apr;5(2):84-97.

Chapter 13: Supplementation

Sayin VI, Ibrahim MX, Larsson E, et al. Antioxidants accelerate lung cancer progression in mice. Sci Transl Med. 2014 Jan 29;6(221):221

Le Gal K, Ibrahim MX, Wiel C. Antioxidants can increase melanoma metastasis in mice. Sci Transl Med. 2015 Oct 7;7(308):308

Kaiser J. Biomedical research. Antioxidants could spur tumors by acting on cancer gene. Science. 2014 Jan 31;343(6170):477

Rutkowski M1, Grzegorczyk K. Adverse effects of antioxidative vitamins. Int J Occup Med Environ Health. 2012 Jun;25(2):105-21.

Maurer HR. Bromelain: biochemistry, pharmacology and medical use. Cell Mol Life Sci. 2001 Aug;58(9):1234-45.

Clark LC, Hixson LJ, Combs Jr GF, et al: Plasma selenium concentration predicts the prevalence of colorectal adenomatous polyps. Cancer Epidemiol Biomarkers Prev 1993; 2:41-46.

Lee IM: Antioxidant vitamins in the prevention of cancer. Proc Assoc Am Physicians 1999; 111:10-15.

Dronfield MW, Malone JD, Langman MJ, et al: Zinc in ulcerative colitis: A therapeutic trial and report on plasma levels. Gut 1977; 18:33-36.

Bandyopadhyay D, Biswas K, Bhattacharyya M, et al: Gastric toxicity and mucosal ulceration induced by oxygen – derived reactive species: Protection by melatonin. Curr Mol Med 2001; 1:501-513.

Azuma J: Long-term effect of taurine in congestive heart failure: Preliminary report: Heart Failure Research with Taurine Group. Adv Exp Med Biol 1994; 359:425-433.

Virtamo J, Pietenen P, Huttunen JK, et al: Incidence of cancer and mortality following alpha-tocopherol and beta – carotene supplementation: A postintervention follow-up. JAMA 2003; 290:476-485.

Lamm DL, Riggs DR, Shriver JS, et al: Megadose vitamins in bladder cancer: A double-blind clinical trial. J Urol 1994; 151:21-26.

Bustamante J, Lodge JK, Marcocci L, et al: Alpha-lipoic acid in liver metabolism and disease. Free Radic Biol Med 1998; 24:1023-1039.

Douban S, Brodsky MA, Whang DD, Whang R: Significance of magnesium in congestive heart failure. Am Heart J 1996; 132:664-671.

Finley JW, Davis CD, Feng Y: Selenium from high selenium broccoli protects rats from colon cancer. J Nutr 2000; 130:2384-2389.

Flagg EW, Coates RJ, Eley JW, et al: Dietary glutathione intake in humans and the relationship between intake and plasma total glutathione level. Nutr Cancer 1994; 21:33-46.

Gurer H, Ozgunes H, Oztezcan S, Ercal N: Antioxidant role of alpha-lipoic acid in lead toxicity. Free Radic Biol Med 1999; 27:75-81.

Levisky JA, Bowerman DL, Jenkins WW, Karch SB: Drug deposition in adipose tissue and skin: Evidence for an alternative source of positive sweat patch tests. Forensic Sci Int 2000; 110:35-46.

Mato JM, Camara J, Fernandez de Paz J, et al: S-adenosylmethionine in alcoholic liver cirrhosis: A randomized, placebo-controlled, double-blind, multicenter clinical trial. J Hepatol 1999; 30:1081-1089.

Neve J: New approaches to assess selenium status and requirement. Nutr Rev 2000; 58:363-369.

Packer L, Witt EH, Tritschler HJ: Alpha-lipoic acid as a biological antioxidant. Free Radic Biol Med 1995; 19:227-250.

Saletu B, Anderer P, Di Padova C, et al: Electrophysiological neuroimaging of the central effects of S-adenosyl-l – methionine by mapping of electroencephalograms and event-related potentials and low-resolution brain electromagnetic tomography. Am J Clin Nutr 2002; 76:1162S-1171S.

Witschi A, Reddy S, Stofer B, Lauterburg BH: The systemic availability of oral glutathione. Eur J Clin Pharmacol 1992; 43:667-669.

Pepping J: Milk thistle: Silybum marianum. Am J Health Syst Pharm 1999; 56:1195-1197.

Zhu M, Lin KF, Yeung RY, Li RC: Evaluation of the protective effects of Schisandra chinensis on Phase I drug metabolism using a CCl4 intoxication model. J Ethnopharmacol 1999; 67:61-68.

Brady LJ, Gallaher DD, Busta FF: The role of probiotic cultures in the prevention of colon cancer. J Nutr 2000; 130(Suppl 2):410S.

Burton JP, Cadieux P, Reid G: Improved understanding of the bacterial vaginal microflora of women before and after probiotic instillation. Appl Environ Microbiol 2003; 69:97.

Campieri M, Gionchetti P: Probiotics in inflammatory bowel disease: New insight into pathogenesis or a possible therapeutic alternative?. Gastroenterology 1999; 116:1246.

Chen CC, Walker WA: Probiotics and prebiotics: Role in clinical disease states. Adv Pediatr 2005; 52:77.

de Vrese M, Stegelmann A, Richter B, et al: Probiotics compensation for lactase insufficiency. Am J Clin Nutr 2001; 73(Suppl):421S.

Gibson GR, Roberfroid MB: Dietary manipulation of the human colonic microbiota: Introducing the concept of prebiotics. J Nutr 1995; 125:1401.

Gibson GR: Dietary modulation of the human gut microflora using prebiotics. Br J Nutr 1998; 80(Suppl 2):S209.

Gionchetti P, Rizzello F, Venturi A, et al: Probiotics in infective diarrhea and inflammatory bowel diseases. J Gastroenterol Hepatol 2000; 15:489.

Goldin BR, Gualtieri L, Moore RP: The effect of Lactobacillus GG on the initiation and promotion of dimethylhydrazine – induced intestinal tumors in the rat. Nutr Cancer 1996; 25:197.

Gorbach SL: Efficacy of Lactobacillus in treatment of acute diarrhea. Nutr Today 1996; 31:19S.

Hooper LV, Gordon JI: Commensal host-bacterial relationships in the gut. Science 2001; 292:1115.

Isolauri E, Arvola T, Sutas Y, et al: Probiotics in the management of atopic eczema. Clin Exp Allergy 2000; 30:1605.

Jenkins B, Holsten S, Bengmark S, et al:: Probiotics: A practical review of their role in specific clinical scenarios. Nutr Clin Pract 2005; 20:262.

Marteau PR, de Vrese M, Cellier CJ, et al: Protection from gastrointestinal diseases with the use of probiotics. Am J Clin Nutr 2001; 73(Suppl):430S.

Miller JL, Krieger JN: Urinary tract infections, cranberry juice, underwear, and probiotics in the 21st century. Urol Clin North Am 2002; 29:695.

Notario R, Leardini N, Borda N, et al: Hepatic abscess and bacteremia due to Lactobacillus rhamnosus. Rev Argent Microbiol 2003; 35:100.

Pirotta M, Gunn J, Chondros P, et al: Effect of lactobacillus in preventing post-antibiotic vulvovaginal candidiasis: A randomised controlled trial. BMJ 2004; 329:548.

Rachmilewitz D, Katakura K, Karmeli F, et al: Toll-like receptor 9 signaling mediates the anti-inflammatory effects of probiotics in murine experimental colitis. Gastroenterology 2004; 126:520.

Rautio M, Jousimies-Somer H, Kauma H, et al: Liver abscess due to a Lactobacillus rhamnosus strain indistinguishable from L. rhamnosus strain GG. Clin Infect Dis 1999; 28:1159.

Reddy BS: Prevention of colon cancer by pre – and probiotics: Evidence from laboratory studies. Br J Nutr 1998; 80(Suppl 2):S219.

Reid G: Instillation of Lactobacillus and stimulation of indigenous organisms to prevent recurrence of urinary tract infections. Microecol Ther 1995; 65:3763-3766.

Reid G: Probiotic agents to protect the urogenital tract against infection. Am J Clin Nutr 2001; 73(Suppl):437S.

Rowlands IR, Rumney CJ, Coutts JT, et al: Effect of Bifidobacterium longum and inulin on gut bacterial metabolism and carcinogen-induced crypt foci in rats. Carcinogenesis 1998; 19:281.

Saikali J, Picard C, Freitas M, et al: Fermented milks, probiotic cultures, and colon cancer. Nutr Cancer 2004; 49:14.

Salminen S, von Wright A, Morelli L, et al: Demonstration of safety of probiotics a review. Int J Food Microbiol 1998; 44:93.

Sllen SJ, Okoko B, Martinez E, et al: Probiotics for treating infectious diarrhoea (Cochrane Review). Cochrane Database Syst Rev (2):CD003048, 2004.

Snelling AM:: Effects of probiotics on the gastrointestinal tract. Curr Opin Infect Dis 2005; 18:420.

Thompson-Chagoyan OC, Maldonado J, Gil A: Aetiology of inflammatory bowel disease (IBD): Role of intestinal microbiota and gut-associated lymphoid tissue immune response. Clin Nutr 2005; 24:339.

Vanderhoof JA, Young RJ: Role of probiotics in the management of patients with food allergy. Ann Allergy Asthma Immunol 2003; 90(Suppl 3):99.

Wollowski I, Rechkemmer G, Pool-Zobel BL: Protective role of probiotics and prebiotics in colon cancer. Am J Clin Nutr 2001; 73(Suppl):451S.

Wood Jr , Sweet RL, Catena A, et al: In vitro adherence of Lactobacillus species to vaginal epithelium cells. Am J Obstet Gynecol 1985; 153:740.

Hardman WE: w-3 fatty acids and cancer therapy. J Nutr 2004; 134:3427S-3430S.

Engel ED: Diabetes mellitus: Impaired wound healing from zinc deficiency. J Am Podiatr Assoc 1981; 71:536-544.

The effect of vitamin E and beta carotene on the incidence of lung cancer and other cancers in male smokers. The Alpha-Tocopherol, Beta Carotene Cancer Prevention Study Group. N Engl J Med 1994; 330:1029-1035.

Hirt M, Nobel S, Barron E, et al: Zinc nasal gel for the treatment of common cold symptoms: A double-blind, placebo-controlled trial. Ear Nose Throat J 2000; 79:778-780.

Lonn E, Bosch J, Yusuf S, Sheridan P, Pogue J, Arnold JM, Ross C, Arnold A, Sleight P, Probstfield J, Dagenais GR; HOPE and HOPE-TOO Trial Investigators. Effects of long-term vitamin E supplementation on cardiovascular events and cancer: A randomized controlled trial. JAMA. 2005 Mar 16;293(11):1338-47.

Sieja K: Selenium (Se) deficiency in women with ovarian cancer undergoing chemotherapy and the influence of supplementation with this micro-element on biochemical parameters. Pharmazie 1998; 53:473-476.

Cathcart RF: Vitamin C: The nontoxic, nonrate-limited, antioxidant free radical scavenger. Med Hypotheses 1985; 18:61-77.

Prasad KN, Kumar A, Kochupillai V, et al: High doses of multiple antioxidant vitamins: Essential ingredients in improving the efficacy of standard cancer therapy. J Am Coll Nutr 1999; 18:13-25.

Simopoulos AP: Essential fatty acids in health and chronic disease. Am J Clin Nutr 1999; 70(Suppl):560S-569S.

Fontham ET, Pickle LW, Haenszel W, et al: Dietary vitamins A and C and lung cancer risk in Louisiana. Cancer 1988; 62:2267-2273.

Lamm DL, Riggs DR, Shriver JS, et al: Megadose vitamins in bladder cancer: A double-blind clinical trial. J Urol 1994; 151:21-26.

Lamson DW, Brignall MS: Antioxidants in cancer therapy: Their actions and interactions with oncologic therapies. Alt Med Rev 1999; 4:304-329.

Ocke MC, Kromhout D, Menotti A, et al: Average intake of anti-oxidant (pro) vitamins and subsequent cancer mortality in the 16 cohorts of the Seven Countries Study. Int J Cancer 1995; 61:480-484.

Gaurav K, Goel RK, Shukla M, Pandey M. Glutamine: A novel approach to chemotherapy-induced toxicity. Indian J Med Paediatr Oncol. 2012 Jan;33(1):13-20.

Chapter 14: Toxins: Where and What Are They?

Ballard KA. The impact of the environment on health. Nurs Adm Q. 2010 Oct-Dec;34(4):346-50.

Tsuchiya M, Asada M, Kasahara E, et al: Smoking a single cigarette rapidly reduces combined concentrations of nitrate and nitrite and concentrations of antioxidants in plasma. Circulation 2002; 105:1155-1157.

Beyersmann D, Hartwig A. Carcinogenic metal compounds: Recent insight into molecular and cellular mechanisms. Arch Toxicol 2008;82(8):493-512

U.S. Department of Health and Human Services, Centers for Disease Control and Prevention: Chronic disease overview: www.cdc.gov/nccdphp/overview.htm/

Danielson P. The cytochrome P450 superfamily: biochemistry, evolution and drug metabolism in humans. Curr Drug Metab. 2002 Dec;3(6):561-97. Review.

Dubey RB, Hanmandlu M, Gupta SK.Risk of brain tumors from wireless phone use. J Comput Assist Tomogr. 2010 Nov-Dec;34(6):799-807.

Hyland GJ. Physics and biology of mobile telephony. Lancet 2000;356(9244):1833-1836

Yakymenko I, Sidorik E. Risks of carcinogenesis from electromagnetic radiation of mobile telephony devices. Exp Oncol. 2010 Jul;32(2):54-60.

Abbott A: Ageing: Growing old gracefully. Nature 2004; 428:116-118.

Cahill Jr GJ, Owen OE, Morgan AP: The consumption of fuels during prolonged starvation. Adv Enzyme Regul 1968; 6:143-150.

Danielson P. The cytochrome P450 superfamily: biochemistry, evolution and drug metabolism in humans. Curr Drug Metab. 2002 Dec;3(6):561-97. Review.

Saudek CD, Felig P: The metabolic events of starvation. Am J Med 1976; 60:117-126.

Sorrentino D, Stump DD, Zhou SL, et al: The hepatocellular uptake of free fatty acids is selectively preserved during starvation. Gastroenterology 1994; 107:1415-1424

Badger C, Preston N, Seers K, Mortimer P: Physical therapies for reducing and controlling lymphoedema of the limbs. Cochrane Database Syst Rev (4):CD003141, 2004.

Hannuksela ML, Ellahham S: Benefits and risks of sauna bathing. Am J Med 2001; 110:118-126.

Hoshi A, Watanabe H, Kobayashi M, et al: Concentrations of trace elements in sweat during sauna bathing. Tohoku J Exp Med 2001; 195:163-169.

Imamura M, Biro S, Kihara T, et al: Repeated thermal therapy improves impaired vascular endothelial function in patients with coronary risk factors. J Am Coll Cardiol 2001; 38:1083-1088.

Little L, Porche DJ: Manual lymph drainage (MLD). J Assoc Nurses AIDS Care 1998; 9:78-81.

Masuda A, Miyata M, Kihara T, et al: Repeated sauna therapy reduces urinary 8-epi-prostaglandin F(2alpha). Jpn Heart J 2004; 45:297-303.

Press E: The health hazards of saunas and spas and how to minimize them. Am J Public Health 1991; 81:1034 – 1037.

Agency for Toxic Substances and Disease Registry: http://www.atsdr.cdc.gov/toxprofiles/index.asp

Brent RL, Tanski S, Weitzman M: A pediatric perspective on the unique vulnerability and resilience of the embryo and the child to environmental toxicants: The importance of rigorous research concerning age and agent.Pediatrics 2004; 113:935-944.

CDC National Report on Human Exposure to Environmental Chemicals http://www.cdc.gov/exposurereport/

Crinnion WJ: Toxic effects of the easily avoidable phthalates and parabens. Altern Med Rev 2010;15(3):190-6

Environmental Working Group: BodyBurden: The Pollution in People: Executive Summary: www.ewg.org

Hites RA, Foran JA, Carpenter DO, et al: Global assessment of organic contaminants in farmed salmon. Science 2004; 303:226-232.

NSF International: Home Water Treatment Devices: www.nsf.org/consumer/drinking_water/dw_treatment.asp?/

Olson ED: Bottled Water: Pure Drink or Pure Hype? NDRC Reports: National Resources Defense Council: http://www.nrdc.org/water/drinking/bw/bwinx.asp

Scorecard: The Pollution Information Site: www.scorecard.org/

Toxicologic consequences of oral aluminum [editorial]. Nutr Rev 1987; 45:72-74.

U.S. Department of Health and Human Services, Centers for Disease Control and Prevention: National Biomonitoring Program: www.cdc.gov/biomonitoring/

U.S. Environmental Protection Agency: Organophosphate Pesticides in Food http://www.epa.gov/pesticides/index.htm

U.S. Environmental Protection Agency: Groundwater and Drinking Water: www.epa.gov/safewater/dwhealth.html

U.S. Environmental Protection Agency: Drinking Water Contaminate Candidate List (CCL): www.epa.gov/safewater/ccl/index.html/

Wiks R, Campbell C: Pesticides in Children's Foods, Washington, DC: Environmental Working Group; 1993. 22. Environmental Working Group: Report Card: Pesticides in Produce: www.foodnews.org/reportcard.php/

Baldwin DN, Suki B, Pillow JJ, et al:: Effect of sighs on breathing memory and dynamics in healthy infants. J Appl Physiol 2004; 97:1830-1839.

Bernardi L, Porta C, Spicuzza L, et al:: Slow breathing increases arterial baroreflex sensitivity in patients with chronic heart failure. Circulation 2002; 105:143-145.

Bernardi L, Sleight P, Bandinelli G, et al: Effect of rosary prayer and yoga mantras on autonomic cardiovascular rhythms: Comparative study. Brit Med J 2001; 323(7327):1446-1449.

Bhargava R, et al: Autonomic responses to breath holding and its variations following pranayama. Indian J Physiol Pharmacol 1988; 324:257-264.

Bjorkqvist M, Wiberg B, Bodin L, et al:: Bottle-blowing in hospital-treated patients with community-acquired pneumonia. Scand J Infect Dis 1997; 29:77-82.

Boron WF, Richerson GB:: The respiratory system. In: Boron WF, Boulpaep EL, ed. Medical Physiology, Philadelphia: WB Saunders; 2003.

Borovikova LV, Ivarova S, Zhang M, et al:: Vagus nerve stimulation attenuates the systemic inflammatory response to endotoxin. Nature 2000; 405(6785):458-462.

Brown RP, Gerbarg PL:: Sudarshan Kriya yogic breathing in the treatment of stress, anxiety, and depression. Part I: Neurophysiologic model. J Altern Complement Med 2005; 11:189-201.

Choliz M: A breathing-retraining procedure in treatment of sleep-onset insomnia: Theoretical basis and experimental findings. Percept Mot Skills 1995; 80:507-513.

Chumillas S, Ponce JL, Delgado F, et al: Prevention of postoperative pulmonary complications through respiratory rehabilitation: A controlled clinical study. Arch Phys Med Rehabil 1998; 79:5-9.

Cohen L, Warneke C, Fouladi RT, et al:: Psychological adjustment and sleep quality in a randomized trial of the effects of a Tibetan yoga intervention in patients with lymphoma. Cancer 2004; 100:2253-2260.

Elliot WJ, Izzo Jr JL, White WB, et al:: Graded blood pressure reduction in hypertensive outpatients associated with use of a device to assist with slow breathing. J Clin Hypertens (Greenwich) 2004; 6::553-559.

Grossman E, Grossman A, Schein MH, et al: Breathing-control lowers blood pressure. J Hum Hypertens 2001; 15:263-269.

Han JN, Zhu YJ, Li SW, et al: Medically unexplained dyspnea: Psychophysiological characteristics and role of breathing therapy. Chinese Med J 2004; 117:6-13.

Hibbert GA, Chan M: Respiratory control: Its contribution to the treatment of panic attacks. Brit J Psychiatry 1989; 154:232-236.

Kwang Jin Kim et al. Efficiency of Volatile Formaldehyde Removal by Indoor Plants: Contribution of Aerial Plant Parts versus the Root Zone. Horticultural Science 2008;133: 479-627.

Lee JS, Lee MS, Lee JY, et al:: Effects of diaphragmatic breathing on ambulatory blood pressure and heart rate. Biomed Pharmacother 2003; 57(Suppl 1):87S-91S.

Manjunath NK, Telles S: Influence of Yoga and Ayurveda on self-rated sleep in a geriatric population. Indian J Med Res 2005; 121:683-690.

Pal GK, Velkumary S, Madanmohan : Effect of short-term practice of breathing exercises on autonomic functions in normal human volunteers. Indian J Med Res 2004; 120:115-121.

Patel C, Marmot MG, Tarry DJ, et al:: Trial of relaxation in reducing coronary risk: Four year follow up. Br Med J (Clin Res Ed) 1985; 290:1103-1106.

Patel C, North WR: Randomised controlled trial of yoga and bio-feedback in management of hypertension. Lancet 1975; 2(7925):93-95.

Perez-Padilla R, Schilmann A, Riojas-Rodriguez H. Respiratory health effects of indoor air pollution. Int J Tuberc Lung Dis. 2010 Sep;14(9):1079-86.

Schein MH, Garish B, Herz M, et al: Treating hypertension with a device that slows and regularises breathing: A randomised, double-blind controlled study. J Hum Hypertens 2001; 15:271-278.

Sydorchuk LP, Tryniak MH: Effect of the special breathing exercises on the autonomic regulation of the functional state of respiration and muscular systems. Likarska Sprava 2005; 3:44-47.

Tsai SL: Audio-visual relaxation training for anxiety, sleep, and relaxation among Chinese adults with cardiac disease. Res Nurs Health 2004; 27:458-468.

Tweeddale PM, Rowbottom I, McHardy GJ: Breathing retraining: Effect on anxiety and depression scores in behavioural breathlessness. J Psychosom Res 1994; 38:11-21.

van Dixhoorn J:: Cardiorespiratory effects of breathing and relaxation instruction in myocardial infarction patients. Biol Psychol 1998; 49:123-135.

Viskoper R, Shapira I, Priluch R, et al: Nonpharmacologic treatment of resistant hypertensives by device-guided slow breathing exercises. Am J Hypertens 2003; 16:484-487.

Vraciu JK, Vraciu RA: Effectiveness of breathing exercises in preventing pulmonary complications following open heart surgery. Phys Ther 1977; 57:1367-1371.

Wolverton BC, McDonald RC, Watkins EA, Jr. Foliage Plants for Removing Indoor Air Pollutants from Energy-efficient Homes. Economic Botany 1984;38(2):224-228

Yan Q, Sun Y, Lin J: A quantitative study on the effect of breathing exercises in improving respiratory muscle contraction. Zhonghua Nei Ke Za Zhi 1996; 35:235-238.

Chapter 15: Detoxification

Andrews GR, Haneman B, Booth JC, et al. Atrophic gastritis in the aged. Aust Ann Med 1967;16:230-235

Babka JC, Castell DO. On the genesis of heartburn: the effects of specific foods on the lower esophageal sphincter. Am J Dig Dis 1973;18:391-397

Faisal MA, Russell RM, Samloff IM, Holt PR, Helicobacter pylori infection and atrophic gastritis in the elderly. Gastroenterology 1990;99:1543-1544

Goldschmiedt M, Barnett CC, Schwartz, Karnes WE, Redfren JS, Feldman M. Effect of age on gastric acid secretion and serum gastrin concentrations in healthy men and women. Gastroenterology 1991;101:977-990

Katelaris PH, Seow F, Lin BPC, Ngu MC, Jones DB. Effect of age, Helicobacter pylori infection and gastritis with atrophy on serum gastrin and gastric acid secretion in healthy men. Gut 1993;34:1023-1037

Lee, SY; Shin, YW; Hahm, KB (2008). "Phytoceuticals: mighty but ignored weapons against Helicobacter pylori infection." Journal of digestive diseases 9 (3): 129–39.

Stoicov, C.; Saffari, R.; Houghton, J. "Green tea inhibits Helicobacter growth in vivo and in vitro" . International journal of antimicrobial agents 2009;33(5): 473–478.

Yanaka et al.; Fahey, JW; Fukumoto, A; Nakayama, M; Inoue, S; Zhang, S; Tauchi, M; Suzuki, H et al. "Dietary Sulforaphane-Rich Broccoli Sprouts Reduce Colonization and Attenuate Gastritis in Helicobacter pylori-Infected Mice and Humans". Cancer Prevention Research 2009;4: 353–360.

Youl Lee and Hae Choon Chang. "Isolation and Characterization of Kimchi Lactic Acid Bacteria Showing Anti-Helicobacter pylori Activity." Korean Journal of Microbiology and Biotechnology 2008;2: 106–114.

Coudray C, Bellanger J, Castiglia-Delavaud C, et al: Effect of soluble and partly soluble dietary fibre supplementation on absorption and balance of calcium, magnesium, iron and zinc in healthy young men. Eur J Clin Nutr 1997; 51:375.

Cummings JH, Bingham SA, Heaton KW, Eastwood MA: Fecal weight, colon cancer risk and dietary intake of non – starch polysaccharides (dietary fiber). Gastroenterology 1992; 103:1408.

Brudnak MA: Probiotics as an adjuvant to detoxification protocols. Med Hypotheses 2002; 58:382.

Chapter 16: Exercise

Walsh NP1, Gleeson M, Shephard RJ, et al. Position statement. Part one: Immune function and exercise. Exerc Immunol Rev. 2011;17:6-63.

Walsh NP1, Gleeson M, Pyne DB, et al. Position statement. Part two: Maintaining immune health. Exerc Immunol Rev. 2011;17:64-103.

Holecek V, Liska J, Racek J, et al: [The significance of free radicals and antioxidants due to the load induced by sport activity]. Cesk Fysiol 2004; 53:76-79.

Bulow J: Adipose tissue blood flow during exercise. Dan Med Bull 1983; 30:85-100.

Impact of Physical Activity on Cancer Recurrence and Survival in Patients With Stage III Colon Cancer: Findings From CALGB 89803

Jeffrey A. Meyerhardt, Denise Heseltine, Donna Niedzwiecki, et al.

JCO, Vol 24, No 22 (August 1), 2006: pp. 3535-3541

Roberts CK, Vaziri ND, Barnard RJ: Effect of diet and exercise intervention on blood pressure, insulin, oxidative stress, and nitric oxide availability. Circulation 2002; 106:2530-2532.

Kanter MM: Free radicals, exercise, and antioxidant supplementation. Int J Sport Nutr 1994; 4:205-220.

Leitzmann M, Powers H, Anderson AS, Scoccianti C, Berrino F, Boutron-Ruault MC, Cecchini M, Espina C, Key TJ, Norat T, Wiseman M, Romieu I. European Code against Cancer 4th Edition: Physical activity and cancer. Cancer Epidemiol. 2015 Jul 15.

Chapter 17: Alternative Cures or Discredited Disproven & Dangerous Therapies?

Milazzo S, Horneber M. Laetrile treatment for cancer. Cochrane Database Syst Rev. 2015 Apr 28;4:CD005476.

Vickers AJ, Kuo J, Cassileth BR. Unconventional anti-cancer agents: a systematic review of clinical trials. J Clin Oncol. 2006 Jan 1;24(1):136-40. Review.

Damyanov C, Gerasimova D, Maslev I, Gavrilov V. Low-dose chemotherapy with insulin (insulin potentiation therapy) in combination with hormone therapy for treatment of castration-resistant prostate cancer. ISRN Urol. 2012;2012:140182.

Damyanov C, Radoslavova M, Gavrilov V, Stoeva D. Low dose chemotherapy in combination with insulin for the treatment of advanced metastatic tumors. Preliminary experience. Journal of B.U.ON. 2009;14(4):711–715.

Ayre SG, Bellon DPGY, Perez Garcia D., Jr. Neoadjuvant low-dose chemotherapy with insulin in breast carcinomas. European Journal of Cancer. 1990;26(11–12):1262–1263.

Laetrile/Amygdalin (PDQ®): Health Professional Version.

PDQ Cancer Complementary and Alternative Medicine Editorial Board.

PDQ Cancer Information Summaries [Internet]. Bethesda (MD): National Cancer Institute (US); 2002-2015 Sep 29.

Song Z, Xu X. Advanced research on anti-tumor effects of amygdalin.

J Cancer Res Ther. 2014 Aug;10 Suppl 1:3-7.

Parrow NL, Leshin JA, Levine M. Parenteral ascorbate as a cancer therapeutic: a reassessment based on pharmacokinetics. Antioxid Redox Signal. 2013 Dec 10;19(17):2141-56.

Allain P, Mauras Y, Premel-Cabic A, et al: Effects of an EDTA infusion on the urinary elimination of several elements in healthy subjects. Br J Clin Pharmacol 1991; 31:347-349.

Lee WL, Huang JY, Shyur LF. Phytoagents for cancer management: regulation of nucleic acid oxidation, ROS, and related mechanisms. Oxid Med Cell Longev. 2013;2013:925804.

Lui GY, Kovacevic Z, Richardson V, Merlot AM, Kalinowski DS, Richardson DR. Targeting cancer by binding iron: Dissecting cellular signaling pathways. Oncotarget. 2015 Aug 7;6(22):18748-79.

Chen HH, Kuo MT. Overcoming platinum drug resistance with copper-lowering agents. Anti-cancer Res. 2013 Oct;33(10):4157-61.

Muehsam D, Chevalier G, Barsotti T, Gurfein BT. An Overview of Biofield Devices. Glob Adv Health Med. 2015 Nov;4(Suppl):42-51

http://www.aetna.com/cpb/medical/data/800_899/0827.html Aetna policies : Accessed March 9, 2016

F Bost, A-G Decoux-Poullot, J F Tanti, S Clavel. Energy disruptors: rising stars in anti-cancer therapy? Oncogenesis (2016) 5, e188

Ahmad A, Ginnebaugh KR, Li Y, et al. Molecular Targets of Naturopathy in Cancer Research: Bridge to Modern Medicine. Nutrients. 2015 Jan; 7(1): 321–334.

SECTION III: SYMPTOM CONTROL & WELLNESS CUREOLOGY

Chapter 18: Complementary Support Modalities

Weeks L, Balneaves LG, Paterson C, Verhoef M. Decision-making about complementary and alternative medicine by cancer patients: integrative literature review. Open Med. 2014 Apr 15;8(2):e54-66.

Chaoul A, Milbury K, Sood AK, Prinsloo S, Cohen L. Mind-body practices in cancer care. Curr Oncol Rep. 2014 Dec;16(12):417.

Dickerson SS, Connors LM, Fayad A, Dean GE. Sleep-wake disturbances in cancer patients: narrative review of literature focusing on improving quality of life outcomes. Nat Sci Sleep. 2014 Jul 12;6:85-100.

Nakamura Y, Lipschitz DL, Kuhn R, Kinney AY, Donaldson GW. Investigating efficacy of two brief mind-body intervention programs for managing sleep disturbance in cancer survivors: a pilot randomized controlled trial. J Cancer Surviv. 2013 Jun;7(2):165-82.

Mayden KD. Mind-body therapies: evidence and implications in advanced oncology practice. J Adv Pract Oncol. 2012 Nov;3(6):357-73.

Chapter 19: Symptom Control

Moore HC. An Overview of Chemotherapy-Related Cognitive Dysfunction, or 'Chemobrain' Oncology (Williston Park). 2014 Sep 15;28(9). pii: 201376.

Wagdi P, Fluri M, Aeschbacher B, et al: Cardioprotection in patients undergoing chemo – and/or radiotherapy for neoplastic disease: A pilot study. Jpn Heart J 1996; 37:353-359.

Donaldson MS, Speight N, Loomis S: Fibromyalgia syndrome improved using a mostly raw vegetarian diet: An observational study. BMC Complement Altern Med 2001; 1:7.

Kaartinen K, Lammi K, Hypen M: Vegan diet alleviates fibromyalgia symptoms. Scand J Rheumatol 2000; 29:308-313.

Dobrzyńska MM. Resveratrol as promising natural radioprotector. A review. Rocz Panstw Zakl Hig. 2013;64(4):255-62. Review.

Maclean CH, Issa AM, Newberry SJ: Effects of omega-3 fatty acids on cognitive function with aging, dementia, and neurological diseases. Evid Rep Technol Assess (Summ) 2005; 114:1-3.

Gaurav K, Goel RK, Shukla M, Pandey M. Glutamine: A novel approach to chemotherapy-induced toxicity. Indian J Med Paediatr Oncol. 2012 Jan;33(1):13-20.

Cassileth BR, Keefe FJ. Integrative and behavioral approaches to the treatment of cancer-related neuropathic pain. Oncologist. 2010;15 Suppl 2:19-23.

Hack CC, Voiß P, Lange S, Paul AE, Conrad S, Dobos GJ, Beckmann MW, Kümmel S. Local and Systemic Therapies for Breast Cancer Patients: Reducing Short-term Symptoms with the Methods of Integrative Medicine. Geburtshilfe Frauenheilkd. 2015 Jul;75(7):675-682.

CPSIA information can be obtained
at www.ICGtesting.com
Printed in the USA
BVOW03s0436311017

499015BV00002B/93/P